Phonetics for Communication Disorders

PHONETICS FOR COMMUNICATION DISORDERS

by

Martin J. Ball & Nicole Müller
University of Louisiana at Lafayette

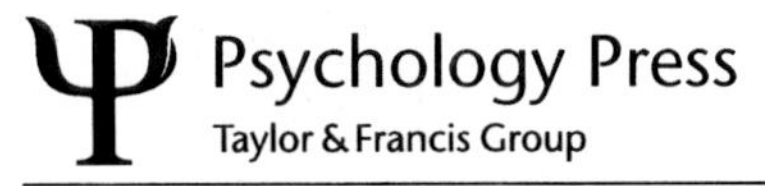

New York London

This edition published 2011 by Routledge

Routledge
Taylor & Francis Group
711 Third Avenue
New York, NY 10017

Routledge
Taylor & Francis Group
27 Church Road, Hove
East Sussex BN3 2FA

Library of Congress Cataloging-in-Publication Data

Ball, Martin J. (Martin John)
Phonetics for communication disorders / by Martin J. Ball & Nicole Müller.
p. cm.
Includes bibliographical references and index.
ISBN 0-8058-5363-4 (case : alk. paper)—ISBN 0-8058-5364-2 (pbk. : alk. paper)
1. English language–Phonetics. 2. Speech disorders. I. Müller, Nicole, 1963– II. Title.

RC423.B2843 2005
616.85′5—dc22 2005004370

Contents

Foreword

Having taught phonetics to students in communication disorders programs for nearly 20 years, I have sampled a wide variety of textbooks in my time. Although there have been many excellent texts to choose from over the years, I am always pleased to come across new books that offer different approaches to the subject. *Phonetics for Communication Disorders* is an exciting addition to the array of choices. It contains all of the features that to me define a good phonetics text, including thorough and accurate content coverage, relevant and useful examples and illustrations, and a comprehensive set of exercises for transcription practice. But it also goes beyond the scope of many other texts, covering all aspects of general phonetics as well as English phonetics and clinical phonetics.

Teaching phonetic transcription to students with communication disorders is a challenge. Many of them have had limited exposure to languages other than English and find it difficult to perceive and transcribe non-English sounds. But as the authors point out in the preface, clients in the speech clinic often produce non-English sounds, and students need to learn to transcribe them. Whereas many other texts begin with, or restrict themselves, to the transcription of English sounds, *Phonetics for Communication Disorders* follows the premise that it is best to begin learning to transcribe both English and non-English sounds, thereby reducing the transcriber's tendency to filter what they hear through the expectations of their own linguistic system. For example, exercises on the accompanying audio CD begin with non-English and nonsense-word examples to sharpen listening skills, and only later move on to English words.

The organization of *Phonetics for Communication Disorders* provides an ideal structure for courses in phonetics geared to students of communication disorders. Part I provides a comprehensive introduction to phonetics, assuming no previous background on the topic. Integrating information from anatomy, physiology, articulation, acoustics, and perception, it leads the reader through the basics of speech production—airstream mechanisms, phonation, vowels, consonants, and prosody. This provides a context for part II, which focuses on the phonetic and phonological structure of English. Students are thus able to examine the speech sounds of their own language, English, from a broader perspective. Another unique feature of this book is its coverage of both British and American models of English; other phonetics texts focus on one or the other, making it difficult for speakers of the other variety of English to follow, especially when the examples provided do not match their own pronunciation. Recognizing that not all clients speak standard varieties of British or American English, part II also includes a description of other varieties of English. Finally, after a solid grounding in general phonetics and an understanding of the range of variation in typical English speech production, part III introduces phonetic and phonological descriptions of disordered speech and the transcription of atypical and disordered speech. Throughout the book, the latest research and models are incorporated, providing students with the benefits of information obtained from new technologies and theoretical models. Exercises from the text and the accompanying audio CD provide opportunities to apply newly learned transcription skills along the way.

The authors, Martin J. Ball and Nicole Müller, are perfectly suited to write this text, both having had extensive experience teaching phonetics in communication disorders programs in the UK and US. Ball was an influential member of the teams that developed the ExtIPA and VoQS symbols for the transcription of disordered speech in the late 80s and early 90s, and is well-known in the UK as the author of other linguistics textbooks, including a popular 1993 text on general phonetics. He also co-authored a 1996 text on phonetic transcription of disordered speech geared toward instructors of applied phonetics courses, which included excellent overviews of the history of phonetic transcription, including recent developments in the transcription of disordered speech, and a range of methods for training students in phonetic transcription. Many of these methods are integrated into the current text.

Finally, although *Phonetics for Communication Disorders* is intended for students in professional training programs, the thorough and current coverage of phonetics and transcription practices may also be of interest to practicing speech-language pathologists wanting to review or upgrade their skills. Those who use it will find themselves well prepared for the challenges of transcribing disordered speech.

—Karen E. Pollock
University of Alberta

Preface

This book is about phonetics, the science of speech, and it has been designed specifically for students following communication disorders programs. It assumes no prior knowledge of the topic, and leads the reader from the basics of human spoken communication, through the mechanics of speech and the analysis of English pronunciation (concentrating on American and British standards, but also including other varieties of English), to the application of phonetics to the description and analysis of disordered speech. It also introduces phonetic transcription and, with the use of the accompanying audio CD, allows the reader to gain proficiency in the transcription of speech into phonetic symbols—a vital skill for clinicians. This text and CD, therefore, will act as a sourcebook for students throughout their undergraduate and graduate programs and in their careers as speech-language pathologists.

There are a few preliminary points we wish to make to aid the reader with the topic and with using the text. First, there are some authors who divide the study of speech, perhaps rather artificially, into *phonetics* (concerned mainly with the description of the articulation of speech sounds) and *speech science* (concerned mainly with aspects such as the anatomy and physiology of speech and the acoustic analysis of speech). Our account offers a more integrated approach, and therefore this book deals with all these aspects of speech, albeit with most emphasis on the production side. This book is deliberately maximal in its coverage. There is no benefit to the student in learning a dumbed-down version of phonetics; the very information you may need to understand the speech production of a particular client may well be missing in such an account. However, the professors teaching from this text may well wish to concentrate on specific aspects of a topic, leaving the student to read the entire chapter to gain further information.

Many texts on phonetics for speech pathology students do not provide a full enough coverage of speech articulation, and restrict themselves to the description of English sounds. Clearly, clients in the speech clinic will often produce non-English sounds, and students need to be equipped to deal with these. For this reason, it is also important that transcription exercises start with syllables and strings of syllables containing both English and non-English consonants and vowels. In this way, the tendency to listen to speech through the sieve of one's own sound system is lessened, and the transcriber enabled to concentrate on the sounds themselves rather than the expected words of his or her own language. The items on the CD for part I of the book, therefore, are mainly examples constructed by the authors or taken from languages other than English. In part II we concentrate on the transcription of English, and in part III we move on to deal with typical patterns of disordered speech.

Although this is a text on *phonetics,* it is impossible to avoid dealing also, to some extent, with the related field of *phonology.* The difference between these two areas is described in detail in chapter 10, as a prelude to the chapters in part II of the book that deal with the phonetics and phonology of English. Nevertheless, it will be helpful to readers to touch on the distinction here also. Phonetics is concerned with the description of the production, transmission, and reception of speech. It describes the required movements of the vocal organs to produce consonants, vowels, intonation, and so on. It is not concerned, however, with how such speech sounds are organized and used in specific languages. Phonology, on the other hand, is concerned with exactly these matters. So phonology will allow us to see, for example, which sounds in any given language are used *contrastively* (that is to say, to contrast one word with another), and which sounds are just variants of each other (where, for example, one variant may be used syllable-initially, and another syllable-finally, but both behave as members of a single sound unit). In part I we will occasionally need to refer to contrastive function of sounds; therefore readers should recall that this refers to the phonological status of a sound.

This difference between phonetics and phonology is also reflected in transcription, whereby symbols in a purely phonetic transcription are placed in square brackets (e.g., [p]), whereas symbols denoting the contrastive units of a phonological analysis are placed within slant brackets (e.g., /p/). In part I we use only phonetic symbols, but in parts II and III both phonetic and phonological transcriptions will be in use.

Many people have helped in the production of this book and audio CD. We would like to especially thank Linda Shockey, Alan Cruttenden, and Joan Rahilly for their helpful suggestions on parts of the text; Kristie Guillory for her work on the illustrations and Ben Rutter for his help with the index; Paul Warren and Peter Loschi for their help with both English and non-English examples; and colleagues and students who helped in the preparation and recording of the audio CD: Francisca Alonso, Linda Bryan, Holly Damico, Marlise Huys, Baha Kardosh, Sharon Williams, Ryan Nelson, Judith Oxley, Tom Powell, Joan Rahilly, Ben Rutter, Mitch Trichon, Ruixia Yan, and Brent Wilson.

Phonetics for Communication Disorders

I

General Phonetics

1

Phonetic Description

INTRODUCTION: THE SPEECH CHAIN

This book deals with the scientific study of speech. However, before we can start investigating speech, we need to consider the context of spoken utterances. In other words, we need to consider the chain of events that occur when a spoken message is transmitted from a speaker to a listener. We assume that the speaker requires some kind of creative ability to think of a message she or he wants to utter (whether it be a formulaic greeting such as "hello," or a complex scientific notion), and we also assume that the listener must have a similar kind of creative ability in order to decode and understand the message. Clearly, this creative ability is found in various parts of the brain and will include, among other things, linguistic meaning, vocabulary items, syntactic arrangements, and the patterns of sounds required to utter the string of words decided upon.

Next, we assume there must be an ability to convert the abstract patterns of sounds in the speaker's brain into neuromuscular commands and that these neuromuscular commands will result in the movement of the various vocal organs, so that speech sounds are produced by the speaker. These speech sounds are transmitted through the air that separates the speaker from the listener (as patterns of movement of the air molecules), until they impinge on the eardrums of the listener. Then there must be a system that allows these movements of air molecules to be converted into movements of the various parts of the middle and inner ear, and the conversion of this activity into neural impulses that travel from the inner ear to those parts of the brain that can decode and interpret the message.

This speech chain is shown diagrammatically in Fig. 1.1. You will notice that production ability (P), which is active in the speaker, is passive in the listener. However, this doesn't mean that it plays no part at all; there is evidence that listeners do actually use their speech production abilities to help in decoding spoken messages. Also, whereas the hearing ability (H) is active in the listener, it is passive in the speaker, though again, we know that speakers do listen to the speech they produce as a feedback mechanism to ensure accuracy. The creative ability (C) is active in both speaker and listener throughout the communication process.

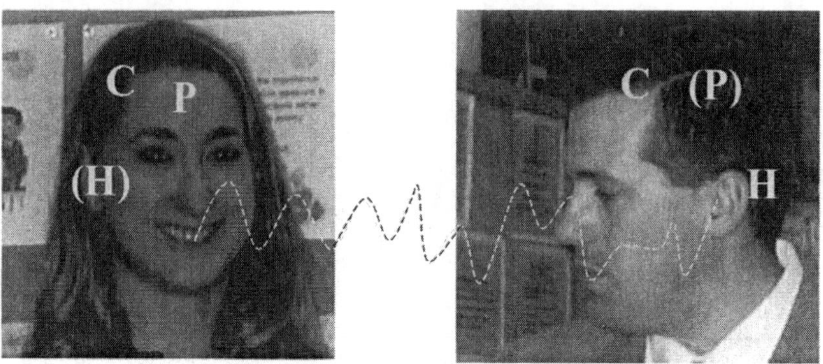

FIG 1.1. The speech chain (with thanks to Holly Hawley and Ryan Nelson).

> The speech chain model highlights the three main areas of study within phonetics: the study of speech production, the study of speech transmission, and the study of speech reception (or perception).

The technical labels given to these three areas of phonetics are, respectively, *articulatory phonetics, acoustic phonetics,* and *auditory phonetics.* Specialist subareas, such as *neurophonetics* (the study of neurological commands in speech production and reception), also exist, but these are outside the scope of our discussion here. The main focus of this book is on speech production, the articulation of speech sounds. However, an analysis of speech acoustics can often be very helpful in clarifying our understanding of speech and in undertaking descriptions of samples of both normal and disordered speech, and we include this area too. The basics of auditory phonetics are normally covered within audiology, whereas more advanced aspects of the area (such as psychoacoustic experimentation) belong in higher level courses.

Naturally, the sounds of speech can be described in different ways depending upon whether we are adopting an articulatory approach or an acoustic one. In articulatory phonetics we are interested in the movements and combinations of the various vocal organs. In order to understand such descriptions we need to have a knowledge of the vocal organs (see chap. 2) and of their activities (the remaining chapters of part 1). In acoustic phonetics we are interested in the nature of sound transmission in air. In order to understand acoustic description we need a basic grounding in the relevant physical concepts. We will deal with these in the next section, providing enough information so that you will understand the acoustic information provided throughout the remainder of the book. This is not, however, intended to replace a full course in speech acoustics, which will allow students to make in-depth acoustic investigations of normal and disordered speech.

BASICS OF ACOUSTICS

Sound Waves

Sound waves are disturbances in the positions of air molecules. For speech, of course, these disturbances originate in the production of a flow of air in the vocal tract and the modifications of this airflow by phonation and articulation. Speech communication can be seen as a process

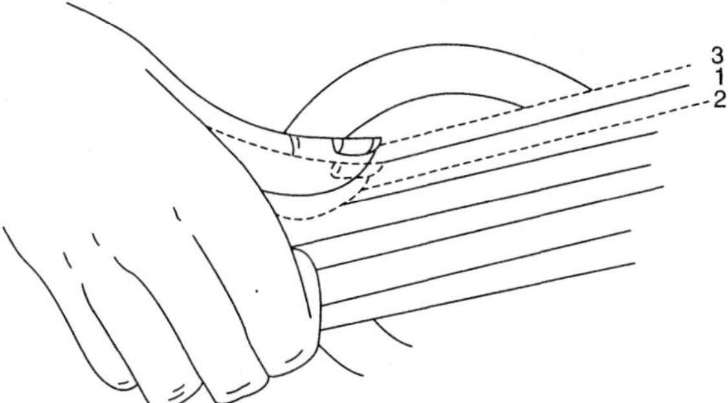

FIG 1.2. The movements of a plucked string.

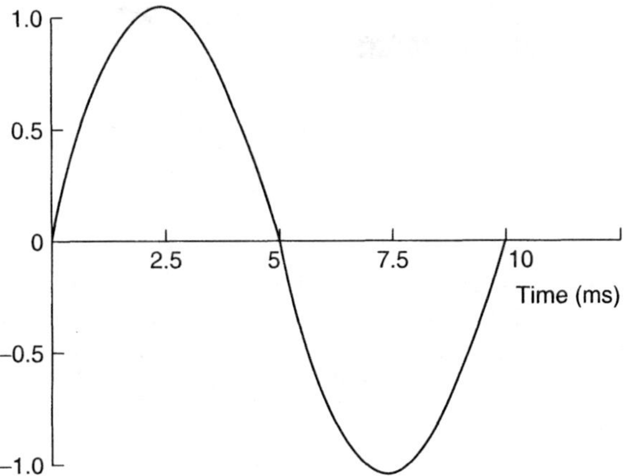

FIG 1.3. A simple sine wave.

in which language in the brain is converted to neural commands, then to muscle activity, and finally to sound waves. At the other end of the speech chain these sound waves are converted back to physical movement, neural commands, and then mental images in the listener's brain.

To understand how sound waves are produced and transmitted, we can take the example of a simple sound producer: a guitar string. If the string is plucked it will move away from its position of rest, position (1) in Fig. 1.2, to a new position (2). Depending on the force used to pluck the string, (2) will be a greater or lesser distance away from (1). However, a fixed object, when moved, will always try to return to its rest position, so having reached (2), the string will move back toward (1). As it moves, it builds up momentum and so overshoots (1) and reaches a position (3), about as far to the other side of (1) as (2) was in the first direction. As we can see in Fig. 1.3, this motion is of a waveform and the guitar string will continue this wave until the motion decreases (or is "damped") by the gradual absorption of energy by the string and the guitar itself.

Now, if we consider what happens to air in the vicinity of the guitar string, we can see that the wave motion of the string sets up a wave motion of air. The movements of the string set up alternate high and low air pressures, affecting particles (or molecules) of air in different ways. The pressure changes ripple through the air in a way similar to the ripples on a pond that spread out from wherever a stone has been thrown in. Of course, these sound waves do not continue

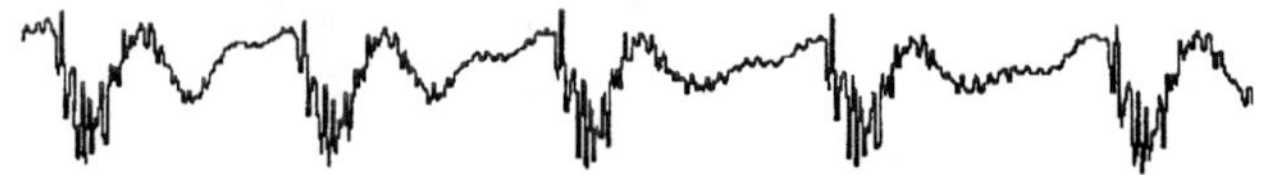

FIG 1.4. The complex waveform of the sound [i].

forever. The length of time the sound continues before dying out depends to some extent on the amount of energy expended in setting the wave in motion initially. Most importantly, it depends on the resistance of the physical forces that oppose the vibratory motion that causes the sound. These include the surrounding air, the metal in a tuning fork (for example), the body of a guitar, and so forth. Some things damp down sound waves faster than others, and in acoustics we refer to this as the property of *damping*.

A waveform such as that in Fig. 1.3 is known as a simple *sine wave*, but in speech there is not a simple, single source of the sound waves such as there is with a tuning fork. The various components of the vocal tract all add their own characteristics to the airflow, and we are left with a complex waveform, that is, a waveform made up of several simple waveforms (see below for discussion of periodic and aperiodic waves). An example of a complex waveform is given in Fig. 1.4; it shows the waveform used in pronouncing the vowel [i], of "tea."

> There are various ways to observe the waveforms of sounds; perhaps the most useful of these is the sound spectrograph, which will be discussed later in some detail.

Frequency

Frequency is an important aspect of sound waves, and one that we will need to study in relation to speech sounds. Let us return to our guitar string. We saw in Fig. 1.2 and 1.3 that by plucking the string we create a wave movement and thereby a sound wave. The movement of the string (or, of course, the air particle) from position (1) to (2) and then to (3) and back again to (1) is called a *cycle*. To find out the frequency of this sound, we need to know how many cycles will be completed in a given time, that is, how frequent is the movement from the starting position through the displacement positions and back to the starting position.

In acoustics the period of time we take for measuring purposes is 1 s: frequency is expressed in cycles per second, more commonly called *hertz* (Hz). Therefore, if we say a sound wave has a frequency of 100 Hz, we mean that in 1 s there will be 100 complete cycles or, in other words, a cycle is completed every 10 ms. Figure 1.5 shows simple sine waves of varying frequencies.

As noted earlier, the sounds of speech are not simple waves of the type shown in Fig. 1.5, but complex waveforms, built up from a bundle of simple forms. Even so, the frequency of the various component parts of these sounds can be measured and used to classify these sounds. Although many speech sounds are *periodic* (in that, however complex, the same regular pattern keeps recurring), others (including voiceless fricatives such as [s] and [f]) are *aperiodic* (in that the sound shows no discernible repeated aspects). A contrast between these two types is shown in Fig. 1.6.

Any complex periodic waveform has a fundamental frequency. In fact, our guitar string will have a complex waveform, and we have only been investigating the fundamental frequency so far. The other frequencies that occur above the fundamental frequency are termed *harmonics* and are multiples of that fundamental. For example, a fundamental frequency of 100 Hz will

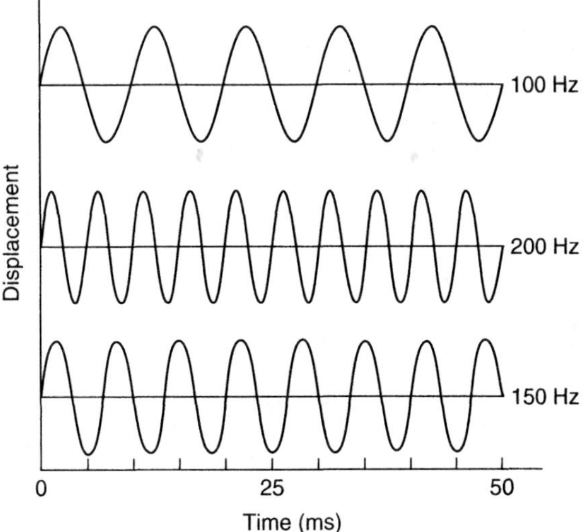

FIG 1.5. Sine waves of varying frequencies.

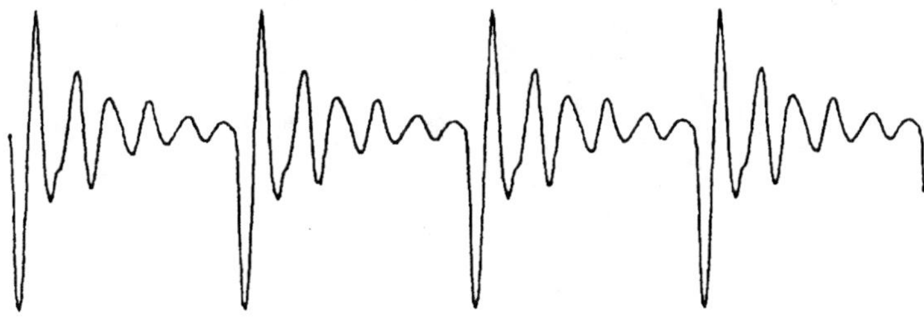

(a)

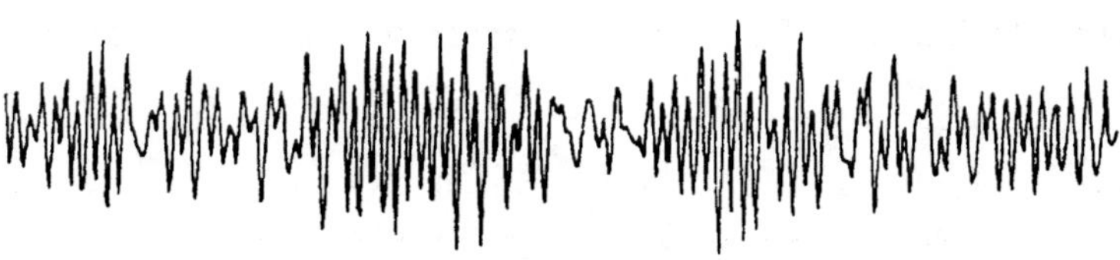

(b)

FIG 1.6. Periodic and aperiodic waveforms: (a) [a]; (b) [s].

have a second harmonic at 200 Hz, a third at 300 Hz, and so on. If the fundamental frequency were 160 Hz, the second harmonic would be 320 Hz, the third 480 Hz, and so on.

> In speech, the fundamental frequency is provided by vocal fold vibration (voiceless sounds are aperiodic in that they lack this feature) with a harmonic series based on that rate, which is constantly changing in speech.

We return to the acoustic makeup of individual sounds in later chapters, but we turn our attention next to the main role of the fundamental frequency in speech: pitch.

Pitch

One of the main linguistic uses of *pitch* is intonation. Acoustically we have to remember that, although related, frequency and pitch are not the same. Frequency is a physical property of sound waves, whereas pitch is the auditory realization (i.e., impression) of that property. In other words, we *produce* frequencies, but we *hear* pitch.

As we noted above, pitch is derived from the fundamental frequency of vocal fold vibration, which is continually changing through speech. The average fundamental frequencies in speech are 120 Hz for adult males, 225 Hz for adult females, and 265 Hz for children. The total range of fundamental frequencies found in speech extends from 60 Hz to 500 Hz or more.

Whereas frequencies are measured in hertz, perceived pitch is measured in either mels or barks, or via the Koenig scale, all of which are scales of perceptual values. These scales are logarithmic, in that they increase not in a linear fashion, but by multiplication of units. This reflects the fact that we perceive high and low pitch differently: the ear is more sensitive to pitch changes at lower frequencies than at higher and the scales reflect this.

Amplitude

Another important aspect of the sound wave concerns the characteristics of the cycle itself. The *amplitude* of a sound wave is the amount of variation in the air pressure from normal that is occasioned by the sound-making device. To return to our example of the guitar string: if this is plucked with great force, it will move further away from its rest position than if it is plucked with less force (Fig. 1.7). The sound waves resulting from such actions will differ in a similar

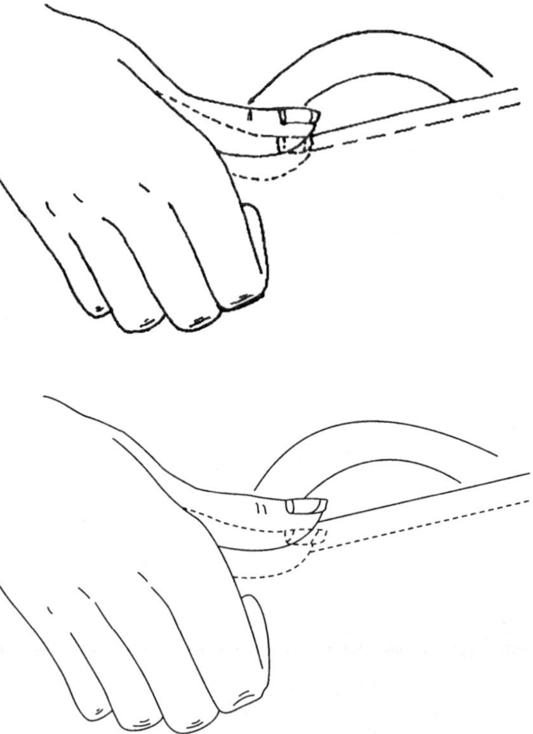

FIG 1.7. String plucked with differing force: (top) slight force; (bottom) greater force.

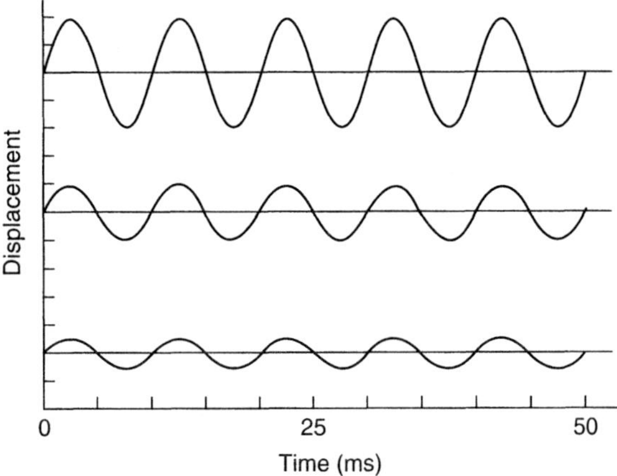

FIG 1.8. Waves of the same frequency but different amplitudes.

way, in terms of greater or lesser disturbance of the air pressure. Amplitude, then, is directly dependent upon physical actions. Figure 1.8 illustrates sound waves of identical frequencies, but with different amplitudes. To measure amplitude one would need to use the system employed for measuring changes in air pressure: the barometric scale. However, for speech purposes, it is much more common to measure differences in *intensity*, rather than amplitude.

Intensity

In the same way that we perceive differences of frequency as pitch changes, so we perceive intensity as loudness. But what exactly is intensity? If we increase the amplitude of a sound it appears louder: for example, if we displace our guitar string more than usual (i.e., we pluck it harder), then we get a louder note. However, amplitude is independent of frequency, in that we can have sound waves of the same amplitude but different frequencies (as well as of the same frequency but different amplitudes as in Fig. 1.8). When two waves have the same amplitude, but different frequencies, the wave with the lower frequency requires less energy, because it completes its cycle less often than the higher frequency wave. Indeed, the sound wave with the higher frequency will be perceived as being louder than the first, despite the fact that their amplitudes are the same.

It appears, then, that loudness is derived not from amplitude or from frequency separately, but from what we might call the energy input into a sound: a combination of the amplitude and the frequency. The term given to this combination in acoustics is *intensity*.

The relationship between the components of intensity (i.e., amplitude and frequency) is a somewhat complicated one. This is because intensity is in a proportional relationship to its components: to the square of the frequency and the square of the amplitude. For example, if we double the amplitude of a 100-Hz sound, we increase the intensity by a factor of 4; if we treble it we increase the intensity by a factor of 9. Similarly, if we keep the amplitude static, but compare sounds of different frequencies, we find that a 200-Hz sound has four times the intensity of a 100-Hz sound, and a 400-Hz sound has 16 times the intensity of the 100-Hz sound. Of course, combinations of frequency and amplitude differences will result in changes of intensity involving the product of both squares. As we noted earlier, speech sounds are all complex sound waves, and it is difficult to work out individual frequencies and amplitudes. Therefore, the concept of intensity is a useful single comparison measure.

Loudness

Loudness is, as we have noted, the perceptual correlate of intensity, and in acoustic phonetics we are often interested in how loud one sound (or indeed one speaker) is compared to another. The important point here is the words *compared to.* Rather than an absolute measure of intensity/loudness, we are interested in a relational measurement. This measurement system is the *decibel* (dB) scale. This scale is both ratio-based and logarithmic. Decibel values do not belong to an absolute scale, but express a difference between two previously noted sounds.

> In giving decibel measurements, it is important to note how far from the source of the sound the measurement takes place. This is because as we increase our distance from the sound source the intensity falls off.

Speakers vary in the loudness of their voices and naturally their speech will become louder or softer dependent upon circumstances. Furthermore, within speech certain sounds have greater intensity than others. For example, the "th" sound in English "thin" has the lowest, whereas the vowel sound in "court" has the highest intensity of all English speech sounds.

Sound Source Differences

We have looked so far at two important areas of acoustics: frequency and intensity. We have seen that frequency (perceived as pitch) refers to the number of times the sound wave completes its cycle in a second, and that intensity (perceived as loudness) refers to the amount of acoustic energy involved in the production of the sound wave. As far as speech is concerned, both these features are eventually derived from the source of sound in the vocal tract, (usually) an airstream flowing outward from the lungs modified by the laryngeal voice source. However, we know that individual speech segments sound different. Further, we know that individual speakers sound different. We need now to consider what causes these differences.

Free Vibrations and Forced Vibrations

The example we have been using of the sound wave produced by plucking a guitar string is termed in acoustics a *free vibration.* This implies that the sound is produced through the application of a force (in our case the plucking motion of the finger) that is then removed. Free vibrations may result in simple sound waves (such as those produced from tuning forks) or complex waves (for example, that produced by our guitar string) having a fundamental frequency and a range of harmonics.

However, there is another way in which sound can be produced, termed *forced vibration.* Unlike free vibration, where the force that starts the vibration is removed, with forced vibration that force is constantly applied. This results in a system (the *driven system*) that is forced to vibrate by being brought into contact with a *driving force* (usually an already vibrating system).

The usual example employed to demonstrate this difference is the tuning fork. If we strike a tuning fork (let us assume the usual musical type, tuned to A) we hear a pure tone of 440 Hz frequency. However, this sound is not very loud, and can only be heard if we position the fork near the ear. It is easy, however, to make the sound louder: We can simply press the foot of the fork onto a table top or desk top. By pressing the fork onto the table we are driving the table top with the vibrations of the fork: we are in effect setting up a forced vibration. The table then is emitting a sound wave caused by the tuning fork. Its frequency will be that of the driving force, 440 Hz for an A fork, 264 Hz for a C fork, and so on. Note that in these instances the table is responding to the driving force; the frequency emitted is not that of the table itself. If we strike the table top to produce free vibration, we find that the resultant sound dies away swiftly and is completely unlike what happens with our tuning fork experiment.

The principle of forced vibrations is utilized in many musical instruments. Our guitar string does not by itself cause sound waves of great intensity when plucked, but (in acoustic guitars at least) the vibrations of the string are the driving force that drives the body of the guitar and this results in much louder sounds. Solid-body electric guitars do not rely on this process, and if a string is plucked when the guitar is not turned on, you will hear how quiet the sound of the string alone is.

Resonance

Resonance is the term used to describe the phenomenon of one system being set in motion by the vibrations of another: one system *resonates* the other. However, the end result of this action depends on the acoustic properties of the driving force and of the driven system. The loudness of the forced vibration depends on two main factors. First we need to consider how closely coupled the driving force and the driven system are. With the tuning fork and the table top we will get a louder forced vibration when the fork is pressed against the table than when it is held just slightly above it. Even in the latter case, however, the vibrations will pass through the air to the table.

Perhaps more important, however, is the relation between the natural frequencies of the two systems. We will get the greatest amplitude of the forced vibrations when the natural frequency of the driving force is the same as the natural frequency of the driven system. (A natural frequency is that which would occur if the system were subject to free vibrations.) In this condition, the two systems are in sympathy, and even when the frequencies are close to each other, and not identical, we still find a greater amplitude in the forced vibrations than when they differ considerably. This aspect of resonance can be seen in a *resonance curve*, as in Fig. 1.9. Figure 1.9 shows that a lightly damped system produces forced vibrations of great amplitude, but only near the point of resonance: that is, where the frequencies of the two systems are in sympathy. On the other hand, although a highly damped system produces a lesser amplitude, this is spread out over a great range of frequencies. The former type is often

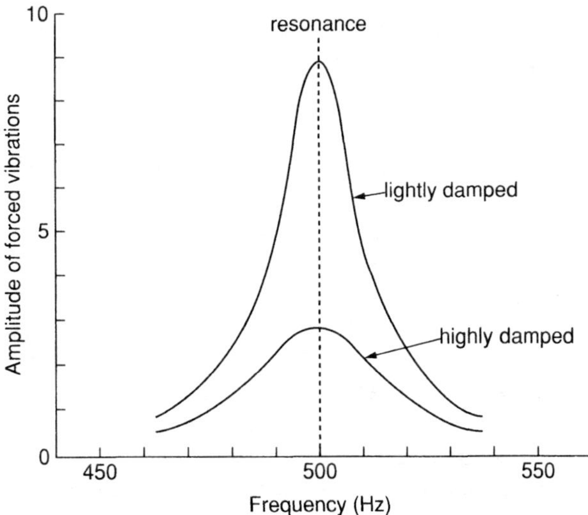

FIG 1.9. Resonance curves for lightly damped and highly damped systems.

described as *sharply tuned.* (Recall that damping is the absorption of energy to overcome the force of friction in a vibrating system. The amount of damping that occurs depends on the physical properties of the system concerned.)

Resonance and Complex Waves

We have seen how forced vibrations are most effective when the natural frequencies of the two systems coincide. But what happens when the driving force, as in speech, is not a simple tone of one natural frequency but a complex tone having more than one frequency and associated harmonics? The answer is straightforward: As long as the natural frequency of the driven system is included in the complex tone of the driver, this frequency will be selected by the resonator and amplified. (Obviously, if it is not included, then the nearest frequency will be amplified to a lesser extent, as seen in Fig. 1.9.)

> In many instances, such as the vocal tract in speech, or a wind instrument in music, the resonator is adjustable. This means that it can be altered so that particular frequencies in the driving force can be maximally amplified by the resonator.

Another important property of resonators is that many have multiple modes of vibration. These are related to different wavelengths, which means that a complex tone in the driving force may well result in resonance in the driven system at a series of different wavelengths (or frequencies), though the amplitude of the forced vibrations decreases with the higher frequencies. This is illustrated in Fig. 1.10 and is particularly important in speech, where the normal noise source is a complex tone, rich in harmonics (see *formants* in the following section). The fact that a resonator amplifies certain frequencies also means that it "ignores" (or "absorbs") others, as it were. In this respect resonators act as filters, reducing the amplitude of ranges of frequencies. This again is an important feature of the acoustics of speech production.

Sound Spectra

Work on resonance allows us a method of classifying speech sounds acoustically. We can do this by examining the *frequency spectra* of the sounds, that is a description of what frequencies are to be found in the mixture and their relative amplitudes. Acoustic analysis of this sort is normally done via speech spectrography, but the results can be set out diagrammatically as in

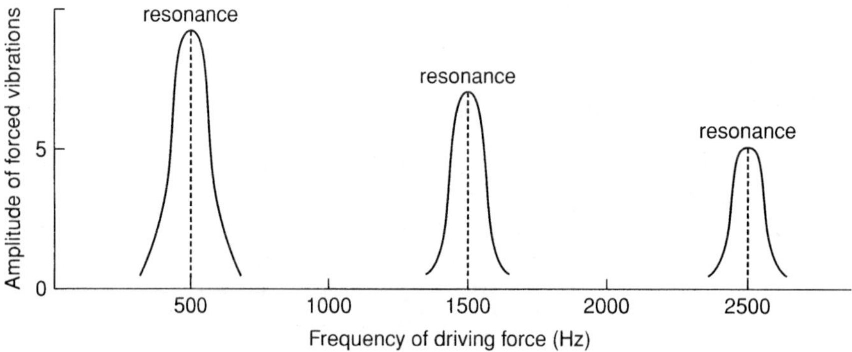

FIG 1.10. Multiple resonances.

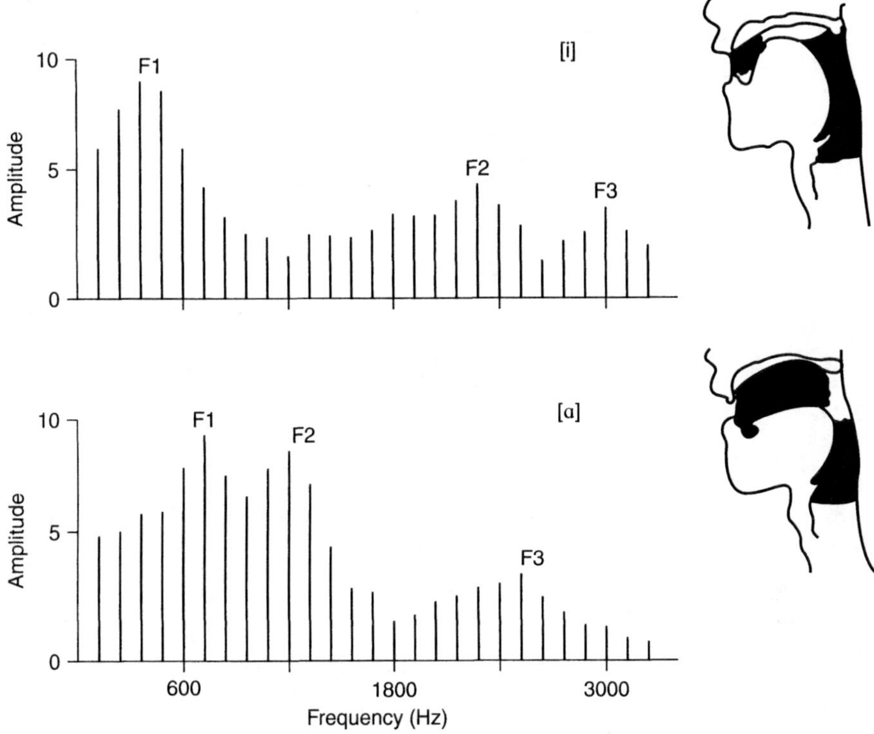

FIG 1.11. Spectra of two vowels: [i] and [ɑ].

Fig. 1.11. We can see that in speech sounds, although the fundamental frequency of speech alters from moment to moment (to create differences in pitch, for example), the overall shape (or *envelope*) of each sound is more or less constant.

Figure 1.11 also shows three of the resonances of the vocal tract (see previous section) for the sounds concerned. In speech acoustics we refer to these peaks of amplitude as *formants.* Because the vocal tract can alter shape, these formants will occur at different frequencies for different sounds. The identification of formant structure is an important part of the acoustic analysis of voiced speech sounds.

Sound Spectrography

Sound spectrography is the way in which we can analyze speech to discover its frequency, intensity, and temporal characteristics. Spectrography can be undertaken with dedicated computer hardware–software combinations or through software programs (often available free) loaded onto a PC that has sound capabilities. Recorded samples of speech taken (either from tape or CDs, or through direct microphone input) can be analyzed in various ways. The results can be displayed on screen and be printed out for a permanent record. Most commonly encountered in acoustic work is the *sound spectrogram*, which plots time against frequency, with intensity also shown by the darkness of the markings. This is a useful technique if we wish to examine stretches of continuous speech. The spectrograph can also provide frequency spectra from a single point in time (which can clearly reveal formant structure), pitch traces, and intensity traces.

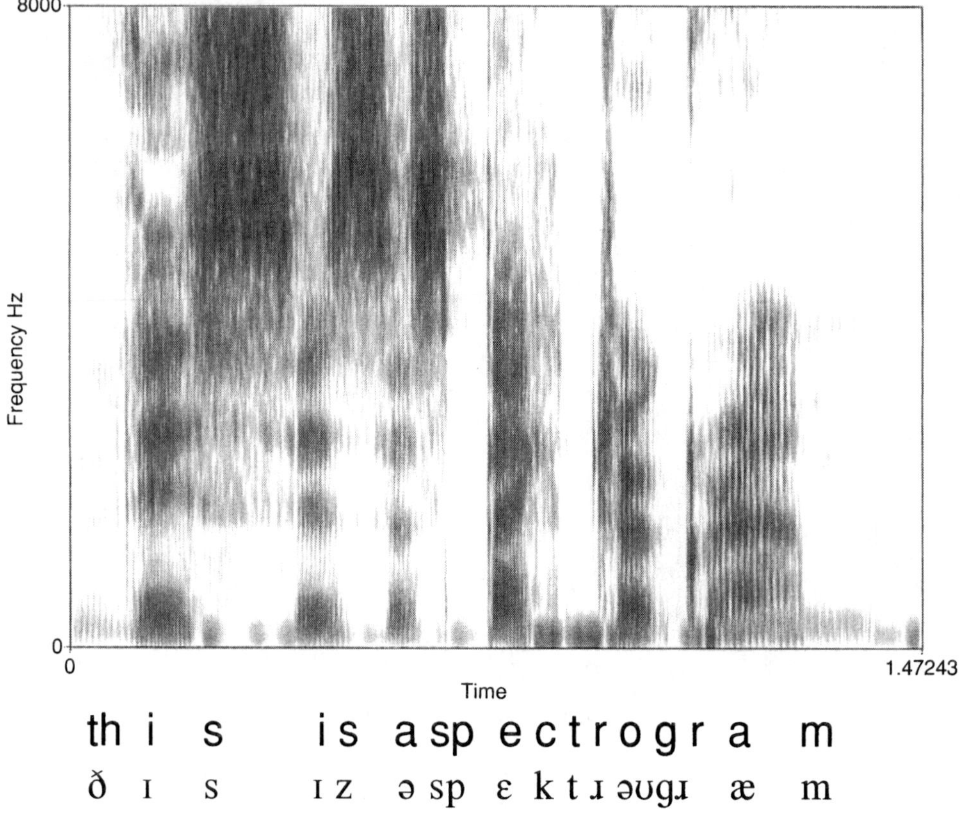

FIG 1.12. Wideband spectrogram of "this is a spectrogram" (annotated in ordinary orthography and phonetic symbols).

We illustrate different sounds and stretches of sounds with spectrographic printouts throughout the book. To give an idea of what a spectrogram looks like we include here as Fig. 1.12 the phrase "this is a spectrogram," analyzed via a broad band (or wideband) spectrogram.

> Spectrograms can utilize a range of different filter settings, most usually a narrow band filter of 45 Hz, which gives maximum frequency information, or a broad band filter of 300 Hz, which maximizes temporal information.

For connected speech purposes, the broad band setting is ideal. If we wish to concentrate on detailed frequency information, we can access this from a broad band analysis through the use of algorithms designed to obtain sound spectra at a chosen moment of time.

Note that the time axis of the spectrogram (along the bottom) indicates milliseconds (i.e., thousandths of a second); we need this degree of accuracy in speech work. The frequency scale is the vertical axis; this scale can be adjusted depending on how high you wish to have frequency marked. Here the settings allow the highest frequency shown to be 8000 Hz. The spectrogram shows the aperiodicity of the sound [s] in "this" and in "spectrogram" in that the frequency markings are spread randomly across a wide range of frequency levels. On the other hand, the periodic sounds of the vowels show their distinctive formant bands running horizontally at different frequency levels. Finally, you should also be able to see the short blank gaps in the spectrogram that coincide with the sounds [p], [k], [t], and [g] (all in the word "spectrogram"), which demonstrate that these sounds all involve a brief shutting off of the airflow during their production. In later chapters we will examine these features in greater detail.

BACKGROUND READING

The idea of the speech chain is taken from Denes and Pinson (1973), and the description of the basics of acoustics is derived from Ball (1993). Many introductory books on acoustics are available that will provide further details in this area: Kent and Read (1992), Borden, Harris, and Raphael (1994), Johnson (1997), Pickett (1999), and Speaks (1999), among others.

EXERCISES

Review Questions

1. Define *articulatory*, *acoustic*, and *auditory phonetics*.
2. What is the fundamental frequency of a complex waveform?
3. How is frequency related to pitch?
4. What is the difference between amplitude and intensity?
5. What is loudness, and how do we measure it?
6. What are free and forced vibrations?
7. Explain how resonance works.
8. What are sound spectra?
9. How do spectrograms distinguish periodic and aperiodic sounds?

Study Topics and Experiments

1. Use any available acoustic analysis package (either one provided by your instructor, or one that you can download free from the Internet) and compare spectrograms for the following samples: (a) the sound of tearing up a piece of paper, (b) a telephone ringing, and (c) a single note produced on a keyboard.
2. Given what you have read about the acoustics of speech, can you explain how sound travels under water, and why speech produced under water sounds so odd, compared to normal speech?

CD

The examples and exercises on the CD for this first chapter are designed to help you distinguish between written letters and spoken sounds. This will be of great help for the chapters to come. Answers to test items are at the end of the book.

2

The Organs of Speech

THE VOCAL TRACT

The expression "the vocal organs" is one that nonspecialists often use without considering which organs, exactly, they have in mind. If you ask them what they mean by the term, you may get answers ranging from the tongue alone, through all the structures of the mouth, and sometimes even including the nose as well. For the phonetician, these answers are not precise enough. Indeed, if we wished to include all those structures that play a part in the production of speech sounds, we would need to start with the brain, look also at the central nervous system, and carry on from there. However, we normally concentrate on the *vocal tract*: that is, those structures through which air is drawn ("tract" is cognate with "tractor," and refers to pulling something) when we speak.

> The vocal tract is here defined as the entire respiratory system from the lungs up to the oral cavity (mouth) and nasal cavity (nose). As we will see, the vocal organs within the vocal tract all have primary functions that are not connected to speech.

The lungs, for example, are for breathing, so that oxygen can be brought into the body and carbon dioxide expelled; the larynx's primary function is to regulate the intake of food and drink and prevent accidental inhalation of these into the lungs; the tongue has functions connected with taste and the movement of food particles in the mouth. However, these organs all have secondary functions connected with speech, and some of them have evolved to be better suited for their speech tasks. Because many of the clients we see in the clinic have speech disorders that derive from a problem within the vocal tract (for example, clients with cleft palate), we need to know how this system operates in some detail.

The main functions of the vocal tract in speech are setting a column of air into motion and then modifying this moving airstream in a number of ways to produce the sounds of speech. We can therefore view the vocal tract as an aerodynamic system, with the individual vocal organs contributing to this system. To initiate a moving column of air we need one of two types of device: a bellows or a piston. The vocal tract has a very efficient bellows-like organ (the lungs) and also a piston-like structure (the larynx), and both of these can be used to initiate an airstream for speech. The larynx can also act in a valve-like manner, allowing free flow of air from the lungs, or metering it in small bursts to produce what we term *voice* (a term we will return to in some detail later).

Furthermore, we have a series of cavities above the larynx that can act as resonating chambers. The pharynx and the oral and nasal cavities can all be used to modify the moving airstream and so produce differences in speech sounds. We can modify the shape of the pharynx and oral cavity, in the case of the latter through movements of the tongue, lips, and jaws, and so all of these must be considered as part of the anatomy and physiology of speech. The soft palate can act as a valve, allowing or stopping air from flowing through the nasal cavity. The soft palate, together with the back of the tongue, can also act in a piston-like manner and so be yet another source of an airstream for speech.

As we can see in Fig. 2.1, the vocal tract extends from the two lungs, via the trachea, the larynx, and the pharynx, to the oral and the nasal cavities. We will examine these structures in turn, commencing with the lungs.

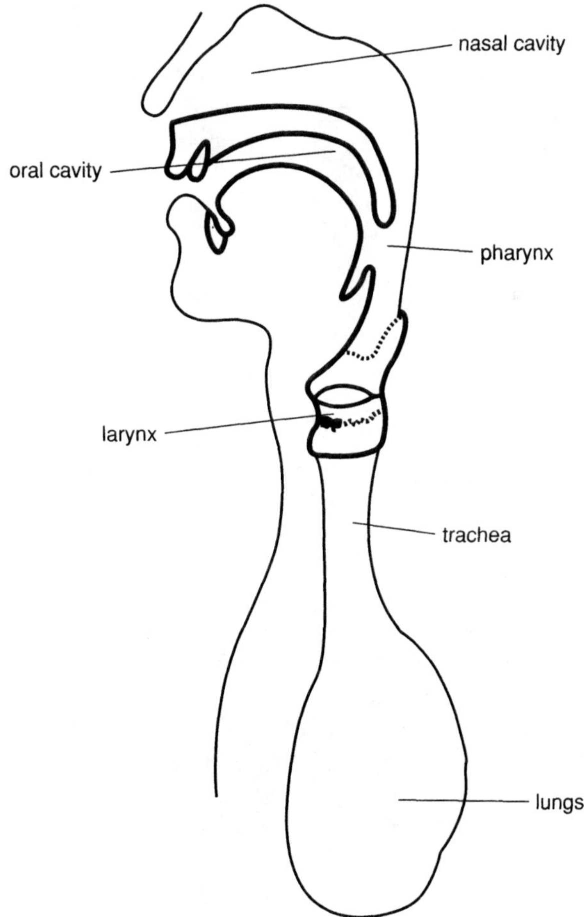

FIG 2.1. The vocal tract.

THE RESPIRATORY SYSTEM

The *lungs* are a pair of organs of an elastic or spongy nature. Although we can characterize them as equivalent to a pair of bellows in their function of drawing air into the body and then expelling it again, they are unlike bellows in their makeup, because they do not consist of two balloon-like structures. It is more accurate to think of them as branching structures, consisting of many air-filled *alveoli* (around 300 million tiny air sacs) that open into *alveolar* ducts, and then into larger tubes (*bronchioles*), all of which come together in the two *bronchi.* These unite at the base of the *trachea* (or windpipe). This arrangement can be seen in Fig. 2.2.

> The lungs are contained within the *pleura,* which consists of one sac (the *visceral pleura)* within another (the *parietal pleura),* the whole making up an airtight entity within the thoracic cavity.

The outer boundary of this arrangement consists of the ribs, whereas the lower one consists of the *diaphragm.* The diaphragm is a large, dome-shaped muscle that separates the thoracic from the abdominal cavities. Apart from the diaphragm, the other important muscles concerned with lung activity are the *intercostals.* The ribs are interconnected by two sets of intercostal muscles: the *external intercostals,* which, among other things, help to expand the thoracic cavity, which creates a negative pressure within it, thus causing air to flow into the lungs to help equalize pressure; and the *internal intercostals*, which, among other things, aid in the contraction of the ribs, thus creating positive pressure, leading to the expulsion of air from the lungs. Other muscles are also involved in breathing (for example, the *pectoralis minor* muscles, which connect the ribs to the shoulder blade, and other abdominal and thoracic muscles), but we do not have the space here to go into all the muscular interactions needed for breathing and speech.

Stated simply, then, the breathing cycle of inspiration and expiration involves first the expansion of the rib cage and lowering of the diaphragm (causing negative air pressure as noted above), resulting in air flowing into the lungs (or *inspiration).* This is followed by a

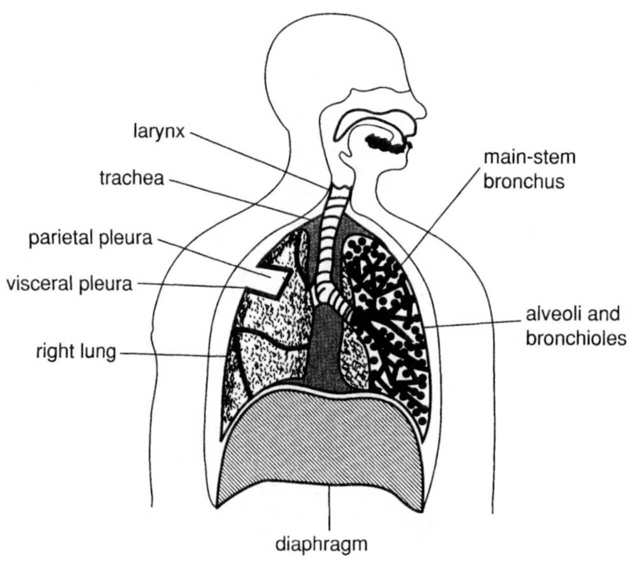

FIG 2.2. The lungs.

combination of gravity and muscular activity to expel air from the lungs. After filling with air, the lungs collapse under their own weight, causing air to start to flow outward again (*expiration*). This is combined with raising of the diaphragm and activity by the internal intercostal muscles to create positive pressure and outward airflow. The lungs never empty completely (see chap. 3 for discussion of amounts of air contained in the lungs at different points in the breathing cycle), but the speed with which they empty can be controlled. This is especially useful for speech, because we normally speak on an outward flowing airstream. By using the external intercostals as a kind of brake during expiration, we can slow this part of the cycle down to allow speech to take place over 2–10 seconds or, exceptionally, up to 25 seconds.

As noted above, the trachea commences at the union of the two bronchi of the lungs. It is a semiflexible tube that is about 11 cm long and consists of a series of rings of cartilage, open at the back, connected by membranes; the top ring of the trachea is also the base of the larynx.

THE LARYNGEAL SYSTEM

The *larynx* also consists of cartilage (in fact, nine separate cartilages), with connective membraneous tissue and sets of intrinsic and extrinsic laryngeal muscles (see Fig. 2.3). For the purposes of speech production, we are mainly interested in the *cricoid* and *thyroid* cartilages and the pair of *arytenoid* cartilages. The *epiglottis* can also have a speech function; this is described in chapter 7.

The cricoid cartilage is the base of the larynx and, as noted above, also functions as the top ring of the trachea. Unlike the other tracheal rings, the cricoid cartilage is a complete ring, which has sometimes been compared to a signet ring, in that the rear portion is flattened out into a large plate. Located above the cricoid cartilage is the thyroid cartilage. This is joined to the cricoid at the cricothyroid joint and the relevant ligaments allow the thyroid cartilage to move in a rocking or gliding motion against the cricoid cartilage.

The thyroid cartilage has been likened to a snowplow, with the front part of the plow being what we call the Adam's apple (or *laryngeal prominence*). This prominence is more marked

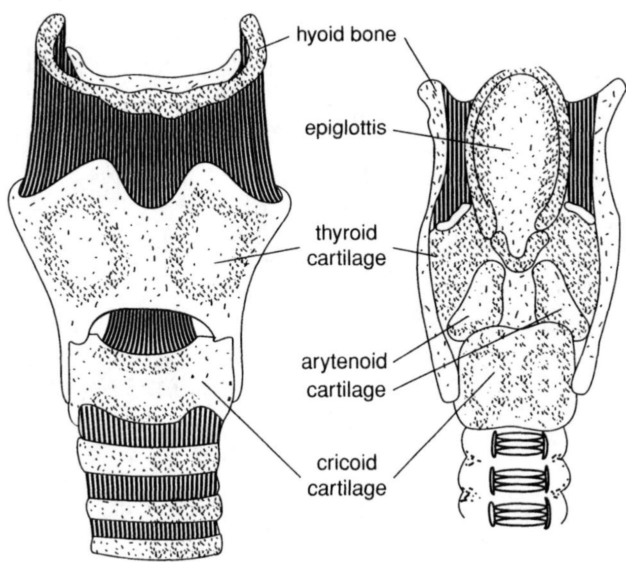

FIG 2.3. The larynx.

in men than in women, partly because the angle of the two thyroid lamina (or blades of the snowplow) is sharper in men than in women (90° as opposed to 120°).

Situated on the signet part of the cricoid ring are the two arytenoid cartilages, which resemble a pair of small pyramids (note that they are a mirror-image pair). They are attached to the cricoid via the cricoarytenoid joint, which allows both forward and backward movement and side-to-side movement. This ability is important for speech because it allows us to adjust the tension of the vocal folds. The arytenoids have a series of small projections, which allow muscular attachments (the *muscular processes*), the cricoarytenoid joint just discussed, and (at the *vocal processes*) the attachments for the *vocal folds.*

The vocal folds run from the arytenoids forward to the interior of the front of the thyroid cartilage (see Figs. 2.3 and 2.4). Each of the folds themselves (the older term *vocal cords* is generally no longer used by phoneticians) consists of a muscle (the *vocalis muscle)* covered by various layers, including the *vocal ligament* (there are different ways of classifying these layers that need not detain us here). The inner edges of the vocal folds, which come into contact when vocal fold vibration takes place (to produce *voice*), are called the margins. These margins are usually divided into the upper and lower (or superior and inferior) margins: in vocal fold vibration the inferior margins make contact first and separate first.

Backward–forward movement of the arytenoids allows us to adjust the tension of the vocal folds (the more tense the vocal folds are, the higher pitch the speaker can produce), whereas side-to-side movement allows us to bring the vocal folds together and move them apart.

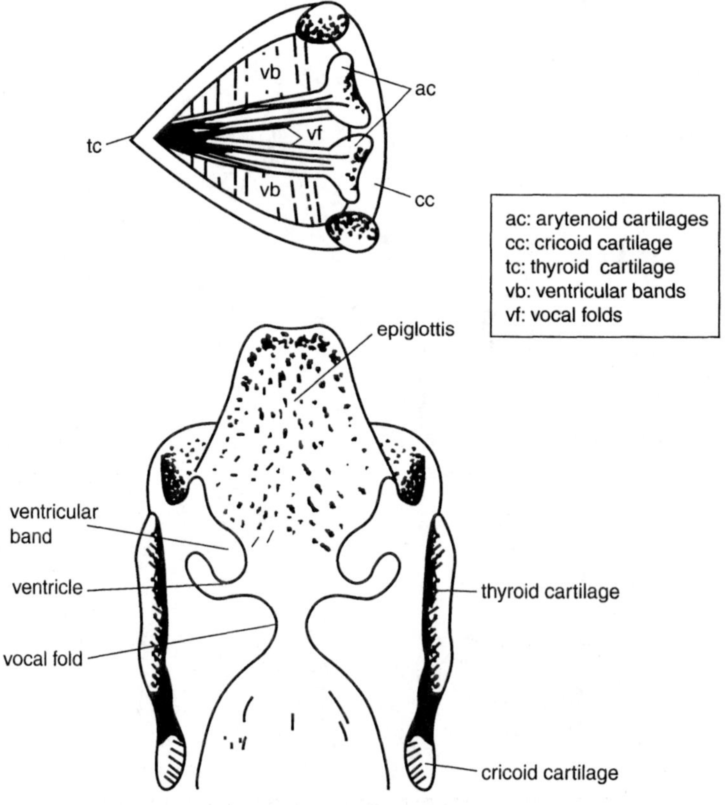

FIG 2.4. The vocal folds.

Above the vocal folds (sometimes termed the *true vocal folds*) are the false vocal folds, or *ventricular bands* (see Fig. 2.4). These are two shelves of tissue situated above the true vocal folds, and although they may be used by themselves or together with the true vocal folds in voice production for special effect, their use normally implies that the speaker has a voice disorder.

The space between the vocal folds is called the *glottis*. Although it may seem strange to have a term for a space, rather than a structure, the glottis is important for speech, because the shape of the space between the folds determines many aspects of voice quality (see chap. 4). The glottis can be open or closed (and various degrees in between), although there is always some resistance to airflow from the lungs, because the maximal glottal opening still covers just under half of the cross-sectional area of the trachea. This resistance to airflow actually causes it to accelerate, and can cause a certain amount of turbulence: the sound [h] is in fact turbulent airflow through an open glottis. Further aspects of glottal shape related to phonation and articulation are dealt with in future chapters.

Finally, we can also note that the larynx itself can be moved slightly upward or downward through the use of the laryngeal muscles. This aids in airflow initiation (see chap. 3) by acting as a piston, but a raised or lowered larynx also plays a role in certain aspects of voice quality (see chap. 4). Above the larynx is the pharynx, which in turn leads to the oral and nasal cavities: it is these supralaryngeal (or supraglottal) structures that we will examine next.

THE SUPRALARYNGEAL SYSTEM

The *pharynx* reaches up from the top of the larynx to the rear of the oral and the nasal cavities. The inferior part can be termed the *oropharynx*, with the superior called the *nasopharynx*. The term *laryngopharynx* has sometimes been used to denote that portion immediately above the larynx. As noted above, all the cavities described in this section are used as resonating chambers in speech production, which increase loudness and alter sound quality. The pharynx is less versatile in this regard than the oral cavity, because there are not many ways to alter the size or shape of the chamber. Nevertheless, certain changes can be made: The larynx may be raised, thus reducing the overall volume of the pharynx; the tongue root and epiglottis can be retracted into the oropharynx, again reducing its volume but also adding an obstruction to the airflow; and finally, the faucal pillars at either side of the back wall of the pharynx may be drawn toward each other, contracting the back wall. This last modification generally results in an alteration to voice quality.

The *nasal cavity* is accessed through the *velopharyngeal port,* and this opening is effected through the lowering of the *velum* (or *soft palate*): see Fig. 2.5. In normal breathing, the velum is lowered all the time, so that air can flow freely through the nose down to the lungs and back out again. However, in speech the majority of sounds are purely oral (that is, the outward flowing air on which speech is produced does not enter the nasal cavity), so the velum must be raised. Nevertheless, a minority of speech sounds in most languages may involve the nasal cavity (for example, [m] and [n] in English), and for these sounds the velum is lowered and the air flows through the nasal cavity (it may also flow through the oral cavity at the same time; this is discussed further in chap. 4). The nasal cavity cannot be modified in size or shape, and the airflow exits through the *nares* or nostrils.

The oral cavity is the most versatile of the three supralaryngeal cavities. The important oral structures for speech are shown in Fig. 2.5. At the front of the oral cavity, the lower jaw (or *mandible*) may be raised or lowered, thus closing or opening the mouth. Linked to this, the upper and lower lips may be brought together or held apart. Also, the lips can adopt a rounded position (different degrees of rounding are possible), spread apart, or be in a neutral shape (see Fig. 5.3 for illustrations of lip shapes). The tongue is the most flexible of the structures within

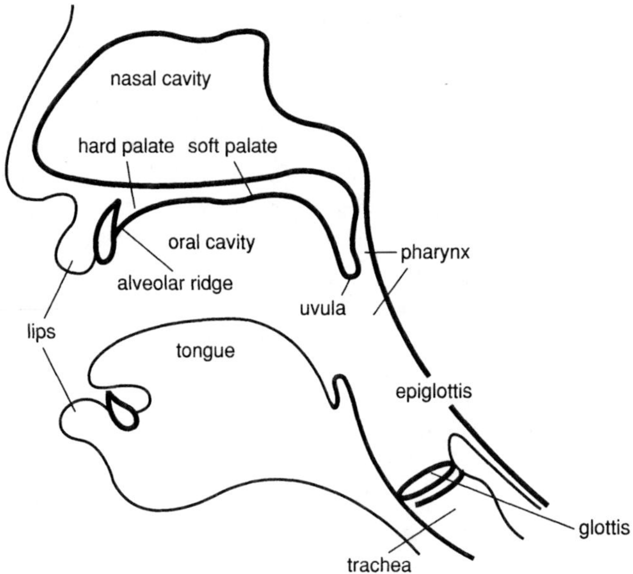

FIG 2.5. The oral cavity.

the supralaryngeal system. Its tip and blade can articulate against the upper teeth or the alveolar ridge; its front section can articulate against the hard palate, and its back against the velum and the uvula; and its root can be retracted into the pharynx (see Fig. 7.1 for a diagram of tongue divisions). The tip and blade are so flexible that they can be bent upward and backward so that the underside of tip and blade articulate against the roof of the mouth. Articulations at these places within the oral cavity can also be of different types (e.g., the tongue firmly touching the alveolar ridge, or leaving a small gap between the tip and the ridge), and these types are described in chap. 6. All these articulations are used in the languages of the world to make individual sounds, and are described in detail in chaps. 5–7.

The modifications to the shape and volume of the oral cavity just described result in a large number of different sound qualities, which go to make up the vowels and consonants of language.

We turn to look at this array of speech sounds in the next few chapters, but before that we also need to consider how the anatomy and physiology of speech allow us to monitor our speech as well as produce it.

MONITORING SPEECH

In previous sections of this chapter we have been interested in the anatomy and physiology of speech production, but here we turn our attention to aspects of the monitoring of speech while it is being produced. It is clear from listening to the speech of hearing-impaired people who learned to speak before experiencing hearing loss (*postlingual hearing loss*) that monitoring of speech through hearing plays an important role. This *auditory feedback* is clearly used to monitor our accuracy in the production of prosodic aspects of speech such as intonation, loudness, tempo (see chap. 9), and voice quality (e.g., harsh, breathy, or modal [= normal];

see chap. 4), because these are among the most obvious disruptions in the speech of postlingually hearing-impaired individuals, especially when their hearing loss occurred some time previously.

Phonetic disruptions also occur at the level of individual speech sounds with these speakers. We find inaccuracies in the vowel system, and precision in the production of many consonants may also deteriorate over time. We can even test the role of auditory feedback with non-hearing-impaired speakers by temporarily blocking it (usually through the use of padded headphones to block most sound from the ears). If you attempt this experiment, remember to record your own speech on a tape recorder, or ask a colleague to let you know how you speak with the headphones on. Certain prosodic features are the first to be affected, loudness and tempo especially. It would appear then that these are under immediate control of auditory feedback, whereas the stored neuromuscular patterns required for intonation, individual sound production, and so on take longer to degrade without this feedback.

However, it has long been known that auditory feedback is not the only monitoring mechanism in speech. For one thing, auditory feedback takes a comparatively long time in speech production terms (see Fig. 2.6 for a simplified model of speech production and feedback); the

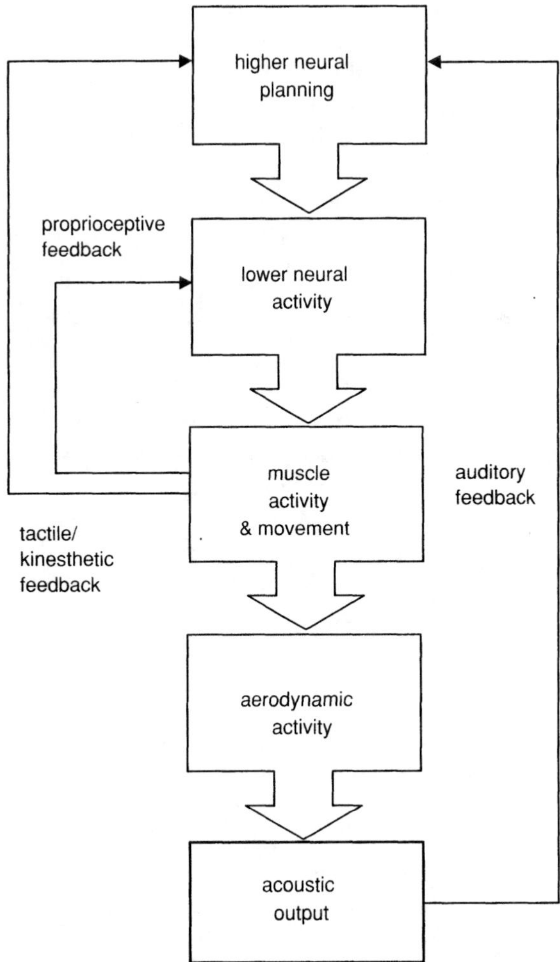

FIG 2.6. Model of speech feedback.

time it takes from the movement of the speaker's articulators until the resultant sound is heard and any necessary alterations can be made is between 160 and 250 msec (= milliseconds, or thousandths of a second). Although this seems a very short time, it is longer than many individual sounds take to utter. Therefore, auditory feedback cannot be used to monitor the production of individual sounds, for even with long segments, such as some vowels, the majority of the sound would be completed before any correction could be made. This is not a problem with features such as loudness, intonation, and so on, which take place over a stretch of segments; and, as already mentioned, these are the very features that often cause the most problems for speakers with postlingual hearing impairment.

Nevertheless, postlingually hearing-impaired speakers very often do experience eventual attrition of the accuracy of consonants and vowels as well as of prosodic features. It appears, then, that although auditory feedback cannot monitor the production of individual segments, it is used to monitor the overall accuracy of classes of vowels and consonants (by testing whether they "sound" correct, presumably). Without it, the stored neuromuscular patterns will deteriorate over time and cannot be corrected even using the other monitoring strategies discussed below.

Another feedback mechanism for speech, and one that might help in monitoring individual segments, is the *tactile/kinesthetic feedback* mechanism derived from the sense of touch and the ability to sense movement. Both tactile and kinesthetic receptors are found throughout the vocal tract. Tactile receptors are responsible for information about touch and pressure; kinesthetic ones inform us about the movement and position of vocal organs. The feedback from these receptors, therefore, can help speakers monitor the accuracy of the movement and placement of the articulators, and this in turn informs speakers about the accuracy of the execution of the neural commands for speech.

The tongue has a large number of tactile and kinesthetic receptors, and this fact helps us to monitor the placement of the tongue, most important for a majority of individual speech sounds. Other parts of the supralaryngeal vocal tract are not so well endowed with receptors: for example, the palate does not have many. This is not a drawback, however, because when the palate is the *passive articulator* for a speech sound, the tongue is the *active articulator,* and so accuracy of articulation can still be monitored by the latter.

The importance of tactile/kinesthetic feedback has been demonstrated through the examination of speakers who lack this mechanism due to an impairment to the receptors (this can be congenital). Alternatively, through the use of a local anaesthetic, the feedback mechanism can be temporarily turned off in experimental subjects and their speech can then be investigated. Such studies show that the lack of this monitoring route results in speech errors, generally in the articulation of individual speech segments. The tactile/ kinesthetic feedback loop is clearly shorter than the auditory one (see Fig. 2.6), but even so it is still too long for monitoring the fine muscle activity required for the correct production of certain speech sounds or parts of speech sounds. We still need to find a quicker route.

Such a very fast feedback system requires that we examine the in-built feedback mechanism found with muscle activation (including, of course, muscle activation for speech). This feedback mechanism has been termed the *proprioceptive* or *gamma loop*. If we simplify this somewhat, we can state that neural impulses originating at higher levels of planning are transmitted via alpha and gamma motor neurons to the muscles. The resultant movement of the muscle is sensed in the *muscle spindle*, and impulses are sent back from the muscle spindles via the gamma system to impinge on the alpha motor neurons again. The returning gamma signal is compared via an automatic process with the original outgoing signal and changes are made to any deviations.

This comparison and emendation process takes place in an area of lower neural activity, and so is a quasi-automatic system, which does not need to be mediated by higher neural functions (unlike the two previous feedback mechanisms discussed). This results in an extremely rapid monitoring procedure, which we assume must be fast enough to control accuracy for even the most rapid and finest articulator movements in speech production (see Fig. 2.6).

Our discussion of feedback mechanisms in speech allows us to propose a simple model of speech production and monitoring. In Fig. 2.6 we show a diagram of this model. The model consists of a series of boxes representing different stages in speech production (we have collapsed several stages into one in many of these boxes). The first of these we call *higher neural planning,* which represents the neural activity required to devise a message, organize it into phonological units needed for speech, and plan the ordering of neural impulses necessary for the final phonetic effect. Both auditory and tactile/kinesthetic monitoring feedback fit into this area, as they have to be decoded before any changes can be implemented.

Lower neural planning concerns the area where the actual nerve impulses are sent and, as mentioned above, where gamma loop feedback operates. The result of action in this box is *muscle activity* and the *physical movement* of articulators and other vocal organs. This is the source of both gamma loop feedback and the tactile/kinesthetic systems, but as the figure shows, they have different destinations. *Aerodynamic activity* is the result of vocal organ activity (see chap. 3), leading to *acoustic output* (i.e., the speech sounds themselves). This last stage of the speech production process is the source of auditory feedback, and the model demonstrates the long path back to higher neural planning (via the hearing system, not included in the diagram) of this monitoring system.

BACKGROUND READING

Perkins and Kent (1986) and Barlow (1999) are texts on the anatomy and physiology of speech that can be recommended for more detailed examination of this area. Further sources are, for example, Kahane and Folkins (1984), Culbertson and Tanner (1997), Kent (1997), and Seikel et al. (2000).

EXERCISES

Review Questions

1. What is the difference between the "vocal organs" and the "vocal tract"?
2. What is needed to set a column of air in motion, and which parts of the vocal tract can fulfill this function?
3. What controls the speed of airflow in speech?
4. Which cartilages of the larynx are the most important for speech production?
5. What is the "Adam's apple"?
6. What controls tension of the vocal folds?
7. What is the glottis?
8. What are the supralaryngeal structures involved in speech production?
9. What is the relation between the position of the velum and breathing?
10. What are the three types of speech feedback mechanisms?

Study Topics and Experiments

1. Use headphones or earplugs to block out most of your own speech. Choose a brief reading passage (such as the "Rainbow Passage") and record yourself reading the passage once

with most of your hearing blocked, and once without headphones or earplugs. Describe in as much detail as you can the differences between the two recordings.

> The Rainbow Passage:
> When the sunlight strikes raindrops in the air, they act like a prism and form a rainbow. The rainbow is a division of white light into many beautiful colors. These take the shape of a long round arch, with its path high above, and its two ends apparently beyond the horizon. There is, according to legend, a boiling pot of gold at one end. People look, but no one ever finds it. When a man looks for something beyond his reach, his friends say he is looking for the pot of gold at the end of the rainbow.

2. Compare the longest duration you can hold a sound with those of three of your colleagues. Record all four attempts on a good quality tape recorder with an external microphone. Tell each person to take a deep breath and then to say the vowel sound "ah" for as long as he or she can. Then measure the recorded vowels in two ways: first, using a stop watch while you play back the tape; then, by inputting the recordings into a computer with any good sound analysis program (your instructor will tell you how to do this) and measuring the vowels in milliseconds from either the sound pressure wave or a spectrogram using the cursors on the screen. Note the difference in measurement between the stop watch and the sound analysis program, as well as the differences between the speakers.

CD

The examples and test items on the CD for this chapter are concerned with the identification of syllables, an important ability for speech-language clinicians. Turn to the end of the book for answers to exercises.

3

Initiation of an Airstream

INTRODUCTION

In the last chapter we looked at the various organs that have been adapted for speech production. We noted that some of these vocal organs can be used in particular ways: as valves, as pistons, and as bellows. In this chapter we will see how these organs and their movement types can be used to initiate speech. For speech to occur, we need a moving stream of air that the articulators can "shape" and so produce the individual sounds of speech. For air in the vocal tract to move we need an airstream mechanism that can alter the air pressures within the vocal tract. Problems connected to incorrect airstream use, airstream initiation, and airstream direction may all be encountered in speech and voice clinics. Although some of the following discussion on aerodynamics is quite complex, it is useful background information.

> In this and the following chapters, we will illustrate individual sounds through the use of *phonetic symbols* (see the Introduction to the book, and the final section of this chapter). We put these phonetic symbols into square brackets to distinguish them from ordinary writing.

AERODYNAMICS OF AIRSTREAM INITIATION

First we need to consider what air pressure is. Pressure is usually defined in terms of force applied to a particular unit of area. In the SI (or metric) system, the unit of force is the *dyne*. A dyne is defined as being the force that produces an acceleration of 1 cm per second per second when applied to a mass of 1 gram. Pressure is then described in terms of *dynes per square centimeter* (dyne/cm^2). This measure is, however, only suitable for very small differences in pressure, and in phonetics we usually take a somewhat different approach. The larger-scale pressure changes recorded in speech initiation can be described in terms of the units used by meteorologists to record air pressure. These include the *bar* (which equals 1 million dyne/cm^2) and the *millibar* (one one-thousandth of a bar). More often, though, phoneticians use a measure that refers to the height of a column of liquid (for example, mercury or water) that a given pressure could hold up. The usual liquid referred to in phonetics is water, so the measure is *centimeters of water* (cmH_2O). At sea level, normal air pressure is about 1030 cmH_2O, so we can use this as a baseline when examining air pressure changes in the vocal tract if the experiment is conducted near sea level. (If the phonetics lab is well above sea level, a new baseline will have to be worked out with the help of a barometer). Air pressure does differ in different parts of the vocal tract due to movement of the lungs and other vocal organs, and we will refer to these in later sections of this chapter.

If our phonetics lab is based in Louisiana, then we can use the sea level measure of 1030 cmH_2O. If, however, we were in Denver, Colorado, then we would need to take a baseline measure of around 850 cmH_2O, and if we were in Mexico City, that would lower to 775 cmH_2O.

How do air pressure changes cause air to flow? Let us consider a pneumatic system (that is, an air-filled system). For our example it doesn't matter whether this system consists of a single chamber or a series of chambers filled with air. Air within a system such as this will normally be at a constant pressure, so if we lower the air pressure at one end of the system, some of the air throughout the remainder of the system will flow toward this spot to bring the overall pressure back to balance. Conversely, if we raise the pressure in one part of the system, air at that point will flow away from this high-pressure point out to the rest of the system—again, in order to bring about an equal pressure throughout. So, if we remember that air in any pneumatic system seeks an equilibrium of pressure, we will understand how increasing or decreasing the pressure will cause air to flow.

If air pressure changes are responsible for the movement of air in a system, what is responsible for causing the air pressure changes? If we increase the volume of the pneumatic system, then we have the same amount of air we started with, but it is spread out through a larger volume container: if you like, we have thinned out the air. This results in lower pressure, as the same amount of air is acting on a larger volume. Conversely, if we decrease the volume of our system—make it smaller—then we have pushed the same amount of air we started with into a smaller space. This increases the pressure, as the air is now acting on a smaller volume than we started with. Air pressure changes, then, come about through the activity of increasing or decreasing the volume of the pneumatic system.

We now need to go back one more step. How do we increase or decrease the volume of our pneumatic system? If this were a mechanical system we could use means such as pistons or bellows to expand or contract the overall volume, but, of course, we are considering in this chapter the aerodynamics of speech. Remember, though, that we saw in the previous chapter how some of the vocal organs can in fact act as pistons and as bellows—they can, therefore, be used to alter the overall volume of the vocal tract and set up pressure changes leading to airflow throughout the tract. The lungs act like a set of bellows, and because of their relatively large volume, can cause large pressure changes (relatively speaking), and thus can set large volumes of air in motion, such that we can speak quite lengthy utterances on a single exhalation from the lungs. The larynx can act as a piston, but its movement is restricted to a few millimeters (mm) up and down. Therefore, it can only cause relatively small pressure changes, and so lead only to minor flows of air through the vocal tract. Even the tongue can, in certain special circumstances which we describe later, act like a piston and produce very small pressure changes leading to just enough airflow to make single sounds of a special type (see *clicks*, later).

In speech, therefore, we must consider several different ways of setting air in motion. First, we must identify the initiator (that is, the organ that is being used to change air pressure); second, we must note whether the initiator is being used to create positive pressure or negative pressure (often termed *compression* and *rarefaction*, respectively); and finally, we must consider the

TABLE 3.1
Types of Airstream

	Pulmonic	*Glottalic*	*Velaric*
Compression	pulmonic egressive	glottalic egressive	*[velaric egressive]*
Rarefaction	*[pulmonic ingressive]*	glottalic ingressive	velaric ingressive

Note: Brackets mark types not found in natural language.

direction of the airflow: out of the vocal tract (egressive) or into the vocal tract (ingressive). The direction of airflow derives from the type of pressure change: compression results in egressive airflow, rarefaction results in ingressive airflow.

In natural language (that is to say, the naturally occurring languages of the world), only three initiators are found (we will discuss other initiators found extralinguistically and in voice clients who have had laryngectomies later): the lungs, the larynx, and the tongue. Each of these initiators is capable of producing compression and rarefaction (thus egressive and ingressive airflow), but only some of these are found in the languages of the world.

Airstreams derived from the three main initiators are termed as follows:

lungs—*pulmonic*
larynx—*glottalic* (or *laryngeal*)
tongue—*velaric* (or *oralic*)

Table 3.1 shows which airstream types can be found in the languages of the world. The airstreams in italics are those that are possible to make, but are not found in natural language.

In the following sections we will examine each of these airstream types in more detail and conclude by looking at airstreams used in clinical situations.

PULMONIC AIRSTREAMS

To a certain extent, using pulmonic airstreams for speech can be thought of as using modified breathing. However, there are some differences. First, we normally speak only on exhaled breath. Although it is possible to use a pulmonic ingressive airstream (i.e., inhaled breath) when speaking, the resultant speech is harsh and unnatural, and it is difficult to maintain the airflow for very long. This leads us to consider the second modification of normal breathing for speech: the exhalation part of the breathing cycle is slowed considerably in speech as compared to quiet breathing, allowing us to speak for several seconds on one exhalation.

We mentioned earlier that the volume of air available for speech using a pulmonic egressive airstream was greater than that in airstreams initiated at the larynx or in the mouth. Probably this is one of the reasons that this airstream is found in all known languages and, indeed, for the vast majority of languages it is the only airstream used in speech. Even for languages that use other airstreams, this one is used for the majority of speech sounds. We consider here the volumes of air associated with normal breathing, so that we can see how these can be exploited in speech. For air volume we use the SI unit of the liter. In normal breathing (termed *tidal*), the volume of air used is termed the *tidal volume*. This volume will differ depending on how much exertion is being used during normal breathing (compare breathing at rest to breathing

TABLE 3.2
Lung Volumes

Lung volume	*Capacity in liters*
Tidal volume	0.5
Inspiratory reserve volume	2.5
Expiratory reserve volume	2.0
Residual volume	2.0
Inspiratory capacity	3.0
Vital capacity	5.0
Functional residual capacity	4.0
Total lung capacity	7.0

Note: Source, Laver, 1994; after Hixon, 1973.

after climbing a flight of stairs). We can work out an average figure, however. Further, we also know the upper and lower limits of the amount of air it is physically possible to breathe in and out; these are termed the *inspiratory* and *expiratory reserve volumes*. These amounts are over and above the tidal volume, so they will, of course, differ from time to time, depending on what the tidal volume is. Again, average figures can be derived from the average tidal volume being assumed. The lungs can never be totally emptied of air, however, so there will always be a *residual volume* in them.

Other air volumes are often referred to in the study of pulmonic airstreams. For example, if the tidal volume is added to the inspiratory reserve volume, we get the *inspiratory capacity*, which is the maximum amount of air that can be breathed in when you have the minimum tidal volume. Conversely, if we add the tidal volume to the inspiratory and expiratory reserve volumes we get the *vital capacity*: that is, the maximum volume of air that can be expelled after a maximum inspiration. If we need to know the amount of air left in the lungs at the minimum of the tidal volume, we add the residual volume to the expiratory reserve volume, which gives us the *functional residual capacity*. Finally, we can derive the maximum amount of air the lungs can hold from these measures, and this is termed the *total lung capacity*. Table 3.2 shows typical amounts for all these measures for a healthy young adult male, standing upright, at sea level.

Apart from air volumes, we can also measure different air pressures involved in normal breathing and in pulmonic speech. There is, of course, *atmospheric pressure*: the pressure of the ambient air (which varies depending on height above sea level). *Vocal tract pressure* will be similar to the atmospheric pressure if measured at a point in time halfway between maximum inspiration and maximum expiration; otherwise it will be higher or lower than atmospheric pressure dependent on which point in the cycle of breathing we examine. It should also be noted that a single pressure does not always hold throughout the vocal tract, and this is especially so during speech. *Pulmonic pressure* (an equivalent term, *subglottal pressure*, may also be encountered) may differ from *supraglottal pressure* because of the activity of the vocal folds in the larynx (see chap. 2). To produce a sound with vibrating vocal folds (such as vowels), there must be a pressure difference of 2 cmH_2O between the subglottal and supraglottal pressures to drive the vibratory system, with the subglottal pressure higher than the supraglottal (this is explained in more detail in the next chapter).

Maximum pressure differentials in inspiration of about –100 cmH_2O (i.e., 100 cmH_2O lower than prevailing atmospheric pressure) have been measured, and with expiration pressure differentials of about 160 cmH_2O have been recorded (that is, 160 cmH_2O higher than prevailing atmospheric pressure). In speech we do not use much of this possible range, even when shouting. For example, a range of *intraoral pressures* of between 3 and 15 cmH_2O (above atmospheric) has been recorded; in shouting, subglottal pressures may be 40 cmH_2O above normal.

> Phoneticians are also interested in velocity of airflow. We can measure *particle velocity* (how fast a particle of air changes position) and *volume velocity* (the volume of air passing through the system in a given time). Both these measures vary depending on the sounds being spoken, how emphatic the speaker is being, and so on.
>
> An average particle velocity in speech is between 1000 and 4000 cm/s (centimeters per second), and an average volume velocity for quiet speech is 100 to 250 ml/s (milliliters per second), though this can rise to 1000 or more for some sounds.

So we now know some of the air volumes involved in pulmonic airstreams, and some of the air pressures. How is this airstream set in motion? Let us first consider normal breathing. As we noted earlier, we need to change air pressure to get air to move. In normal breathing the lungs are expanded (through the action of the diaphragm and the external intercostal muscles). This leads to a lowering of pressure within the lungs, and air flows in to equalize this pressure. At the head of the breathing cycle, the lungs are filled with air and the effect of gravity causes them to start collapsing, and so to expel the air. This is aided by use of the internal intercostal muscles that contract the rib cage and so contract the lungs also (inherent elastic properties of the lungs, rib cage, and diaphragm aid this contraction). At this point the positive pressure in the lungs causes aerodynamic conditions that promote outward-flowing air. When the lungs are emptied (apart from their residual volume), muscle activity takes over once more to expand the lungs and start the cycle all over again. Figure 3.1 shows the pressure changes involved in breathing.

In speech, we need to adapt this quasi-automatic system so that we have enough air and enough time to speak. We use muscle activity to increase the tidal volume by speeding up the inspiration stage and postponing the lung collapse point. To slow down the expiration stage, we use the external intercostal muscles as a kind of braking mechanism. This allows us to speak for several seconds on a single breath. This stage can be maintained for up to 25 seconds, but normally we use between 2 and 10 seconds for speech on one expiration. This airstream is clearly well suited to speech, because it allows many sounds to be uttered on one expiration and allows us to control loudness through the volume of air going through the system.

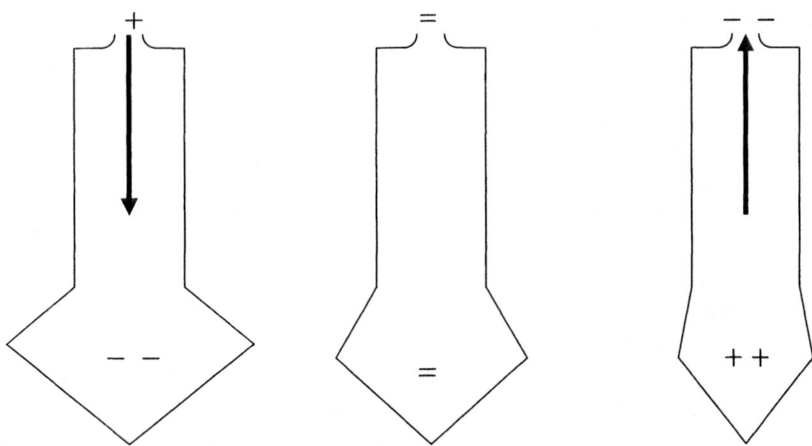

FIG 3.1. Pressure changes involved in breathing.
(+: positive pressure; –: negative pressure; =: equal pressure; arrow shows direction of airflow.)

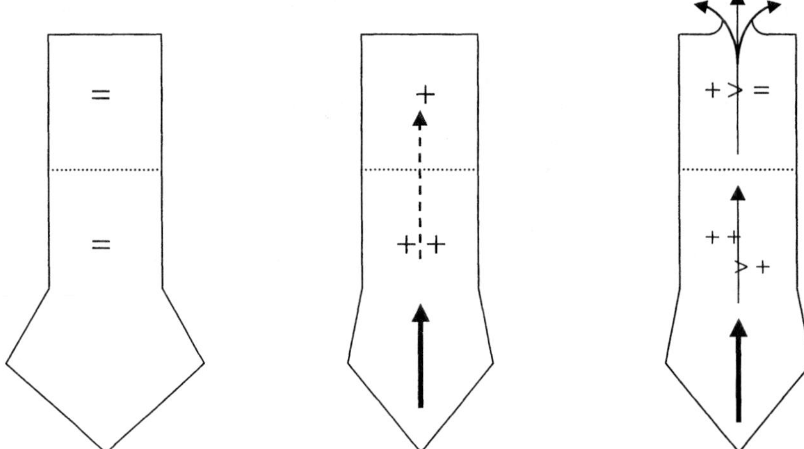

FIG 3.2. Voiced pulmonic egressive airstream.
(Dotted line: vibrating vocal folds.)

Airflow through a pneumatic system can be of different types: laminar (or smooth) and turbulent (or rough). Turbulence is related to velocity (faster velocities tend to produce turbulent airflow) and to the presence of obstacles in the path of the airflow (e.g., in the case of speech, the position of the tongue in the mouth). English sounds such as [f] and [s] have turbulent airflow, whereas vowels such as [i] and [u] have laminar airflow.

It is worth noting that pressure differences in pulmonic egressive speech may not always be as simple as those shown in Fig. 3.1. Where sounds involve vocal fold vibration, as noted earlier, subglottal and supraglottal pressures must also be considered. In Fig. 3.2 we show a diagram of pressure differentials encountered during the production of voiced plosives (sounds such as [b], [d], [g]).

Various types of consonants and vowels can be produced on a pulmonic egressive airstream:

plosives, e.g., [p, b, t, d, k, g]
fricatives, e.g., [f, v, s, z, h]
nasals, e.g., [m, n]
approximants, e.g., [w, l]
vowels, e.g., [i, ɑ, u]

More details of all these sound types are given in later chapters.

It is possible to use a pulmonic ingressive airstream for speaking, though no known language uses this as a regular part of its speech patterns. It is difficult for us to expand the inspiration part of the breath cycle in time, so if we do speak on an ingressive airflow, we can only produce a few syllables at a time. Further, the shape of the vocal folds is especially suited to air flowing through them from below. With ingressive speech, the vocal folds impart a rough quality to the resultant speech sounds. Nevertheless, pulmonic ingressive speech may sometimes be used when we are counting items rapidly, with each second number spoken on an inflowing airstream (e.g., "one, *two*, three, *four*, five, *six*," where the italicized words are spoken ingressively). Pulmonic ingressive speech has also been reported in different cultures as a means of disguising the voice. Pulmonic ingressive speech may also be encountered clinically. People with voice problems may use it, but it has also been reported in the speech of some persons who stutter.

> There are no phonetic symbols especially for pulmonic ingressive sounds. However, we can add a downward arrow after a symbol, or mark an entire stretch of symbols with the downward arrow, to show that this airstream is being used. For example: [s↓], [{↓sɪks↓}] ("six")

GLOTTALIC AIRSTREAMS

Glottalic Egressive

Glottalic airstreams use a piston-like action to create the necessary air pressure changes needed to set air in motion. For glottalic egressive sounds, the vocal folds within the larynx are clamped firmly shut to create an airtight seal, and the whole larynx is jerked upwards a short way using the extrinsic laryngeal muscles. This action compresses the air above the larynx (up to 40 or 50 cmH_2O above normal), and so causes the air to rush out of the mouth. The rapid increase in pressure means these sounds are relatively loud but, as only the amount of air above the larynx is involved, this airstream only lasts short periods of time. This means that only single sound segments are employed at a time on a glottalic egressive airstream in those languages that use it. Sounds produced on a glottalic egressive airstream are termed *ejectives*, and they are found in many Native American languages, and languages of Africa and Asia. Interestingly, some English speakers use ejective versions of [p, t, k] at the end of words, perhaps for emphasis. Such sounds may also occur, though rarely, as articulation disorders. Figure 3.3 shows the pressure changes involved in the production of ejectives.

> Several different types of ejectives are found in the languages of the world:
>
> ejective stops, e.g., [p', t', k']
> ejective fricatives, e.g., [f', s']
>
> and various combinations of stops and fricatives.

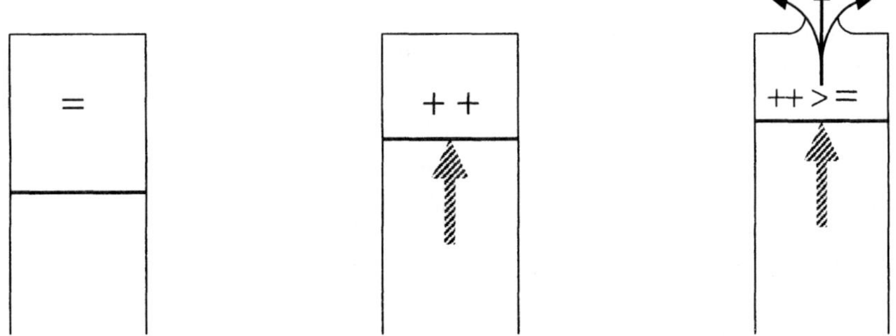

FIG 3.3. Glottalic egressive airstream (ejectives).
(Dark line: closed glottis; shaded arrow: movement of initiator.)

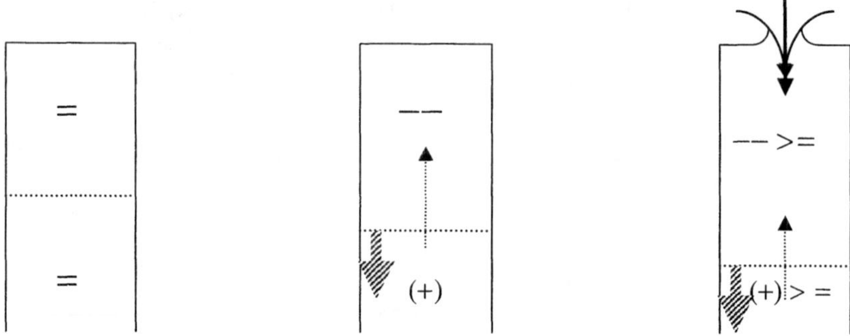

FIG 3.4. Voiced glottalic ingressive airstream (implosives).

Glottalic Ingressive

A glottalic ingressive airstream is produced by bringing the vocal folds together and sealing them, and then jerking the larynx downwards through use of the extrinsic laryngeal muscles. This rarefies the air pressure above the larynx, causing air to flow into the mouth. Sounds produced in this way are termed *reverse ejectives* (or sometimes *voiceless implosives*). It would seem, however, that this process does not produce as much pressure change as with ejectives so the resultant sounds are not only short, but very quiet. In fact, reverse ejectives have been found in very few languages. Much more common are sounds produced on a mixture of glottalic ingressive and pulmonic egressive airstreams. This is achieved by adjusting the seal of the vocal folds so that they are not tightly closed. Then, as the larynx is jerked downwards, the compressed air beneath the larynx can "leak through" the folds, causing them to vibrate. There is, therefore, a combination of air flowing into the mouth and airflow out of the lungs. Together with the sound created by the vibrating vocal folds, this produces enough noise for the resultant speech to be readily audible. Sounds produced this way are termed *voiced implosives* or simply *implosives*. While technically it is possible to produce more than one sound at a time this way (and to produce a variety of consonant types and even vowels), only stop-like consonants seem to occur in natural language. Languages in many parts of the world use implosives, though they are rare in the clinical situation. Figure 3.4 shows the pressure changes involved with implosives.

> It is possible to produce a wide range of implosive consonants and even vowels and sequences of consonants and vowels. However, in the languages of the world, only implosive stops are found, e.g., [ɓ, ɗ, ɠ].
>
> Reverse ejectives/voiceless implosives have been symbolized in two different ways: either using the ejective symbol with a downward arrow ([p'↓, t'↓, k'↓]), or using the implosive symbols with a little circle added to them that stands for voiceless ([ɓ̥, ɗ̥, ɠ̊]).

VELARIC AIRSTREAMS

To produce a velaric ingressive airstream, the back of the tongue makes an air-tight seal against the velum (soft palate). There is also a closure further forward, for example, between the tongue tip and the alveolar ridge. A small pocket of air is trapped between the tongue body and the roof of the mouth, bounded by the two closures mentioned. If the tongue body is lowered (while maintaining the closures), and/or the tongue back slid somewhat further forward, then the air pressure in this pocket is rarefied, as the space between the tongue body and the roof of the mouth has increased. Then, when the forward closure is released (e.g., by lowering the tongue tip in this instance), air will move into the mouth from outside to equalize the pressure difference. There is only enough air pressure differential and air volume to produce short sharp sounds on this airstream, and these sounds are termed *clicks*. Clicks are normal consonant sounds in some languages (mainly in southern Africa), but English speakers use some clicks as extralinguistic sounds; for example, the annoyance sound often written "tut" or "tsk" is a click, as is the sound often used to encourage horses. Clinically, these sounds are not as rare as implosives or ejectives, and clicks have been reported being used for a variety of different target sounds by clients with articulatory disorders. The pressure changes involved in click production are illustrated in Fig. 3.5. We can note that *reverse clicks*, while technically possible, have not been reported for natural language or in clinical data.

Five basic click types occur in natural languages, though combinations of clicks and aspects of pulmonic sounds also occur. The phonetic symbols for clicks do not resemble any letters we're familiar with, partly because the click sounds themselves are so different from pulmonic consonants. The symbols and their places of articulation are [ʘ], bilabial (a kiss-like sound); [ǀ] dental (the "tut" sound); [!], alveolar (a loud hollow-like click sound); [ǂ], palatal (somewhat like the "tut" sound, but pronounced further back in the mouth); and [ǁ], lateral (the encouragement noise for horses).

ESOPHAGEAL AND OTHER AIRSTREAMS

Persons who have had a laryngectomy lose the ability to use the vocal folds to produce *voice* (see chap. 4). Further, the surgery often results in the inlet for breathing being repositioned to a stoma (an artificial opening) in the throat, which means lung air no longer flows out through the mouth. For various types of laryngectomy clients, therefore, a pulmonic egressive airstream

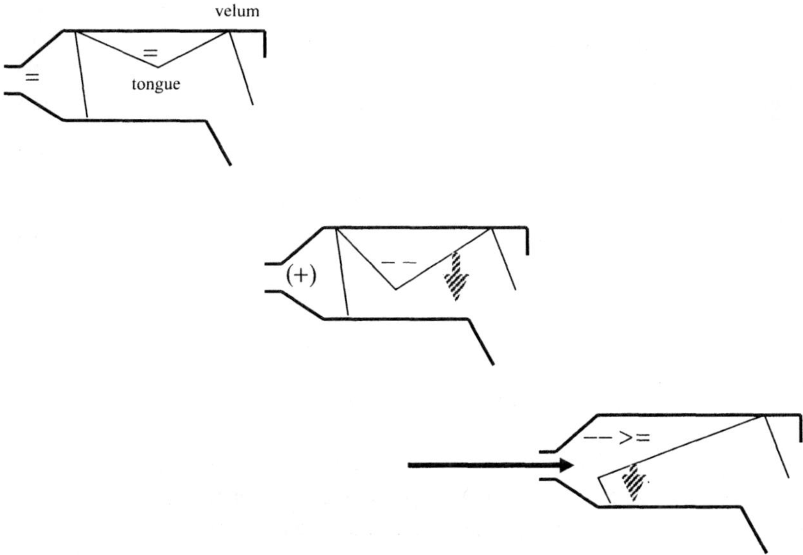

FIG 3.5. Velaric ingressive airstream (clicks).

may no longer be appropriate for speech. An alternative that can be developed by such patients through training is esophageal speech. Here, air is gulped down into the esophagus by the client and regurgitated back up, to flow through the mouth, and so used to produce speech. The equivalent of vocal fold vibration can be brought about as the air is forced past the esophageal sphincter, so serviceable (if somewhat strange-sounding) speech is possible. In clients whose trachea has been attached to the esophagus below the sphincter, tracheo-esophageal speech is used. Here, lung air flows into the esophagus and past the esophageal sphincter, rather than air gulped into the esophagus. Users of these airstreams can develop the ability to produce quite long stretches of speech.

> There are no separate symbols for sounds produced with an esophageal or tracheo-esophageal airstream, although stretches of such speech can be marked with a symbol to show this.
>
> The symbol for esophageal speech is {Œ}, whereas the symbol for tracheo-esophageal speech is {Ю}.

Finally, we can note that a variety of oral airstream mechanisms can be utilized to produce extralinguistic sounds. Perhaps the best known of these extralinguistic sounds is the *raspberry* (or *Bronx cheer*). Here, the cheeks are expanded and filled with air, while the tongue tip is usually protruded between the upper and lower lips. The cheeks are then contracted, forcing the air out between the tongue and the lips, forcing them all to vibrate. Needless to say, if a young client produces this sound, it's not normally a speech error!

TRANSCRIPTION

In this and following chapters of part I you will be required to undertake some transcriptions into the phonetic symbols that we are introducing in these chapters (see exercises for this chapter on the CD). Most of the examples are invented ones that are not intended to be words of any specific language; they are designed simply to develop your ability to perceive speech sound differences (an essential tool for a speech-language pathologist). Because the examples we are using are not from a specific language, the convention is that we put our phonetic symbols into square brackets, for example, [ɬaŋvaɪɹpʊ ɬ]. We always put phonetic symbols into square brackets so that the reader of a report knows when the ordinary orthography ends and the phonetic symbols begin. As we will see in part II, we sometimes use different brackets dependent on the status of the analysis being shown.

BACKGROUND READING

Catford (1977) and Stevens (1998) present more detailed accounts of the aerodynamics of speech. Zajac and Yates (1997) discuss how to measure speech aerodynamics for clinicians. More details on the various airstreams and the languages that use them can be found in standard phonetics texts, such as Laver (1994), and Ball and Rahilly (1999). Studies of click substitutions in disordered speech include Bedore, Leonard, and Gandour (1994), and Heselwood (1997).

EXERCISES

Review Questions

1. How is air pressure measured?
2. How are volumes of air measured?
3. Explain the difference between vital capacity and total lung capacity.
4. What pressure changes are associated with ingressive and egressive airflow respectively?
5. What are the initiators that are used in natural language?
6. What are the main differences between pulmonic egressive speech and all other airstreams (apart from location or direction)?
7. What is the difference between implosives and reverse ejectives?
8. What is the difference between esophageal and tracheo-esophageal airstreams?

Study Topics and Experiments

1. Explain how air is set in motion in a pneumatic system.
2. How have we modified normal breathing to allow the production of speech?

CD

Listen to the examples of sounds using different airstreams, and try to imitate as many as possible. See if you can identify the test examples following the instructions on the CD. Answers to all the exercises are given at the end of the book.

4

Phonation and Voice Quality

INTRODUCTION

In chapter 3 we looked at the different ways in which air for speech can be set into motion within the vocal tract. We also noted that the majority of speech sounds in all languages (and all the speech sounds in most languages) are made on an airstream flowing out of the lungs. Air flowing out of the lungs passes up the trachea and through the larynx before flowing into the pharynx and then into the oral cavity and/or the nasal cavity. As we will see in later chapters, it is in the oral cavity that the articulatory movements take place that are responsible for forming the vowels and consonants of speech. Nevertheless, activity vital for speech occurs before that point, in the larynx. The various positions and movements of the vocal folds within the larynx constitute the process of *phonation*. Further, phonation contributes not just to the differentiation of certain sound segments (which we will describe shortly), but also to the overall *voice quality* of an individual speaker or of particular language or dialect groups. Voice quality, however, can be influenced by factors other than phonation. The overall *articulatory setting* also has a part to play. For example, a hypernasal (i.e., overly nasal) voice quality results if a speaker regularly fails to raise the soft palate completely when speaking.

Both phonatory activity and voice quality are important areas of phonetics for speech–language pathologists. Clients with a variety of communication disorders exhibit problems with phonation, and many clients in the voice clinic, of course, demonstrate difficulties with their voice quality. In this chapter we will examine these issues in some detail.

> As we have noted, pulmonic egressive sounds pass through the larynx, and so undergo phonation. Ejectives are made using air *above* the larynx, and so cannot pass through the larynx. We noted in chap. 3 that implosives were mixed in terms of their airstream, so phonatory activity is possible. Clicks are made in the mouth and so do not themselves undergo phonation; nevertheless, air can still flow up from the lungs during click production, and that air is subject to one or another of the types of phonation.

PHONATION

Main Phonation Types

Phonatory activity occurs in the larynx, as we have noted. In order to understand better how phonation operates we need to look at the structures of the larynx in a little more detail than we did in chapter 1. Figure 4.1(a) is a view of the larynx from above. Of importance for us are the two arytenoid cartilages; these are the triangular-shaped cartilages that sit on the cricoid cartilage and articulate with it. They can move from side to side and forward and backward (controlled by the intrinsic muscles of the larynx, in particular, the arytenoideus muscle and the lateral cricoarytenoid muscle). Attached to the two arytenoid cartilages, and running forward to the interior of the front of the thyroid cartilage, are two parallel muscles with their covering of ligament and tissue: the vocal folds. The inner surface of the folds is sometimes termed the *vocal ligament*. The tension of the vocal folds is controlled by the forward–backward movement of the arytenoids, together with muscle activity from the vocalis and thyroarytenoid.

Because the arytenoids can also move laterally, the folds can be brought close together or moved far apart (in fact, when fully apart the folds still cover about half the opening of the trachea into the larynx). Phonetics has a term for the space between the vocal folds: the *glottis*. The size of the glottis alters depending on whether the vocal folds are together or apart, and so it is convenient for us to refer to the size of the glottis rather than the position of the folds. The various phonation types we will describe in this section depend considerably on the size

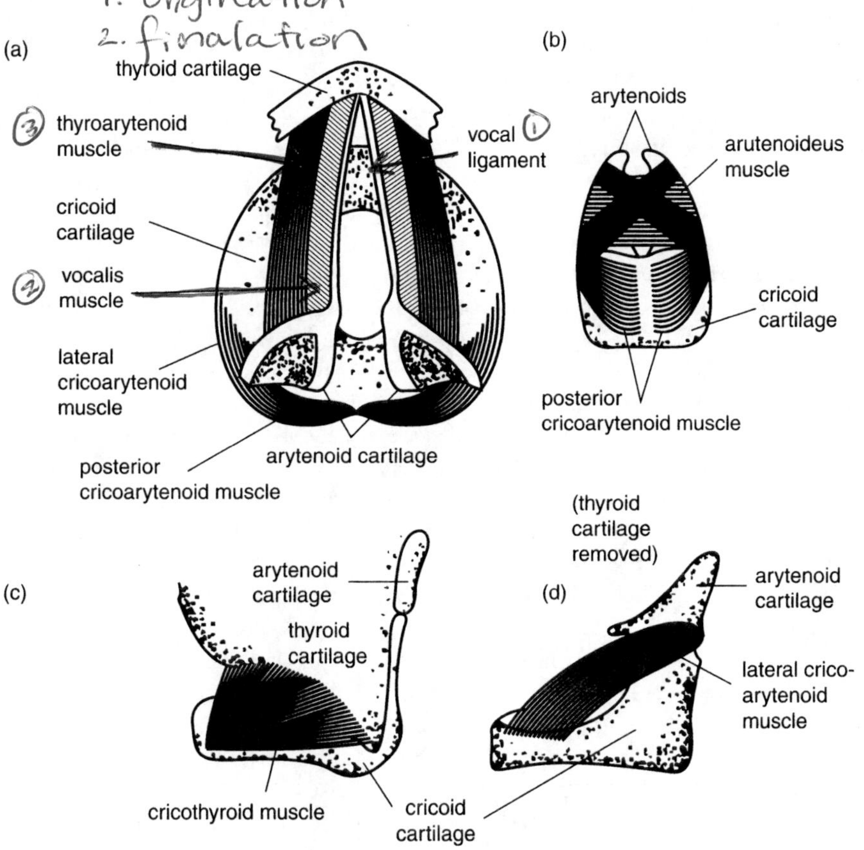

FIG 4.1. Views of the larynx.

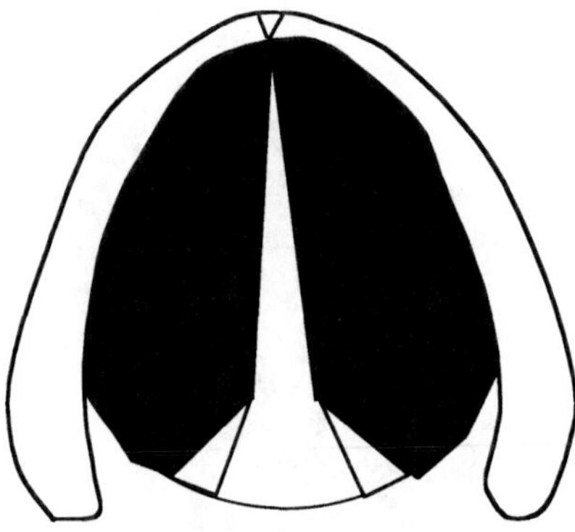

FIG 4.2. Voiceless phonation.

of the glottis, the activity and tension of the vocal folds, and the ever-changing aerodynamic aspects of the vocal tract. We will start by describing the five main phonation types: voiceless, whisper, voice, creak, and falsetto. We will also briefly consider the glottal stop.

Voiceless phonation requires an open glottis (somewhere between 60% and 95% of maximal glottal opening suffices). Air from the lungs flows freely through this open glottis with a minimum of disruption (see Fig. 4.2). However, this does not mean that voiceless phonation has no effect on the airflow at all. Remember that even with the open glottis required for voiceless phonation, at least half (and sometimes more than half) the area of the opening of the trachea is still covered; this means that the lung air will meet some resistance, which will cause acceleration of the airflow. If the volume velocity of the airflow is high, turbulence will occur. Such turbulent airflow occurs in sounds such as [h] and is sometimes called *breath*, or *breathiness*. If volume velocity is low, then a laminar (smooth) airflow results, which is sometimes termed *nil-phonation*: it appears that the quality of the sounds with nil-phonation derives mostly from the articulatory setting rather than being partly derived from larynx activity. English sounds with laminar airflow through the larynx include [f,s,ʃ] ([ʃ] is the sound spelled "sh" in words such as "ship"). All known languages use voiceless phonation, and in English we have many voiceless consonants (it is rare linguistically for vowels to be voiceless): [p, t, k, tʃ, f, θ, s, ʃ, h] ([tʃ] is the sound at the beginning of "chips", [θ] the sound at the beginning of "thin").

Whisper requires a glottis at 25% or less than maximal possible opening. The usual vocal fold setting for whisper is to have the opening at the arytenoid end of the vocal folds, with the anterior portion held together (see Fig. 4.3). This results in an inverted-y shape of the folds. As air passes through this narrow opening it becomes turbulent, causing a rich hushing sound quality. Whisper is used nonlinguistically, for example when speakers wish to disguise their voice or reduce loudness. In such cases, normally voiced sounds are transferred to whisper, but normally voiceless sounds stay voiceless (to maintain the distinction between voiced and voiceless sounds).

Voice requires a more complex laryngeal setting than the previous two types. The glottis needs to be closed by bringing together the two vocal folds. However, the glottis is not closed tightly (see below for the *glottal stop*). Using the intrinsic laryngeal muscles, the folds are subjected to varying degrees of tension which, in conjunction with the varying degrees of air pressure from the air flowing upward from the lungs, cause the folds to vibrate (see Fig. 4.4). This vibration is in the form of slight openings and closings of the folds along their lengths, allowing small puffs of pressurized air to escape through the larynx. In this regard, the vocal folds have been thought of as having a regulating function during voice: metering the amounts of air let through the larynx. The cycle of activity encountered with voice consists of an

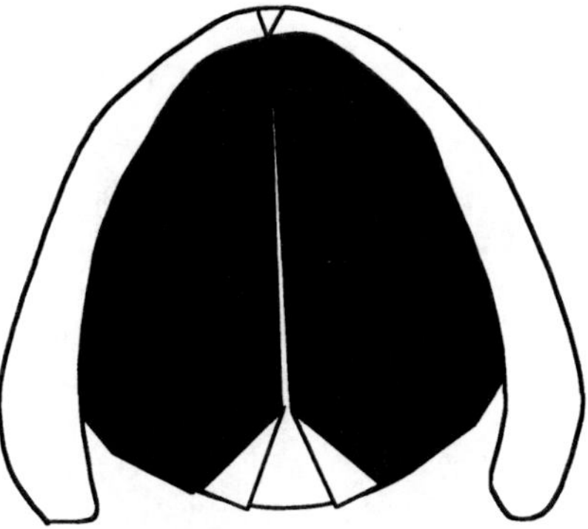

FIG 4.3. Whisper phonation.

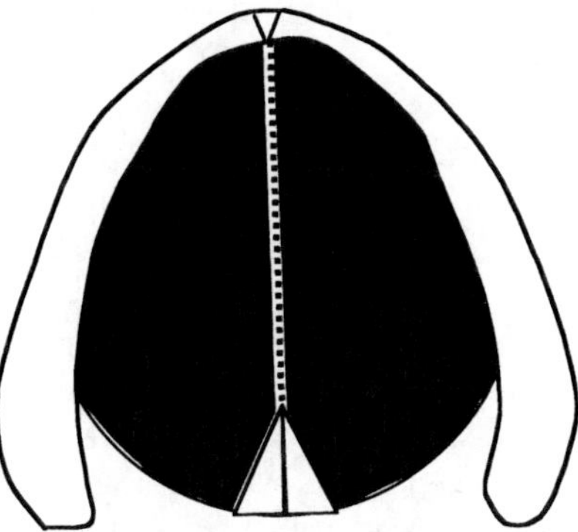

FIG 4.4. Voiced phonation (dashed line represents vibrating vocal folds).

adduction section (where the folds are brought together) and an abduction section (where they move apart). However, this cycle (the *vibratory cycle of voice*) is not wholly under muscular control. At the beginning of the cycle, muscle activity is required to approximate the vocal folds (i.e., bring them together); from then on, aerodynamic factors also have an important part to play. Pulmonic air pressure increases beneath the closed glottis until eventually the folds are forced apart and an amount of air rushes through. However, because the intrinsic laryngeal muscles are still working to hold the folds together, there is only a small gap for the air to pass through. If any gas is forced through a narrow channel, it accelerates and pressure drops (this is known as the *Bernoulli effect*). The drop in pressure causes the folds to be sucked back together again, and a new cycle of voice activity begins. Figure 4.5 illustrates this cycle diagrammatically. All known languages use voiced sounds (and indeed for most languages the majority of sounds are voiced). All vowels in English are voiced, as are the consonants [b, d, ɡ, m, n, ŋ, dʒ, v, ð, z, ʒ, l, ɹ, w, j] ([ŋ] is the sound at the end of the word "ring"; [dʒ] is the sound at the beginning of "jam"; [ð] is the sound at the beginning of "then"; [ʒ] is the sound in the middle of "treasure"; [ɹ] is the sound at the beginning of "red"; and [j] is the sound at the beginning of "yes").

It is worth noting that speed of vibration of the vocal folds during voice production is also important for speech. For adult male speakers the number of vibrations of the vocal folds per second varies from about 80 to 300, whereas for adult females the upper limit will be about 500 (we refer to vibratory cycles per second as hertz, or Hz). The frequency of vibration of the folds (the *fundamental frequency*, or F0) is controlled by the tension of the folds and the amount of

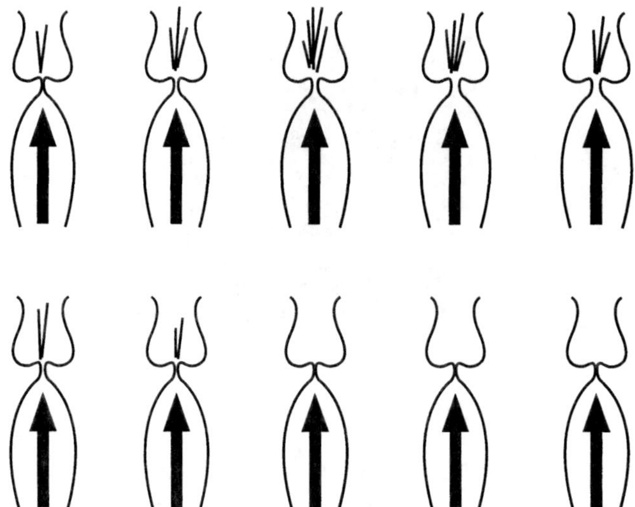

FIG 4.5. Vibratory cycle of voiced phonation.

subglottal pressure. The hertz values of the F0 differ from moment to moment during speech, and these differences are perceived as changes in the speaker's pitch. Languages use pitch changes as part of a system of intonation, and this system has a linguistic role: it can express the difference between statements, questions, and commands. It also has a role in expressing certainty, sarcasm, sincerity, and even features such as tiredness or sadness. Some languages also use pitch as part of a system of word level tones. We return to this area in more detail in chapter 9. Finally, we note that the space between the vocal folds (the glottis) can vary during voice, depending on how far apart the folds move during the abduction phase of the vibratory cycle. A wider glottis is often associated with a louder voice, and in such circumstances the adduction phase may be drawn out somewhat to allow for the extra energy in moving the folds so far apart to be dissipated when the folds come together again. The *opening quotient* and the *closing quotient* of the vibratory cycle can be worked out, and these measures seem to correlate with certain timbres of the voice. For example, if the speaker uses a low opening quotient, the voice is often described as "sharp" or "bright." On the other hand, a high opening quotient is associated with "mellow" voice timbres. A neutral vocal timbre is often called "modal voice."

The fourth basic phonation type is *creak* (also termed *glottal / vocal fry*). Creak is produced with a mainly closed glottis and a low subglottal air pressure. This low pressure is able to cause vocal fold vibrations, but only at the anterior part of the folds (see Fig. 4.6), and the rate of vibration is low (it can be as low as 25–50 Hz according to Laver, 1994). Some speakers of English may occasionally use creak instead of modal voice (particularly towards the end of an utterance), but it is used linguistically in some languages contrasting with voice and voicelessness.

Finally, we can consider *falsetto*. Falsetto can be thought of as a special variety of voice, because the vocal folds vibrate allowing small amounts of air through the larynx. However, the vocal folds are much stiffer for falsetto than for voice. This is achieved by contracting the thyroarytenoid muscle and relaxing the vocalis muscle. At the same time the cricothyroid muscle contracts to leave the vocal ligament very thin. There is relatively low subglottal air pressure, which together with a very slightly open glottis results in extremely rapid vocal fold vibrations (between 275 and 635 Hz). Falsetto is not used linguistically in any known language, but can, of course, be used for special effects such as disguising the voice.

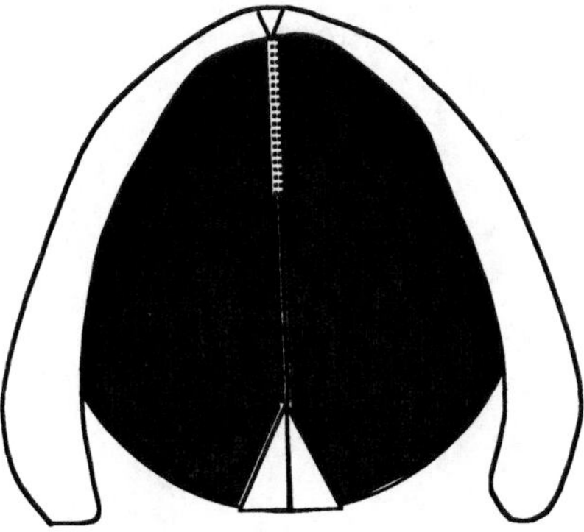

FIG 4.6. Creak phonation (dashed line represents vibrating vocal folds).

As we have seen with these five phonation types, there are various states of the glottis, from fully open through partially open to closed and vibrating. It is also possible to close the glottis tightly so that no air is allowed through at all. We can't do this for too long (for one thing the pulmonic pressure will become too great, and we need to open the glottis at some time in order to breathe!). Nevertheless, many languages allow speakers to produce glottal stops, in other words, to very briefly stop the airflow by snapping the vocal folds together (and causing thereby a brief moment of silence). In some languages, this functions as equivalent to a consonant, while in others, it serves as a word boundary marker when a word begins with a vowel. In English, some speakers use the glottal stop instead of [t] in words such as "better" (for example many speakers from London, England). Other speakers may use it as a word boundary marker, especially if the second word starts with a vowel, as in "go in."

> The five main phonation types have their own phonetic symbols. We can either mark individual sounds, or stretches of speech. Of course, some symbols already stand for voiced or voiceless sounds; therefore voice or voicelessness does not need to be marked by diacritics for these sounds.
>
> Voiceless: [p, m̥]; V̥
> Whisper: [ɑ̣]; Ẇ
> Voice: [z, s̬]; V
> Creak: [ɑ̰]; C
> Falsetto: F (used for stretches of speech; no mark for individual sounds)
> Glottal stop: [ʔ] (no mark for stretches of speech because, with the glottis stopped, speech is impossible).

Combined Phonation Types

Various combined phonation types are possible, although some are encountered more often than others. Voice can be combined with both breath and whisper. *Breathy voice* requires a glottis more open than for whisper but less than for voicelessness. The airflow is of high volume velocity, and the vocal folds are allowed to flap in this fast flowing airstream (see Fig. 4.7). Because the air is flowing at high volume velocity, one cannot speak for very long with this phonation type, as one runs out of breath. *Whispery voice*, also termed *murmur*, is somewhat different. Here the vocal folds are relaxed and vibrating, while a small gap at the arytenoid end of

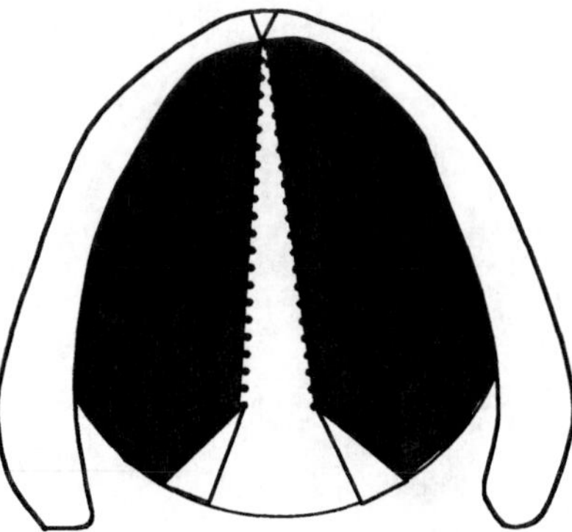

FIG 4.7. Breathy voice (dashed line represents vibrating vocal folds).

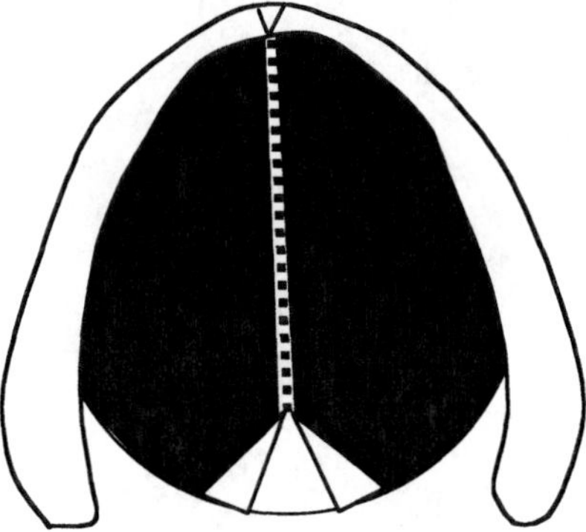

FIG 4.8. Murmur phonation (dashed line represents vibrating vocal folds).

the folds allows air to pass through and become turbulent (see Fig. 4.8). It should be noted that some authorities call this phonation type "breathy voice" (see, for example, Clark and Yallop, 1995), and so confusion may occur if publications do not make clear their definition of this term. Both these voice types may be used for special effects, or may occur in the voice clinic due to some vocal pathology. However, only whispery voice is used linguistically, as in some languages it may contrast with modal voice and with voicelessness.

Creak may be combined with voice and with whisper. *Creaky voice* probably has low-frequency vibrations at the posterior end of the vocal folds and higher frequency vibration at the anterior ends. This combination may be heard from English speakers who use a slow, low-pitched voice quality. *Whispery creak* is similar to murmur, except that the vocal fold vibrations are much slower.

Phonetic symbols are provided for some of these combined phonation types. We can either mark individual sounds, or stretches of speech.

Breathy voice: V^h
Whispery voice / murmur: [ɑ̤]; V̤
Creaky voice: V̰
Whispery creak: Ç̣

Location of Phonatory Activity

As we have seen, some of the phonation types noted above have activity at the anterior portion of the vocal folds, some at the posterior, and some all along the folds (termed *full glottal*). It is not normally necessary to note these differences, but with modal voice the sound quality may differ depending on the location of the phonatory activity. For example, if most of the vibratory action of the vocal folds takes place at the anterior end, a voice quality often called "tense, sharp, tight" or "pressed voice" occurs. There is another location we need to bear in mind, especially because it may occur in the voice clinic: *ventricular*. The *ventricular bands* or *false vocal folds* are situated above the vocal folds and may vibrate separately from them, or together with them. *Ventricular phonation* (which may be in the form of voice, whisper, or creak) sounds harsh and unnatural, although it may be adopted deliberately for certain vocal effects. If both modal voice and ventricular voice occur at the same time (*diplophonia* or *double voice*), the effect is increased. Certain types of jazz singing deliberately use diplophonia, but it can be an unwanted effect needing clinical intervention. Most ventricular voice types sound harsh, but the term *harsh*, when applied to voice quality, may be independent of any ventricular involvement and derives from excessive laryngeal tension, for example by overapproximation of the vocal folds.

> Phonetic symbols are provided to mark stretches of speech for some of these location types:
>
> Pressed voice: V̟
> (Posterior) whisper: W̠
> Harsh voice: V!
> Ventricular phonation: V!!
> Diplophonia: V̬!!

SUPRALARYNGEAL ASPECTS OF VOICE QUALITY

As we have seen, different phonation types play a major part in influencing the quality of a voice that we perceive. However, voice quality is also derived in part from the activity of the vocal organs above the larynx (supralaryngeal aspects). For example, if speakers habitually speak with the tongue body raised toward the hard palate (except of course when the demands of individual sounds preclude this), their voice quality will be generally higher in pitch than for a speaker who does not do this. Conversely, a speaker who habitually raises the back of the tongue toward the soft palate, or pulls the root of the tongue back into the pharynx when possible, will have a lower pitched voice quality. There are a wide range of such settings that derive in part from the normal articulator placements required for making different consonants and vowels, and we return to these in more detail in chapters 7 and 8. We can briefly consider a few other such settings here. First, the position of the larynx itself can play a part in voice quality. The larynx can be raised or lowered slightly using the laryngeal muscles, and different voice qualities result if we speak with a raised larynx or with a lowered larynx. Raised larynx voice is generally high in pitch, whereas lowered larynx voice is low in pitch and even "of a somewhat sepulchral quality" (Laver, 1994, p. 406). The faucal pillars are muscles at the back of the oral cavity running down into the pharynx. When they contract they reduce the volume of the pharynx and, again, affect the voice quality.

Even the position of the jaw can affect voice quality: for example, if speakers consistently clamp the jaw together when speaking, or leave it open, or protrude the lower jaw, or speak with it moved out to the left or the right. In the clinic we may encounter speech-disordered children who leave the tips (and sometimes the blades) of their tongues protruding between their teeth during much of their speech: Clearly this too will have an effect on voice quality.

There are phonetic symbols from the VoQS system to mark stretches of speech for some of these supralaryngeal voice qualities:

Raised larynx: L̝
Lowered larynx: L̞
Faucalized voice: V^{H}
Closed jaw: J̝
Open jaw: J̞
Protruded jaw: J̟
Rightward jaw: J͕
Leftward jaw: J͔
Clenched teeth voice: ⊓
Protruded tongue: Θ

Orality and Nasality

In clinical descriptions of pathological voice quality we often encounter the term *nasal* or *hypernasal*. In order to understand such terms, however, we need to consider in more detail the use of the oral and nasal cavities (or *resonators*) in speech production. When the pulmonic egressive airstream has passed through the larynx into the pharynx there are three different possible further routes. First, the airstream may pass into the oral cavity only (the soft palate being raised blocks any airflow from moving into the nasal cavity) and eventually leave the vocal tract through the mouth opening after the various activities of the articulators (these will be described in the next few chapters). Second, if the soft palate is lowered and the mouth shut, the air will flow into the nasal cavity and leave the vocal tract through the nares (nostrils). Of course, some air will enter the oral cavity, where articulatory activity will take place, but if the mouth is kept closed this will eventually have to flow back up into the nasal cavity to escape. Finally, if the velum is lowered and the mouth is open, then the air will flow through both the oral cavity (where articulation occurs) and the nasal cavity simultaneously. The first type of sound is termed *oral*, the second *nasal*, and the third *nasalized*. Examples of oral sounds in English are [p, d, z, ʃ, l, w] and all the vowels. The nasal sounds of English are [m, n, ŋ]. English does have sounds that are nasalized (for example, vowels before any of the nasal consonants), but these are only positional variants of oral vowels. A language such as French has nasalized sounds that occur irrespective of position, for example, the nasalized vowels in words like *en, un, on, vin* [ɑ̃, œ̃, ɔ̃, vɛ̃]. As can be seen in these examples, nasalized sounds are transcribed with a small curved line (a *tilde*) above the main symbol. It should be noted that, although nasalized vowels are relatively common in the languages of the world as distinctive sounds, nasalized consonants can also occur. Figure 4.9 shows articulations with oral airflow (a), nasal airflow (b), and both oral and nasal airflow (c).

We were concerned in the preceding discussion with types of individual sounds that are either oral, nasal, or nasalized. However, this topic also has implications for voice quality. For example, if for some reason (such as a cleft palate) a speaker is unable to shut off airflow into the nasal cavity, his or her speech is going to be characterized by excessive nasal resonance (in other words, sound segments are always going to be nasal or nasalized, and oral sounds will not be possible). Such a voice quality is termed *hypernasal*. On the other hand, if the

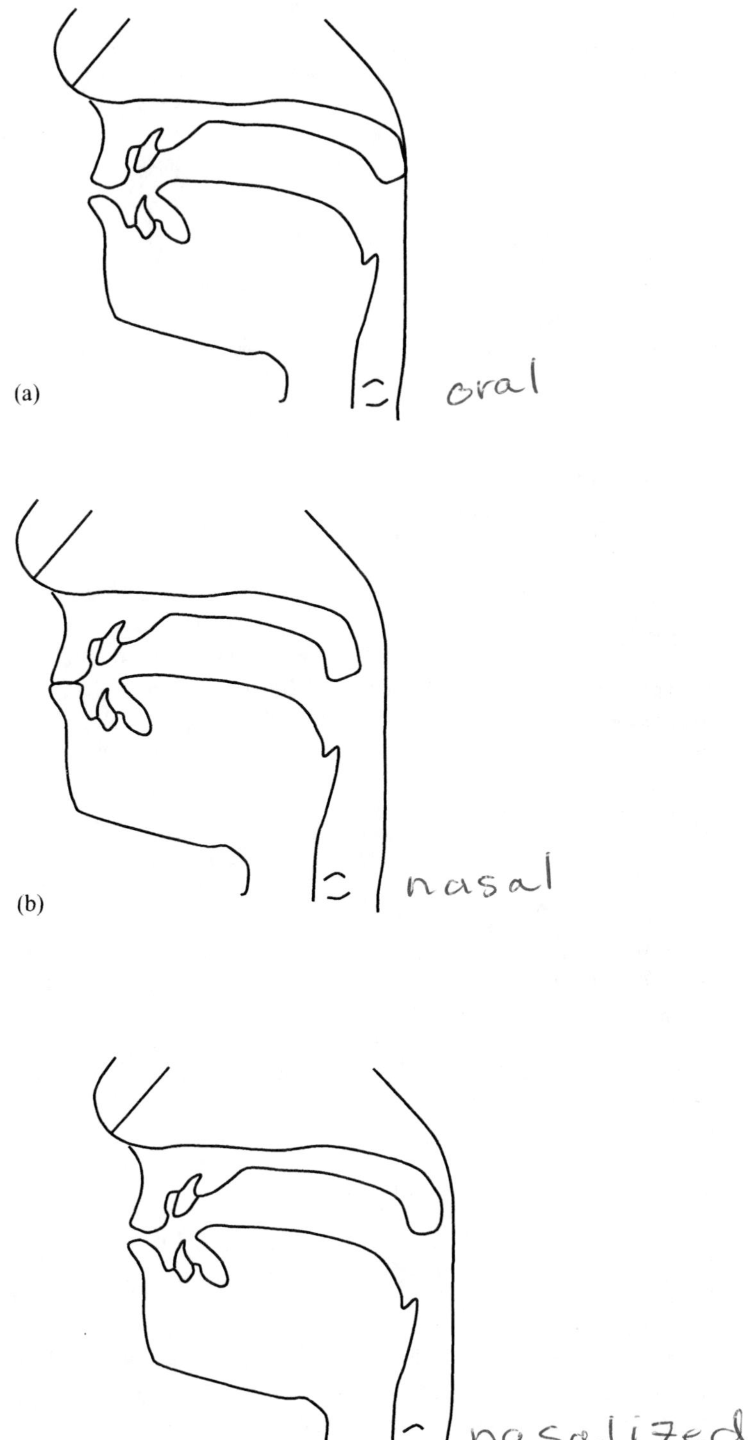

FIG 4.9. (a) Oral, (b) nasal, and (c) nasalized articulations.

speaker has difficulty in lowering the velum (as in some types of dysarthria), so that air very rarely can flow into the nasal cavity and most sounds are fully oral, even those that should be nasal, then the voice quality will be *hyponasal*. This sometimes happens if a speaker's nose is blocked due to a cold. Hypernasality needs to be judged against the norms of the speech community, as some dialects are noted for using more nasal resonance than would be expected in others. Some clients in the voice clinic may demonstrate other voice disorders connected to the airflow through the nasal cavity (such as excessive escape of air through the nose), and such pathological voice qualities are described in chapter 20.

> Phonetic symbols are provided to mark individual sounds and stretches of speech for voice qualities connected to nasal and oral resonance:
>
> (Hyper)nasal resonance, or nasal voice quality: Ṽ
> Hyponasal resonance, or denasal voice quality: V͊

In this chapter we have seen how the airflow from the lungs is shaped in the larynx through the process of phonation, and how aspects of voice quality derive from both phonation and supralaryngeal settings of the vocal organs. In the next four chapters we are going to see how the articulators in the supralaryngeal vocal tract work to make the individual speech sounds: the vowels and the consonants.

BACKGROUND READING

Other accounts of phonation types are available in Catford (1977) and in Stevens (1998). Abberton and Fourcin (1997) describe how to measure phonatory activity for clinicians. More details on phonation type use in the languages of the world can be found in standard phonetics texts, such as Laver (1994) and Ball and Rahilly (1999). These books also discuss supralaryngeal aspects of voice quality, but for more details readers should consult Laver (1980) and Kent and Ball (1999). The symbols provided for voice quality are from the VoQS system, as described in Ball, Esling, and Dickson (1999).

EXERCISES

Review Questions

1. What factors, other than phonation, influence voice quality?
2. What are the main phonation types, and how are they defined?
3. What is the difference between "voice" and "voice quality"?
4. What are opening and closing quotients, and what effect do they have on voice quality?
5. How are breathy voice and murmur characterized?
6. What is the role of the velum in directing, and in initiating, an airstream?
7. What is the difference between oral sounds, nasal sounds, and nasalized sounds?
8. What is the difference between laryngeal and supralaryngeal aspects of voice quality?

Study Topics and Experiments

1. Using library and Internet resources, find as many languages as you can that use murmur linguistically, and as many languages as you can that use creak/creaky voice linguistically. Give examples of words illustrating these phonation types, and give details of the languages concerned.
2. If you have access to a glottograph (also called a laryngograph) in your speech lab, use it to compare different phonation types. See what patterns you get on the screen when you utter a voiced sound (such as [ɑ]), the same sound whispered, murmured, or with creak. Describe the shape of the waves (print them out if possible) and note what each part of the wave signifies in terms of the cycle of vocal fold vibrations.

CD

Listen to the examples of sounds using different phonation types and voice quality types, and try to imitate as many as possible. See if you can identify the test examples following the instructions on the CD. Answers to all the exercises are given at the end of the book.

5

The Description of Vowels

INTRODUCTION

In the previous two chapters we have followed the path of speech production from the initiation of an airstream through phonatory activity and up into the supralaryngeal vocal tract. We now need to consider how individual speech sounds (sometimes called *phones*) are produced. This area of phonetics is known as *articulation*, and because of its importance we devote this and the following three chapters to it.

One major binary division of speech sounds is into the categories of *vowels* and *consonants*. A strictly phonetic definition of the difference between these two classes of sounds would be that consonants involve contact or near contact between the relevant articulators (for example, the tongue body and the hard palate), whereas vowels do not (that is to say, there is a wide gap between the articulators). This definition does not always fit well with how languages actually use speech sounds. In English, for example, sounds such as [w], [j], and [ɹ] (= "r") fit into the phonetic category of vowel, as they have wide gaps between the relevant articulators. Nevertheless, they behave like the other consonants of English, in that they cannot be the nucleus (i.e., center) of a syllable. Further, [w] and [j] are always followed by a vowel, and [ɹ] can be preceded or followed by a vowel. (In some accents of English [ɹ], like [w] and [j], can be followed by a vowel but not preceded by one.) So a phonological rather than a phonetic definition of the difference between the two classes might be that vowels can be syllabic nuclei, whereas consonants cannot (for the difference between phonetics and phonology see the preface and chap. 10). Some authorities use *consonant* and *vowel* for the units defined phonologically, and *contoid* and *vocoid* for those defined phonetically. In this book we adopt the phonological definition. We do need to stress, however, that these terms are used only to refer to sounds, not to letters in the spelling system!

We referred above to the space between the articulators, and this vertical dimension is an important one in describing speech sounds. The widest space is found with the vowel class, which we describe in detail in this chapter. The next widest gap is found with the class of consonants called *approximants*; then we have a class with a very narrow gap between the articulators termed *fricatives*. Finally, *stops* have complete contact between the articulators. These categories and subgroupings of them are explored in the following chapters.

Be careful you don't confuse speech with writing. People often say that the vowels are "a, e, i ,o, u"—but this refers to the letters of our writing system only! Most varieties of English have somewhere between 17 and 20 distinctive vocalic units, depending on dialect.

ARTICULATORY, ACOUSTIC, AND PERCEPTUAL DESCRIPTIONS OF VOWELS

There are various ways in which we can describe individual sounds. We can describe them in terms of how they're made (articulatory description), in terms of the physics of their sound waves (acoustic description), and in terms of how we perceive them (perceptual description). With consonants it is relatively straightforward to adopt the first of these approaches, because the articulators are usually fairly to very close together and we can use our own sense of touch and movement to work out their relative positions and their movements during sound production. Vowels are somewhat more difficult to describe from an articulatory viewpoint, however. This is because there is no contact or near contact between the articulators, and it is difficult for us to sense exactly where they are and how they move. Because vowels can be produced in a comparatively large part of the oral cavity (see Fig. 5.1), even very slight movements of the tongue or the lips can produce different vowel qualities, resulting in an almost impossible task of devising terminology to record these differences.

Therefore, alternatives to articulatory description have been developed, both acoustic and perceptual, and we return to these in later sections of this chapter. Nevertheless, articulatory description need not be completely abandoned. Although it is difficult to use this approach if comparing large numbers of slightly differing vowels across languages, this is often not the case when dealing with one specific language or language variety. This is because individual languages do not normally have a very large number of distinctive vowels. Languages with as few as three or five vowels are commonly reported (Greenlandic, for example, has three,

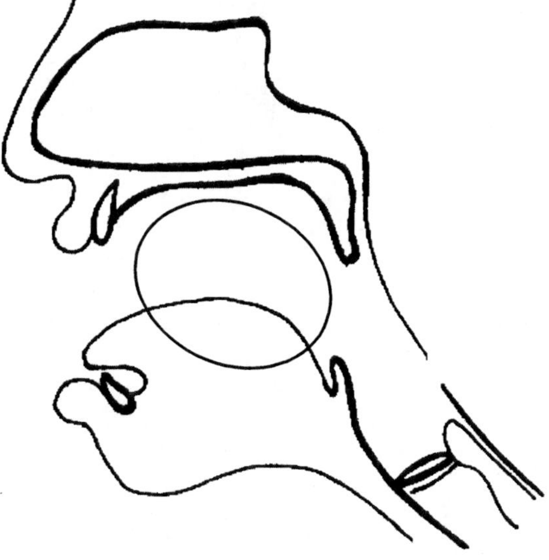

FIG 5.1. The vowel area.

and Spanish has five). English is somewhat exceptional, with as many as 17 to 20 distinctive vowels, but even here, some are diphthongs (see below), some are tense and some are lax (see below for these terms), and within any one subcategory of vowel, there are perhaps no more than half a dozen or so different examples. This means that we can use approximate articulatory labels relatively easily for such small numbers, although recognizing that these labels cannot give precise locations for the tongue and other articulators.

According to Maddieson (1984), one of the languages with the highest number of distinctive vowels in the UCLA corpus is !Xũ (spoken in southern Africa), with 24 plus 22 diphthongs extra; Aleut (spoken in the Aleutian Islands of Alaska) is one of several languages in the corpus with the lowest number of vowels, only 3.

DESCRIBING VOWELS BY ARTICULATION

In describing vowel sounds by their articulation we have to consider several parameters. First, we need to describe the placement of the tongue. This is not, however, a single measure. We need to know the tongue shape (convex or concave), the tongue height on the vertical axis within the vowel area, and the tongue position on the horizontal axis (i.e., in terms of how front or back it is within the vowel area). These parameters will have a variety of values, and the ones we normally use are as follows:

Parameter 1. Tongue shape: (i) convex (usual shape for vowels); (ii) concave (shape for *rhotic*, also known as *r-colored*, or *retroflex*, vowels) (though note that rhotic vowels can also be made with tongue bunching, described in chap. 15).
Parameter 2. Tongue height: (i) high vowels; (ii) half-high vowels; (iii) half-low vowels; (iv) low vowels. (Some phoneticians and textbooks, use only three values: high, mid, and low.)
Parameter 3. Tongue anteriority: (i) front vowels; (ii) central vowels; (iii) back vowels.

Figure 5.2 illustrates these parameters with tongue positions for several vowels set within the vowel area of the oral cavity.

We can use examples for English to illustrate the first three vowel parameters:

1. Tongue shape
   (i) convex—[i], [ɑ], [u], [ə] as in *tea, spa, two, sofa*
   (ii) concave—[ɚ], [ɝ] as in *softer, err*
2. Tongue height
   (i) high—[i], [u]
   (ii) half-high—[e], [o] as in monophthongal versions of *bait, goat*
   (iii) half-low—[ɛ], [ɔ] as in *bet, core*
   (iv) low—[ɑ]
3. Tongue position
   (i) front—[i], [ɛ]
   (ii) central—[ə], [ɚ], [ɝ]
   (iii) back—[ɑ], [ɔ], [u]

Apart from tongue placement, we must also consider lip shape. A different vowel sound is perceived if the lip shape is spread as opposed to rounded, even if the tongue placement is

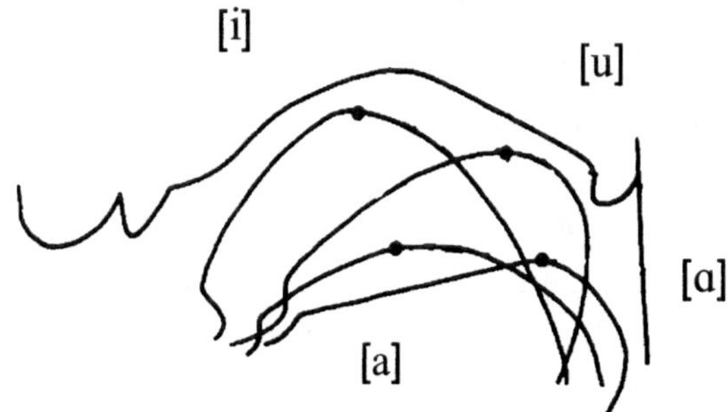

FIG 5.2. Tongue positions for the vowels [i], [a], [ɑ], [u].

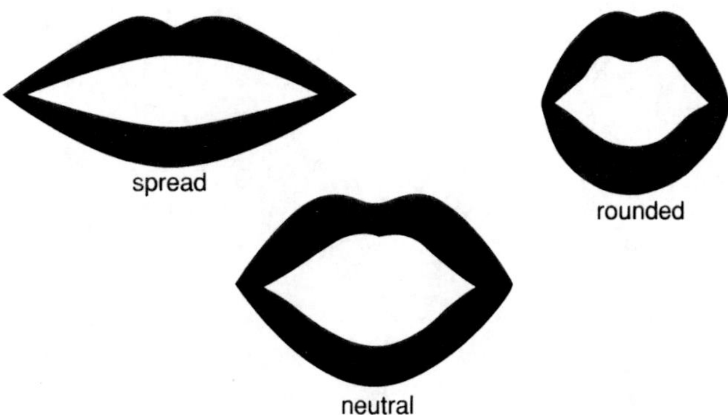

FIG 5.3. Lip shapes.

identical. For example, French *rue* "street," and *rit* "(s/he) laughs," are [ʁy] and [ʁi], respectively, where [y] represents a high front rounded vowel as opposed to the high front unrounded [i]. Although some researchers recognize a wide range of lip shapes in speech (Laver, 1994, note 8), we need only consider two or three as being vital for the contrast of vowels in natural language. These are:

> Parameter 4. Lip shape: (i) spread; (ii) neutral; (iii) rounded. For most purposes, a simple distinction between *rounded* and *unrounded* will suffice. With rounded vowels the lips are closely rounded when the tongue is high, and more open rounded when the tongue is low.

Figure 5.3 illustrates a range of lip shapes.

We can use examples for English to illustrate the fourth vowel parameter:

4. Lip shape
   (i) spread—[i], [ɛ] as in *tea*, *bet*
   (ii) neutral—[ə], [ʌ] as in *sofa* , *hut*
   (iii) rounded—[ɔ], [u] as in *core two*

Finally, we need to consider a set of parameters that have more to do with long-term features of vowel production, such as muscular tension and duration. We recognize three of these:

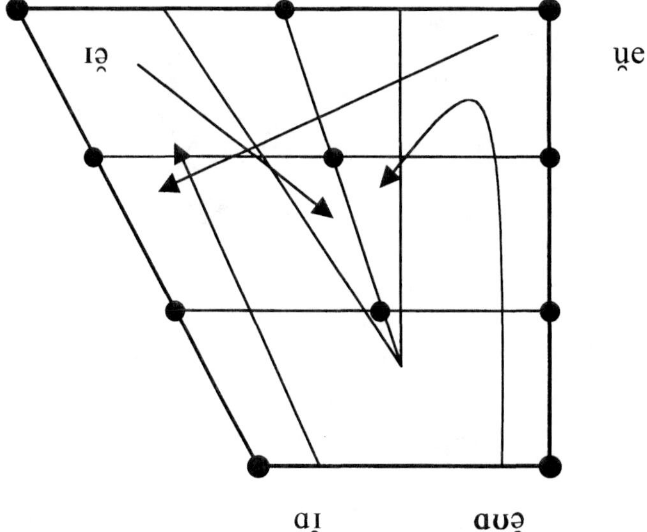

FIG 5.4. Diphthong and triphthong trajectories ([ɪə̯] is a centering diphthong; [aɪ̯] a closing diphthong; [u̯e] an opening diphthong; and [aʊə̯] a triphthong. [u̯e] is a rising diphthong; all the others are falling.)

Parameter 5. Tension: (i) tense; (ii) lax.
Parameter 6. Length: (i) long; (ii) short. (A few languages need a third, *half-long*, value, because they distinguish linguistically three degrees of length.)
Parameter 7. Stability: (i) stable, usually called *monophthongs*; (ii) trajectory, usually termed *diphthongs* (though note that *triphthongs* may also be used in some languages).

Figure 5.4 illustrates some diphthong and triphthong trajectories on the stylized version of the vowel area.

The values given for Parameter 6 suggest that only two, or at the most three, different vowel durations can occur in languages. However, there is a difference in phonetics between *duration* and *length.* Duration refers to the actual time (measured in msec) from the beginning to the end of a segment (in this case, a vowel). A wide range of slightly different values may be measured for the same vowel unit. These differences may be the result of the vowel being followed by a different consonant (for example, it appears that for most languages vowels are slightly shorter when followed by voiceless consonants than before voiced ones), of the tempo of speech, or just due to the slight differences that we see in speech from moment to moment. The term *length,* on the other hand, refers to the contrastive use of time. For example, irrespective of context or tempo, the vowel [i] (as in English "seat") is always considerably longer than the vowel [ɪ] (as in English "sit"). This is one of the ways in which these two vowels are consistently distinguished in English (there are also slight tongue height and position differences, and [i] is tense, whereas [ɪ] is lax), and many languages use length differences alone to distinguish sets of vowels (see chap. 9).

Parameter 7 describes the difference between monophthongs and diphthongs. The term *diphthong* is sometimes used to refer to a particular combination of symbols in spelling, so we need to emphasize that in phonetics this term applies to a vocalic segment that changes its quality (i.e., alters its tongue height and position, and sometimes also its lip shape) while remaining a single syllable. So, for example, the [ɔɪ] in English "toy" is a diphthong, because "toy" is a single syllable word, whereas the [iæ] in English "react" is not, as the [i] is in one syllable, and the [æ] is in the following syllable.

Diphthongs can be classed into several different categories. Diphthongs have most of their duration either on their first element (*falling diphthongs*) or on their second element (*rising diphthongs*). English diphthongs are all falling, although some researchers classify combinations such as [w]+vowel as rising diphthongs. We can also class diphthongs in terms of the direction of tongue movement: *closing diphthongs* have the tongue rising, *opening diphthongs* have the tongue lowering, and *centering diphthongs* have the tongue moving toward the center of the vowel area. Finally, we should note that triphthongs are comparatively rare and, even in those languages (including dialects of English) that have them, they tend to simplify to diphthongs in rapid speech. For example, nonrhotic accents of English may pronounce "fire" with a triphthong [aɪə], though this often simplifies to [aə] in rapid speech, or is spoken as two syllables ([aɪ.ə]).

We can use examples for English to illustrate the last three vowel parameters:

5. Tension
   (i) tense—[i], [ɑ], [u] as in *teal, spa, boot*
   (ii) lax—[ɪ], [æ], [ʊ] as in *till, spat, book*
6. Length
   (i) long—[i], [ɑ], [u]
   (ii) short—[ɪ], [æ], [ʊ]
7. Stability
   (i) monophthongs—[i], [ɑ], [u], [ɪ], [æ], [ʊ]
   (ii) diphthongs—[aɪ], [ɔɪ], [aʊ] as in *sky, toy, now*

DESCRIBING VOWELS BY PERCEPTION

Of all the parameters we have just examined, only tongue height and tongue position are essential for denoting where the tongue actually is during the production of a vowel sound. The number of values for these two parameters is relatively small (4 and 3, respectively), allowing a total of 12 possible tongue locations. Even if we double this by adding the rounded and unrounded lip shapes, this still only allows us 24 basic vowel locations for monophthongs. Although we can increase this number through the use of diphthongs, long and short vowels, and so on, we only have a small number of vowel categories in the articulation approach. Comparing the slight differences in realizing vowel units in different dialects, comparing vowels across languages, or examining the misarticulation of vowels in the speech clinic may well require a set of finer distinctions than this approach allows.

The limitations of an articulatory approach to vowel description prompted the famous phonetician Daniel Jones to devise a perceptual scale of vowel description, nearly 100 years ago. Although Jones was not working with disordered speech, he was interested in describing the differences between the vowels of different languages and in providing a tool for those working on the analysis of the subtle differences between accents of the same language. He came to realize that the limited number of articulatory terms we considered in the previous section did not suffice for these tasks. Further, it was clear that instrumental phonetic analyses at the time were not exact enough to allow more precise labels of articulatory position. (In fact, the use of x-rays to examine speech had already taken place, with some of the earliest studies in the 1890s. However, it was impractical—as well as dangerous—to x-ray every speaker in a study uttering all the vowels being investigated.)

Jones was attracted to the notion of a set of cardinal perceptual values for vowels, much in the same way as there are cardinal points of the compass. We can describe any direction in terms of how close it is to north, south, east, or west (e.g., northwest, east by southeast, and so on). In a similar way, phoneticians could describe the vowels they heard in real languages in terms of how close they perceived them to a set of previously learned values. Instead of having to guess the physical position of the tongue within the vowel area, phoneticians could use a "vowel compass" and their perceptual abilities to describe a vowel's position with reference to the cardinal compass points.

Jones decided to establish a small set of *cardinal vowels* that could be used in this manner. He decided that his cardinal vowels would be independent of any particular language, and that they should be situated around the periphery of the vowel area. This last point was partly to make it easier for users to learn how to produce the vowels (because being able to produce them aids considerably in learning to perceive them correctly), and partly because he felt it would be more straightforward to be able to describe nonperipheral vowels in terms of peripheral cardinal values, rather than vice versa.

He set up two anchor points for his system using articulatory criteria: cardinal vowel 1 was the highest, frontest vowel that one could make without the sound becoming a consonant, and cardinal vowel 5 was the lowest, backest vowel one could produce without pulling the tongue back into the pharynx. Then he added at the front of the vowel area three more vowels between 1 and 5 that were auditorily equidistant from one another and from the anchor points. So vowels 1 through 5 were separated by equal amounts of auditory or perceptual distance, rather than physical distance. These first five vowels were all unrounded. Finally, Jones added three vowels along the back edge of the vowel area, again all auditorily equidistant from each other and from the anchor points. These cardinal vowels 6 through 8 are all rounded vowels. Figure 5.5 shows a stylized version of the vowel area, with Jones's cardinal vowels plotted on it: Remember that in this instance the diagram represents an auditory map of the vowel area, rather than a physical one. Shown on the diagram are the cardinal numbers and the phonetic symbols normally used to denote those cardinal values.

We can illustrate these primary cardinal vowels from a variety of languages. In these examples the vowels are near (but not necessarily exactly) the relevant cardinal value.

C.V. 1 [i] Italian [si] "yes"	C.V. 8 [u] Tibetan [nuː] "west"
C.V. 2 [e] Welsh [hen] "old"	C.V. 7 [o] Galician [koro] "I run"
C.V. 3 [ɛ] French [mɛtʁ] "put"	C.V. 6 [ɔ] Amharic [gʷɔrf] "flood"
C.V. 4 [a] Spanish [kapa] "cloak"	C.V. 5 [ɑ] Hungarian [hɑt] "six"

Jones's choice of unrounded and rounded vowels for cardinal vowels 1 through 8 derives, at least in part, from the way vowels work in English and many other European languages. However, it is to an extent an arbitrary division, and many languages do have front rounded vowels (as in the French example quoted earlier) and/or back unrounded ones. Further, some languages have important vowel distinctions in the central region of the vowel area: both rounded and unrounded ones. For these reasons, Jones augmented what he termed his *primary cardinal vowels* with a set of *secondary cardinal vowels*. Secondary cardinal vowels 9 through 16 have exactly the same position on the auditory chart as 1 through 8, except that the lip shape is reversed. So 9–13 are rounded vowels, whereas 14–16 are unrounded. Cardinal vowels 17–22 are pairs of unrounded and rounded central vowels (the last four of these were not part of Jones's original scheme, but are now generally accepted by the International Phonetic Association, the IPA). Figure 5.6 shows the secondary cardinal vowels charted on the auditory vowel map, together with their IPA symbols.

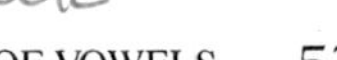

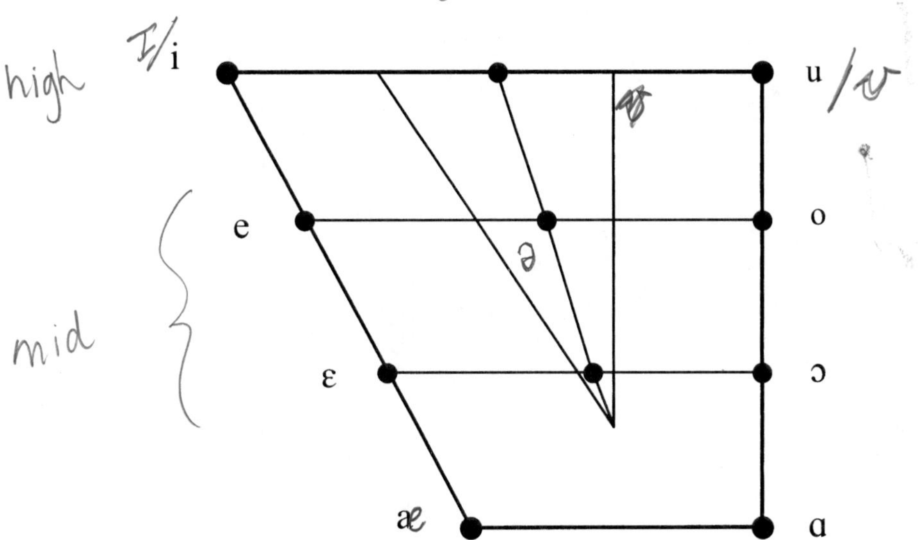

FIG 5.5. Primary cardinal vowels.

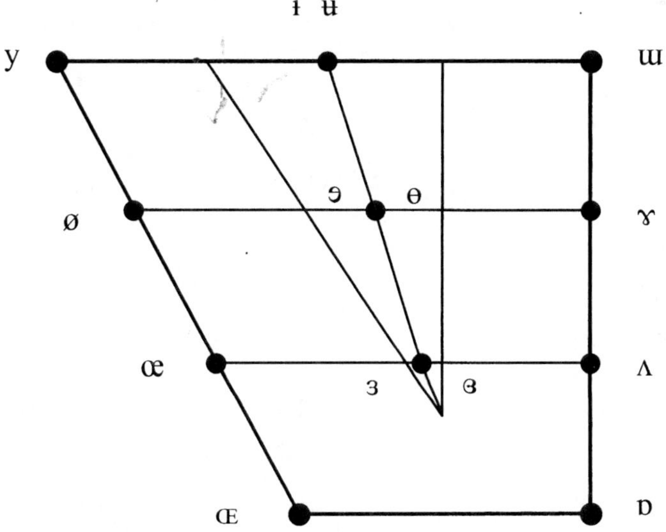

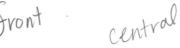

FIG 5.6. Secondary cardinal vowels.

We can illustrate these secondary cardinal vowels from a variety of languages. In these examples the vowels are near (but not necessarily exactly) the relevant cardinal value.

C.V. 9 [y] German [myde] "tired"
C.V. 10 [ø] Dutch [bøk] "beech"
C.V. 11 [œ] French [sœʁ] "sister"
C.V. 12 [ɶ] Austrian German [sɶ] "rope"
C.V. 17 [ɨ] Welsh [tɨ] "house"
C.V. 19 [ɘ] New Zealand Eng [kɘt] "kit"
C.V. 21 [ɜ] S. Brit Eng [wɜd] "word"

C.V. 16 [ɯ] Scots Gaelic [ɫɯɣ] "calf"
C.V. 15 [ɤ] Marathi [mɤg] "afterwards"
C.V. 14 [ʌ] Korean [bʌ:l] "bee"
C.V. 13 [ɒ] Farsi [nɒn] "bread"
C.V. 18 [ʉ] Scots English [tʉ] "two"
C.V. 20 [ɵ] Swedish [dɵm] "stupid"
C.V. 22 [ɞ] S. Welsh Eng [bɞd] "bird"

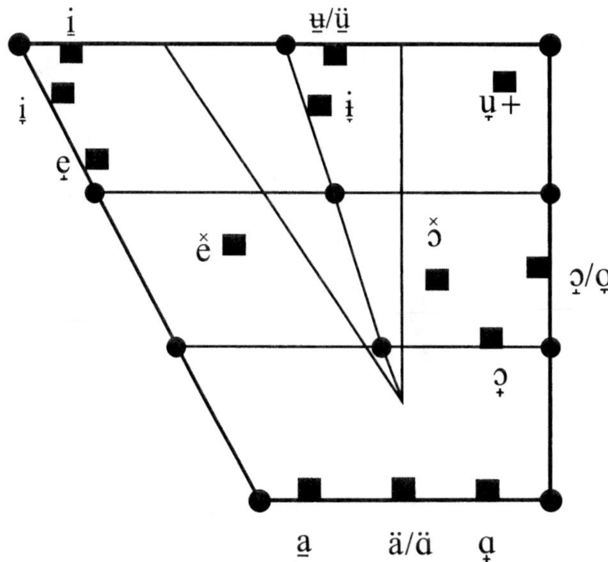

FIG 5.7. Diacritic use.

With reference to cardinal compass points, we can give precise directions, such as north-northeast, northeast, east-northeast, and so forth. In using the cardinal vowel system, Jones wanted to achieve the same precision. While we can describe verbally any specific vowel in terms of how close it is to a cardinal value, there needed to be also a method of showing these relationships in phonetic transcription. For this purpose, over the years, the IPA has developed a series of diacritics (small marks added to phonetic symbols) to express notions such as (auditorily) higher or lower than a cardinal value; more advanced or retracted; more or less lip-rounded; spoken with nasal resonance; long, half-long, and short versions of a vowel; and centralized and mid-centralized versions. With these diacritics, the transcription of the auditory percept of a vowel sound can be made quite fine-grained. The use of the diacritics when charting vowel values on the auditory diagram can be seen in Fig. 5.7.

A system such as this, however, can only gain wide currency if it is learned properly by those using it. Intensive training in producing and perceiving the cardinal values is required before one can become proficient, and, because some people seem to be better at dealing with perception tasks than others, the danger is that what one person describes may not correspond with the percepts of another. There is a tendency these days, therefore, to retain the symbols and diacritics of the cardinal vowel system, but to assume that they refer to approximate physical positions of the tongue rather than precise perceptual values.

It should be noted that Jones did not provide diacritics or symbols for lax as opposed to tense vowels, but the IPA has developed a set of such vowel symbols. They do not represent either precise physical tongue position or perceptual value and, as seen in Figure 5.8, can cover a relatively wide area of the vowel diagram. They are, however, very useful in the transcription of languages (such as English) that have a good number of lax vowels.

We can illustrate these lax vowels symbols from a variety of languages.

[ɪ] Irish [ɪlʲe] "all"	[ʊ] Sindhi [sʊrə] "tunes"
[ʏ] Swedish [nʏtta] "use" (noun)	[ə] Catalan [blaβə] "blue" (fem)
[æ] Hindi [bæʈ] "cricket bat"	[ɐ] Palatinate German [ʀidɐ] "knight"

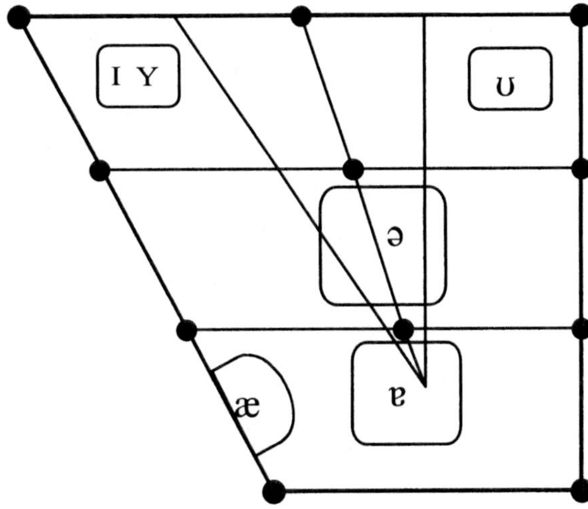

FIG 5.8. Lax vowels.

Over the past 40 years, instrumental phonetics has become more and more sophisticated, so that today acoustic analysis can be undertaken using free software on an ordinary PC. To some extent, this approach has overtaken auditory perceptions as a means of providing finely detailed descriptions of vowel sounds. In the next section we will look at this in more detail.

> We can return to diphthongs and illustrate some of these in a variety of languages.
>
> | | |
> |---|---|
> | [ai] German [ais] "ice" | [au] Dutch [lau] "lukewarm" |
> | [ei] Catalan [rei] "king" | [ɛu] Slovene [lɛu] "lion" |
> | [ɔi] Cantonese [sɔi˥] "gill" | [ou] Czech [mouxa] "fly" (noun) |
> | [uɪ] Welsh [uɪ] "egg" | [ɪu] Welsh [ɪu] "is" |
> | [ɪə] S. Brit Eng [pɪə] "peer" | [ʊə] N. Brit Eng [pʊə] "poor" |

DESCRIBING VOWELS BY ACOUSTICS

The introduction to this book provides a brief account of the acoustic parameters important for the description of speech. In terms of vowel analysis, the analysis packages available today allow us, for example, to measure the duration of a vowel in thousandths of a second (milliseconds, msec). Perhaps more important, when we wish to distinguish one vowel from another and obtain information on tongue height and position, are the frequency and intensity characteristics of a vowel sound. All vowels have bands of frequency (measured in hertz, Hz) that are particularly intense, and it is the arrangement of these bands of intense frequency across the frequency range that constitutes the acoustic "fingerprint" of the particular vowel. These bands are termed *formants* (see discussion in chap. 1). (We'll see later that some consonant sounds also have distinctive formants.)

To see how we can use formants to describe vowels, we can consider the first three formants (counting from the lowest part of the frequency range) of the vowels [i] and [ɑ] in American English (Petersen and Barney, 1952). The lowest formant (F1) for [i] was 270 Hz, F2 was 2290 Hz, and F3 was 3010 Hz. On the other hand, the values for [ɑ] were F1—730 Hz, F2—1090 Hz, F3—2440 Hz. There are formants higher in the frequency range of speech, but the first three are all that are normally used in speech analysis. By analyzing many different vowel sounds, acoustic phoneticians have determined that raising the front of the tongue during vowel production lowers the F1 and raises the F2; raising the back of the tongue lowers the F2; using lip-rounding lowers all formants somewhat; and retracting the tongue root into the pharynx raises F1. Front vowels have a higher F2 than back vowels, and using a concave tongue shape (r-colored vowels) lowers the F3 (in fact, what seems to happen is that an extra formant—F_R—is produced by the concave tongue shape, and this intervenes between F2 and F3 and sometimes merges with the latter).

We can illustrate these differences in formants with the following examples (recorded by the first author) measured in Hz.

	F1	F2	F3
Front vowel [i]	212	2555	3595
Back vowel [u]	303	710	2139
High vowel [i]	212	2555	3595
Low vowel [æ]	710	1524	3668
Unrounded vowel [i]	212	2555	3595
Rounded vowel [y]	240	2162	2474
Nonrhotic vowel [ə]	443	1285	2452
Rhotic vowel [ɚ]	466	1235	1597

There are two main ways in which we can access information about vowel formants when doing acoustic analysis: through measuring spectrograms, or through a spectral analysis. Spectrograms, as we noted in chapter 1, chart time along the horizontal access and frequency on the vertical, with intensity shown by the darkness of the markings.

Figure 5.9 shows a spectrogram of several sample vowels ([i], [u], [æ], and [y]) uttered in succession. We can clearly see the formants of the vowel sounds, and can measure them by

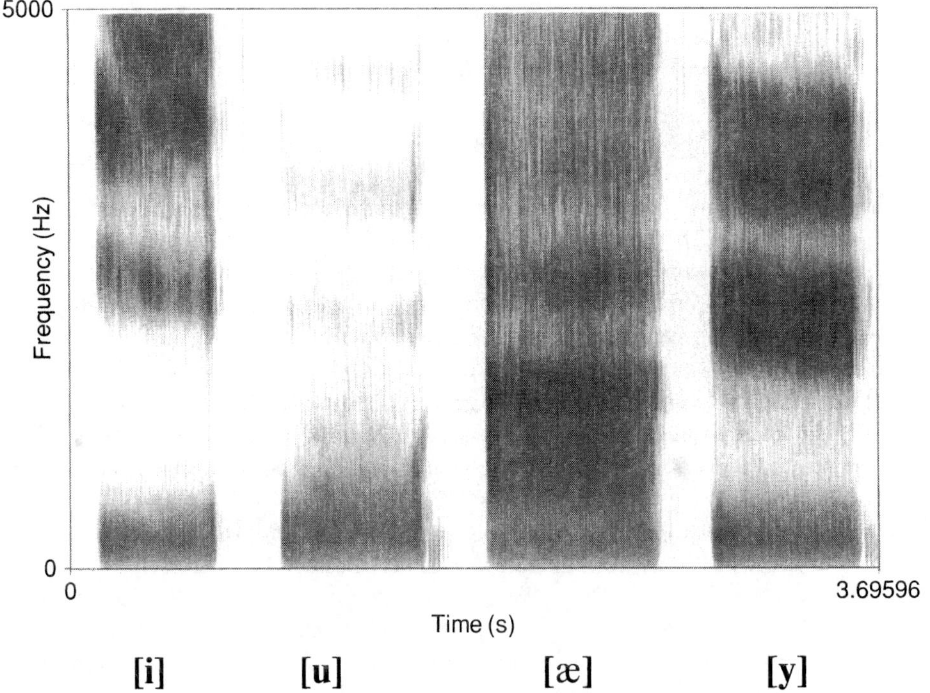

FIG 5.9. Wideband spectrogram of sample vowels [i], [u], [æ], and [y].

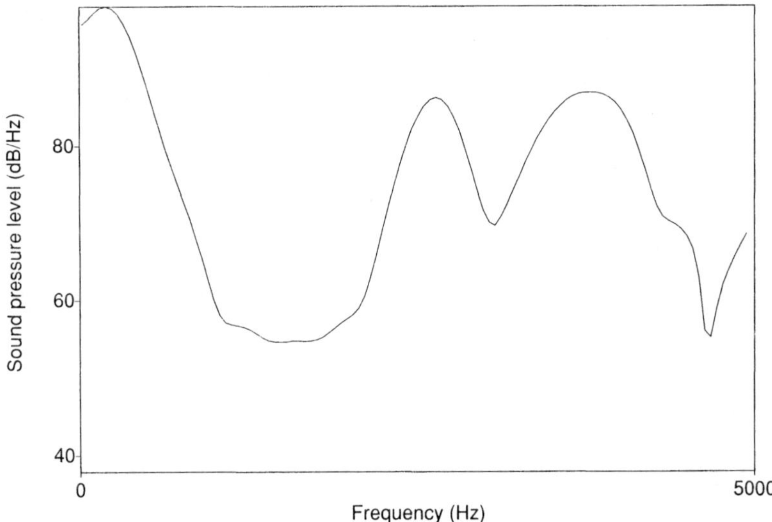

FIG 5.10. Spectrum of the vowel [i] obtained via LPC.

placing the cursor provided by the software onto that vowel sound. When doing this, we normally chose a point midway through the vowel to avoid the *coarticulatory* effects of neighboring sounds, and about halfway up the dark markings of the formant. To examine a spectrum of a sound, on the other hand, we have to choose a single point in time (usually, as before, halfway through the vowel) and instruct the software to undertake either a LPC (linear predictive coding) or an FFT (fast Fourier transform) analysis. (These two procedures are different methods of producing a similar result: LPC usually provides a simpler graphic display.) In Fig. 5.10 we can see a spectrum of the vowel [i], with the frequency on the horizontal axis and the intensity on the vertical (compare this with the drawn example in Fig. 1.11). The peaks of intensity correspond to the formants and are labeled on the diagram; remember that this illustrates the formant values at a single point in time. Of course, if we wish to analyze formant values of diphthongs, we will need to select more than one point in time in order to chart the formant changes over time reflecting the tongue (and possibly lip shape) changes during diphthong production. We will return to more examples of acoustic analyses of both monophthongs and diphthongs when we examine the vowel system of English in part II of this book.

BACKGROUND READING

The examples of vowels from different languages come from various sources: Maddieson (1984), Laver (1994), Ladefoged and Maddieson (1996), the *Handbook of the IPA* (1999), Ball and Rahilly (1999), and the authors' own experience. We would also like to acknowledge Paul Warren's help with the example from New Zealand English.

EXERCISES

Review Questions

1. Give a phonetic definition, and a phonological definition, of vowels and consonants.
2. What do the terms *articulatory*, *acoustic*, and *perceptual* description of speech sounds refer to?

3. Would a person with a severe hearing impairment be more likely to have problems with consonant or vowel production, and why?
4. Name and define the articulatory parameters and their variables that we use in the description of simple vowels.
5. Name and define the categories that are used to classify diphthongs.
6. What is the cardinal vowel system?
7. Why is it important to keep in mind that the cardinal vowel diagram is an auditory/perceptual, rather than an articulatory map?
8. What is the relationship between primary and secondary cardinal vowels?
9. What are formants, and what is their significance in the acoustic description of vowels?
10. How do formants relate to articulatory characteristics of vowels?

Study Topics and Experiments

1. Discuss the advantages and disadvantages of a purely articulatory system of vowel description and of the cardinal vowel system.
2. Record your and a fellow student's production of the sample vowels used in this chapter, and do a formant analysis, using an acoustic analysis package. How similar are your productions, and how much do they differ from the values given in the chapter? What might account for the differences?

CD

Listen to the examples of vowels, and try to imitate as many as possible. Try to identify the test examples following the instructions on the CD. Answers to all the exercises are available at the end of the book.

6

Articulation: Consonant Manner Types

INTRODUCTION

Unlike vowels, consonants are articulated with a close or fairly close constriction between the articulators. In fact, the proximity of the articulators to each other is going to provide us with the classification of consonant classes, or manners of articulation. Before we look at this classification, however, we have to consider the phonetic parameters we use for describing consonants. As with vowels, we need to take the vertical (or height) dimension into consideration: this deals with the distance between the articulators we have just mentioned. Second, we have to examine the horizontal dimension: Where are the articulators making their constriction in terms of front to back through the oral cavity and beyond? We will look at this feature in the following chapter. Then we need to examine the lateral dimension: whether the airflow is central across the tongue body, or directed to flow over the side of the tongue. We also need to note whether the airflow during the production of the consonant is oral or nasal. We can also distinguish between strong (*fortis*) and weak (*lenis*) sounds in terms of the muscular effort and resultant amount of airflow. Finally, there is the temporal characteristic of the consonants: are they prolongable, or instantaneous?

Examining the vertical dimension gives us three main categories of consonants:

1. Stops. These are made with the articulators (e.g., the two lips, or the tip of the tongue against the alveolar ridge) brought so closely together that an air-tight seal is caused, and the air is *stopped*.
2. Fricatives. These are made with the articulators very close together, but a narrow channel remains open through which air can flow. Because the channel is narrow, the resultant air flow is turbulent. We hear this as a noisy quality that is called *friction* or *frication* in phonetics.
3. Approximant. These consonants are made with a relatively wide space between the articulators and there is no turbulence in the resulting airflow.

There are also some hybrid manners of consonant articulation: *affricates* (a combination of stop and fricative); *trills* (swiftly repeated brief stop-like contacts between articulators); and *flaps* or *taps* (a single brief stop-like contact). For each of the manner types we will look at below, we examine their lateral, temporal, and oral/nasal characteristics in addition to the basic description.

> As with the vowels, be careful you don't confuse speech with writing. People often imagine, for example, that "sh" consists of a combination of [s] and [h] (of course, it's a single sound in its own right); or that the words "thin" and "then" start with the same sound because they're both written the same (they do in fact differ: the first is voiceless and the second voiced). With consonants, as with vowels, there are more distinctive sounds in English than there are single letters available in the Latin alphabet.

Speech disorders often show problems with consonants, with both manner and place of articulation disrupted. If we wish to describe these errors properly, it is vital that we know the full range of manner and place types that can be used in speech.

STOPS: PLOSIVES AND NASALS

The production of a stop consonant requires a complete closure between the articulators so that airflow through the oral cavity is stopped. The seal must be air-tight, and this can be achieved by pressing one articulator firmly against the other. An example of this might be the movement of the tongue tip and blade up to the alveolar ridge resulting in a firm contact there. However, for air to be fully stopped, the side rims of the tongue must also make a seal against the insides of the upper side teeth. Stops can be made at a wide variety of places within the oral cavity (and even in the pharynx and at the glottis), and we explore these different places in the next chapter.

If airflow is stopped in the oral cavity, there are two possible outcomes: The air is eventually allowed to leave the oral cavity with the removal of the articulatory closure (oral release of the air), or the air can escape through the nasal cavity if the velum is lowered at the time the articulatory closure is made (nasal release of the air). This means that there are, in fact, two categories of stop sounds: oral stops, or *plosives*, and nasal stops, or simply *nasals*.

Plosives

As the name suggests, these stops are characterized by a popping quality that sounds a little like a very small explosion! (Interestingly, many of our words for explosions start with plosive consonants: *pop, bang, crash, boom.*) How do these mini-explosions come about? Oral stops, as we have just noted, require the airflow to be literally stopped in the oral cavity. Further, they also require that the velum be raised, so that no air can escape through the nasal cavity. This means that the air flowing up from the lungs is trapped in the oral cavity behind the closure of the articulators, and this inevitably results in a buildup of pressure. We do not keep the articulators closed for very long (usually about 40–150 ms), but this is long enough to create sufficient pressure so that when we move the articulators apart, the trapped air rushes out with the popping sound we've noted (see Fig. 6.1).

Plosives appear to be very basic sounds in human languages, because almost all known languages have them. However, although English has both voiceless and voiced plosives, it seems as if the voiceless ones are more basic, because not all languages have voiced plosives. (Other varieties, such as plosives with creak or murmur, may also be found.) We can consider plosives as having three main stages: phase 1, when the articulators draw close together; phase 2, when the closure is in place and held; and phase 3, when the articulators are moved apart to let the air flow out again. As we'll see in chapter 8, phases 1 and 3 can be modified (and this happens often in English), but let us for now just consider these phases in relation to phonation. If a plosive is fully voiced, then vocal fold vibration continues throughout all the stages we've

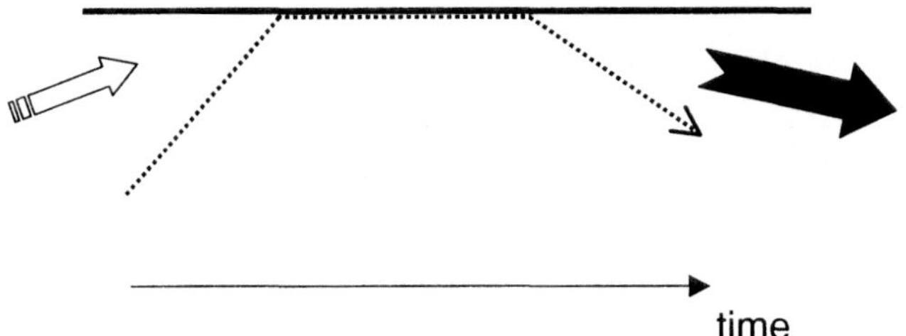

FIG 6.1. Plosive stop production (solid line: passive articulator; dotted line: active articulator; arrows: airflow).

just outlined. However, maintaining voicing during phase 2 is difficult, because we need air flowing through the vocal folds to maintain voicing, yet the air is now trapped in the oral cavity. This means that as more air is let through the folds up into the mouth, the pressure differential between subglottal and supraglottal air is lowered, making it hard to maintain the pressure needed to force the folds into action. Therefore, voiced plosives tend to have a shorter closed phase, and in many languages (English being one), voicing may not be maintained all through phase 2, but may cease partway through and be resumed in phase 3.

Voiceless plosives, on the other hand, are characterized by silence during phase 2, when the closure is complete (no air is escaping to make noise), whereas voiced plosives do still emit the buzz from the vocal fold vibrations. On the release of a voiceless plosive, phase 3, vocal fold vibration starts up again. It can either start more or less immediately, or after a brief pause, called the *voice onset time* or VOT (for example, of about 40 ms). In the latter case, we hear a brief puff of voiceless air, called *aspiration*. In English, many word-initial voiceless plosives are aspirated, whereas in a language such as Spanish or French, they are not.

> Plosives are easier to produce than many other types of consonants—probably because as long as there is full contact between the articulators, it doesn't matter how precise the articulator movement is: A very firm contact is as good as a less firm one.
>
> Possibly for this reason, plosives are often found as substitutions for other sound types (fricatives, affricates, liquids), both in normally developing speech, and in the disordered speech we encounter in the clinic.
>
> Voiceless unaspirated plosives can be transcribed as [p⁼, t⁼, k⁼]
>
> Voiceless aspirated plosives can be transcribed as [pʰ, tʰ, kʰ]
>
> Normally, we don't add these diacritics if the presence or absence of aspiration is predictable.

Because phase 3 can be prolonged to a certain extent, plosives are considered to be prolongable sounds; however, because they require a total closure of the articulators, the distinction between central and lateral articulations is deemed not to apply to them. (We return in a later chapter to the distinction between central and lateral release of plosives.)

NASAL STOPS

Nasal stops differ from plosives because throughout the production of the sound the velum is lowered. This means that while air cannot escape through the oral cavity, it can flow quite freely through the nasal cavity (see Fig. 6.2). So no air pressure builds up, and there is no plosion. However, even though airflow is through the nasal cavity, the constellation of articulators in the oral cavity is still important. Because the oral and nasal cavities are linked via the pharynx and

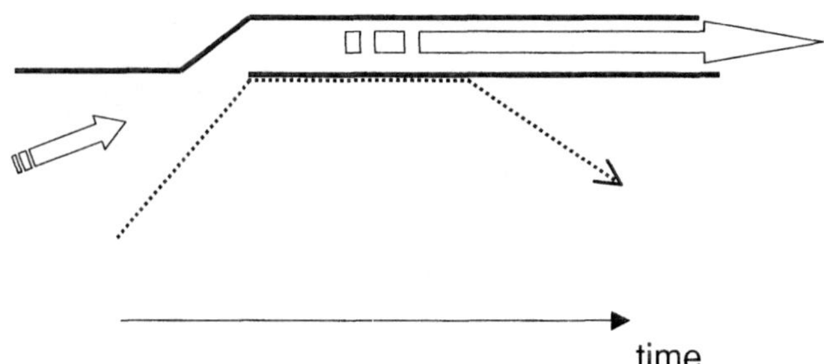

FIG 6.2. Nasal stop production (solid line: passive articulator; dotted line: active articulator; arrows: airflow).

the velopharyngeal port, the sound quality of the nasal stop is made up of all the resonances imparted to the airflow as it passes through all these cavities. This can be heard if we hum a long, prolonged [m] sound and compare that with an [n] sound. They differ. This difference can only come from the effect of the altered size of the oral cavity: [m] has a larger oral cavity than [n], because for [m] the closure is at the lips, whereas for [n] it is between the tongue tip and the alveolar ridge.

When we make nasal stops, we tend to lower the velum a little in advance of the beginning of the stop itself (i.e., the closure of the articulators). This results in any sound coming before the nasal stop becoming somewhat nasalized. If you listen closely to the [i] vowel in the word "seed" and compare it with the same vowel in the word "seen," you should be able to hear the somewhat nasalized quality of the latter. At the end of the nasal stop, there may also be an amount of nasalization on the following sound, as it takes a certain amount of time to raise the velum again. This does not appear to be so strong, however, and phoneticians generally consider that *anticipatory coarticulation* (as they call it) is stronger than *persevatory coarticulation* (see also discussion of coarticulation in chap. 9).

In the languages of the world, nasal stops are very common (though there are a few languages that lack them, including Rotokas—an Indo-Pacific language). However, in the overwhelming majority of languages, only voiced nasal stops are found. This is probably because voiceless nasals are not very loud, and those languages that have them may well add voicing toward the end of the sound in order to add to the sound's salience. Some southeast Asian languages, such as Burmese, have voiceless nasals.

> Because voiceless nasals are relatively uncommon, the IPA has no separate symbols for them in transcription. When we need to transcribe them we add the voiceless diacritic to the symbol for the voiced nasal. For example, [m̥] is a voiceless version of the normally voiced [m].
>
> Clients who have, or have had, a cleft palate may use voiceless nasals for target voiceless plosives.

Nasal stops are prolongable but, as in the case of the plosives, the central/lateral distinction does not apply to them, because the oral closure is complete.

FRICATIVES AND AFFRICATES

Fricatives

If stops are the "strongest" articulation type on the strength of articulation hierarchy (because they involve total closure between the articulators), then fricatives are the next strongest. This

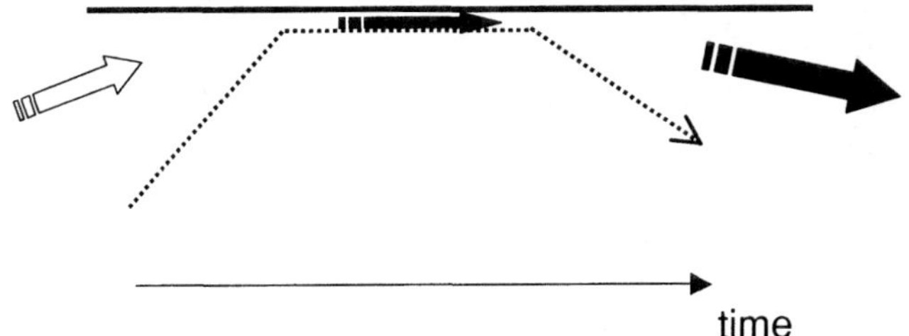

FIG 6.3. Fricative production (solid line: passive articulator; dotted line: active articulator; arrows: airflow; black arrow: turbulent airflow).

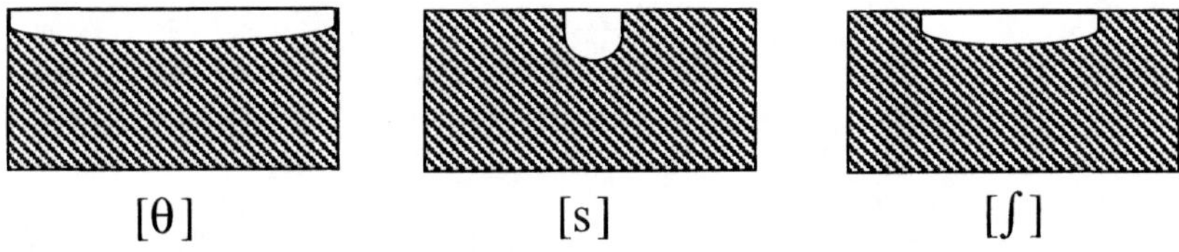

FIG 6.4. Fricative channel shapes.

is because they require articulators that are very close together (indeed, maintaining closure at some points), but with a small gap left in one area to allow the air coming up from the lungs to escape. Because the gap that is left is so small, the escaping air is put under increasing pressure as it is forced through the air channel. This results in turbulent airflow, and this turbulence is perceived by listeners as having a hissy, or noisy quality (see Fig. 6.3). Phoneticians likened the production of these sounds to the creation of friction when two surfaces rub against each other, so the term *fricative* came into being. The noise component of these sounds is sometimes termed *frication*, or *friction*.

The exact quality of the frication differs from sound to sound depending partly on which articulators are involved, but also on the shape and size of the narrow channel through which the escaping air is forced. For example, there are several different fricatives that are made with the tip and/or blade of the tongue up against the back of the front teeth or the alveolar ridge. Other sounds made at these areas, for example, stops, are very similar to each other. However, with fricatives it is possible to alter the air channel as well as the exact location of the articulation. Let us compare the fricative sounds at the beginning of the English words "sin" and "shin." The [s] in "sin" is made with the tongue tip on the alveolar ridge, and with a very narrow air channel, such that the resultant sound is termed a *grooved fricative*. On the other hand, the [ʃ] in "shin" is produced with the tip and blade of the tongue against the back part of the alveolar ridge, but with a flatter, broader channel shape, and the resultant sound is called a *slit fricative*. We can also look at the fricative at the beginning of the English word "thin," which is articulated between the tongue tip and the back of the front upper front teeth (or for many speakers, between the upper and lower front teeth). The [θ] sound in this word is made with a slit channel shape also, but this is broader than the one we noted for [ʃ]. These various channel shapes can be seen diagrammatically, as if from the front, in Fig. 6.4.

These different channel shapes produce different qualities of frication. This has led some phoneticians to propose a division of the fricatives produced toward the front of the mouth into two different categories (back fricatives do not exhibit these differences in the shape of the air channel). *Sibilants* are those fricatives with a grooved or narrow-slit air channel, which produces high-pitched frication (the narrow-slit fricatives are sometimes assigned to a third category: *shibilants*); *nonsibilants* are those with a wide-slit air channel and a lower pitched frication. In English, sibilant fricatives are [s, z, ʃ, ʒ] (as in "*s*ue," "*z*oo," "*sh*oe," and "trea*s*ure"), whereas nonsibilants are [f, v, θ, ð] (as in "*f*an," "*v*an," "*th*in," and "*th*an"). You may also come across a division of these fricatives into the categories of *strident* and *nonstrident*. This categorization is derived from the acoustic characteristics of the frication, and it classes [f, v, s, z, ʃ, ʒ] as strident, and [θ, ð] as nonstrident. Such a classification is not especially useful, however, because in terms of articulation, pitch analysis of the frication, and patterns of disordered speech, there appears to be little to recommend having [θ, ð] in a separate category from the other fricatives, and classing together the noisy and less noisy fricatives [f, v, s, z, ʃ, ʒ].

Fricatives can be both voiceless and voiced in natural language, although voiceless fricatives tend to be longer and louder (because part of the energy required to produce frication is used up in making vocal fold vibration in voiced fricatives). Languages may have voiceless fricatives but not voiced ones, but if they do have voiced ones then they also have voiceless ones.

As we have seen, many fricatives require very precise articulator movement to produce the correct air channel shape and location. For this reason, fricatives are among the sounds acquired late in normal phonological development, and fricative problems are often encountered in the clinic.

Not surprisingly, in languages with fricatives made at the back of the mouth (where channel shape is not so important) it is reported that these fricatives are acquired relatively early, and seem less problematic.

Fricatives are prolongable, and they may also occur with central or lateral airflow. Lateral fricatives are made when the air is directed over the side edge of the tongue rather than centrally across the surface of the tongue. To do this, the speaker needs to produce a gap for the air to flow out at the side. English has no lateral fricatives, but voiceless and voiced lateral fricatives are not very rare sounds in the languages of the world. For example, Zulu has both a voiceless and a voiced lateral fricative, and Welsh has a voiceless one.

Lateral fricatives are frequently encountered as substitutions for sibilant fricatives in young children. This usage is sometimes termed a *lateral lisp,* and may require intervention in the clinic if it persists.

Affricates

Affricates are often described as combinations of a plosive and a fricative. However, this does not mean a cluster of two separate consonants, but a merging together of the characteristics of each sound type into a single consonant. How is this brought about? When we reach the release phase of a plosive, we normally move our articulators apart to allow the compressed air to escape freely (with the characteristic popping sound). However, if we move the articulators only slightly apart, leaving just a narrow gap, the pressurized air will be forced along this narrow channel and become turbulent; remember, we hear this turbulence as frication. Therefore, an affricate has a closure stage like a plosive (silent for voiceless affricates, and just the voicing buzz for voiced ones) and a release stage like a fricative. Affricates are not twice as long as plosives or fricatives, however, because the fricative portion is shorter than a full fricative (this is one way of distinguishing between affricates and clusters of plosives plus fricatives). Affricates are made at a single place of articulation; the plosive part and the fricative part are *homorganic* (articulated at the identical place).

Many languages have affricates; for example, in English, the sounds at the beginning and end of the words "church" and "judge" are affricates, both voiceless in "church" and both voiced in "judge."

In IPA we transcribe affricates with a combined symbol: one to represent the plosive part and the other to denote the fricative part. Sometimes a tie-bar is placed over the symbols to show they are a single sound, but it is not really necessary to include that. The English affricates, therefore, can be shown as [t͡ʃ, d͡ʒ] or [tʃ, dʒ].

Affricates are prolongable in two different ways. First, the closure phase of the stop component can be prolonged somewhat, and second, the fricative part can also be drawn out a little. The fricative part of the affricate can also be lateral (though this is less usual than central release). Some of the native American languages of the northwest Pacific coast area have laterally released affricates (for example, in Tlingit the word [tɬaa] means "to be big").

APPROXIMANTS

The third main grouping in the consonant strength hierarchy is the approximant type. These sounds have a wide air channel, which does not produce turbulent airflow. Voiceless approximants are rare, but when they do occur their airflow is stronger (because less of the air pressure is expended in the production of vocal fold vibration), so that some turbulence does occur (see Fig. 6.5). Laterals can have central or lateral air flow.

Phoneticians generally recognize two categories of approximants; *liquids*, and *glides* or *semivowels*. Liquids generally fall into three subtypes: *laterals, frictionless continuants,* and *rhotic approximants*.

Liquids

Frictionless continuants are those approximants made with air flowing over the central surface of the tongue and this term can be applied to all approximants that do not have lateral airflow. However, we are restricting the term here to deal with nonlateral and nonrhotic liquids. One of the very common nonstandard pronunciations of English /ɹ/ is a central approximant articulated between the lower lip and the upper teeth ([ʋ]). Other misarticulations of this target include an approximant articulated between the upper and lower lips (but differing from [w] in that no raising of the back of the tongue occurs). Most of the voiced fricatives we describe in chapter 7 can also occur as frictionless continuants if the air channel is made somewhat wider than required for frication.

Lateral approximants are much more common, and some languages have two or three of these. In English we just have [l], produced by placing the tongue tip and/or blade against the alveolar ridge and leaving a wide gap at one side rim of the tongue (some speakers may have

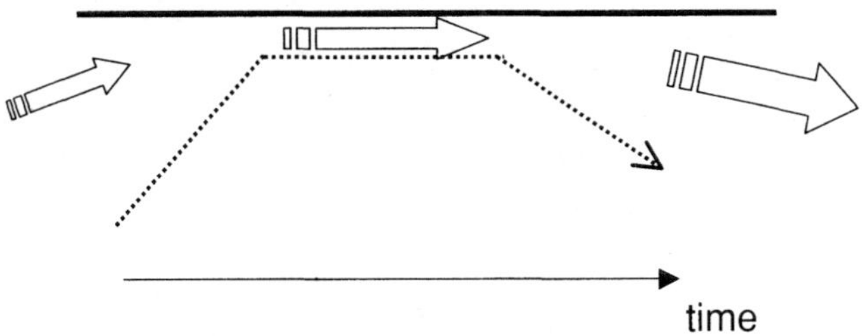

FIG 6.5. Approximant production (solid line: passive articulator; dotted line: active articulator; arrows: airflow).

gaps at both sides; these differences are not important). The air flows over the side rim of the tongue and through the gap to create the lateral approximant sound.

Rhotic approximants are those made with some degree of tongue tip retroflexion (i.e., curling the tongue tip up and sometimes also back). The "r" sound in most English dialects is usually a rhotic approximant, though some Scottish varieties use a trill or a tap (see *Trills and Taps*). Rhotics have central airflow. As noted in chapter 5, vowels can also be produced with retroflexion, and it is not always easy to determine whether speakers are producing a vowel followed by a rhotic approximant, or an r-colored vowel. We return to this question in chapter 15, where we also examine the so-called bunched-r that some English speakers use instead of the retroflexed rhotic.

> To transcribe those frictionless continuants that are "weak" versions of voiced fricatives, the IPA allows the addition of a diacritic marking "more open" (to show the opener/wider air channel), unless there is a dedicated approximant symbol already approved:
>
> | | |
> |---|---|
> | bilabial approximant: | β̞ |
> | dental approximant: | ð̞ |
> | alveolar approximant: | z̞ |
> | palatal approximant: | j |
> | velar approximant: | ɰ |
> | uvular approximant: | ʁ̞ |

These three types of liquids are all prolongable, though in normal speech they tend to be relatively short sounds.

Glides

As their alternative name—semivowels—suggests, these sounds are similar in many respects to vowels. In fact, each glide is the approximant counterpart to one of the vowels we examined in chapter 5 (though only high vowels have a glide equivalent). So the English glide [w] is equivalent to the vowel [u]; the English glide [j] (as in "*y*es") is equivalent to the vowel [i]; and the French glide [ɥ] (as in "*hu*it," *eight*) is equivalent to the French vowel [y].

> The glide symbols are even designed to resemble the equivalent high vowels:
>
> | | | | | | |
> |---|---|---|---|---|---|
> | front unrounded | [j] | [i] | back unrounded | [ɰ] | [ɯ] |
> | front rounded | [ɥ] | [y] | back rounded | [w] | [u] |
> | central unrounded | [ɉ] | [ɨ] | central rounded | [w̶] | [ʉ] |

The name *glide* suggests the main characteristics of these approximants: They consist of a rapid glide from the relevant vowel position to the following sound in the word in question. Because they require this rapid glide, they are not prolongable. If you try to prolong an English [w] or [j] it will just sound like the vowel [u] or [i]. It is the actual gliding movement of the articulators that distinguishes these sounds. Like the other approximants, then, these sounds are comparatively short.

TRILLS AND TAPS

These two types of consonants are sometimes classed as varieties of stops, because they both involve complete closure of the articulators and thereby stoppage of the airflow. However, these closures are very brief, and no air pressure buildup occurs. A trill is made when one moveable articulator is repeatedly and rapidly struck against another, static one. A trill requires at least two such strikes in a very short time, and because these sounds are prolongable in terms of the number of strikes but not in the duration of their contact, numerous strikes are in theory possible. Languages that use trills will often restrict the contacts of the articulators to two or three times, unless they are using emphasis. A common trill (found, for example, in Spanish and Italian) requires the rapid contact of the tongue tip against the alveolar ridge and, indeed, Scottish accents of English may use this *apical trill* (apical means "tongue tip") for "r," at least in some contexts. Standard European French and German normally use a trill involving the trilling of the uvular at the back of the oral cavity. Interestingly, in Canadian French some speakers use the apical trill (reflecting an earlier standard in French, and current southern varieties) and some use the back trill.

Taps (also known as flaps) are single-strike versions of trills. In other words, if you make a very rapid strike of the tongue tip against the alveolar ridge, and do not repeat this strike, you have made a tap. Because you cannot repeat the strikes (as you'd then make a trill), and because you cannot prolong the contact (or you'd make a plosive), taps are not prolongable. In American English taps are commonly used for intervocalic /t/. So, for example, the /t/ in "better" is made with a single-strike tap of the tongue tip against the alveolar ridge, rather than with a full voiceless plosive (this latter pronunciation is used in many other varieties of English, such as British English). Taps of this type are used in Spanish as well, where they are represented in writing by a single "r," as opposed to the double "rr," which denotes the trill. Thus, Spanish "pero" *but* and "perro" *dog* differ through the choice of tap over trill. Compare trills and taps in Figs. 6.6 and 6.7. The term *flap* is generally applied to the sound made when the underside of the tongue blade strikes the alveolar ridge as the curled tongue is uncurled and brought back to the rest position. This sound is common in some Indian languages.

> Because both trills and taps are often used to represent various "r"-spellings, and because in some languages they may vary in this role with the rhotic approximants, some phonologists use an overall category of *rhotic* to cover all these types. In terms of their articulations, however, we feel that this is somewhat confusing, and we avoid that grouping in this book.

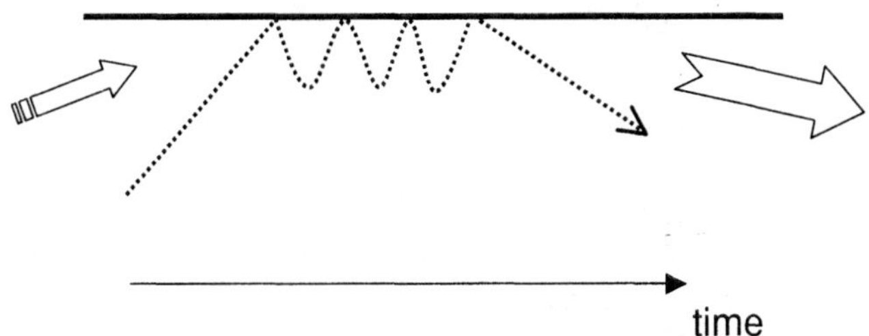

FIG 6.6. Trill production (solid line: passive articulator; dotted line: active articulator; arrows: airflow).

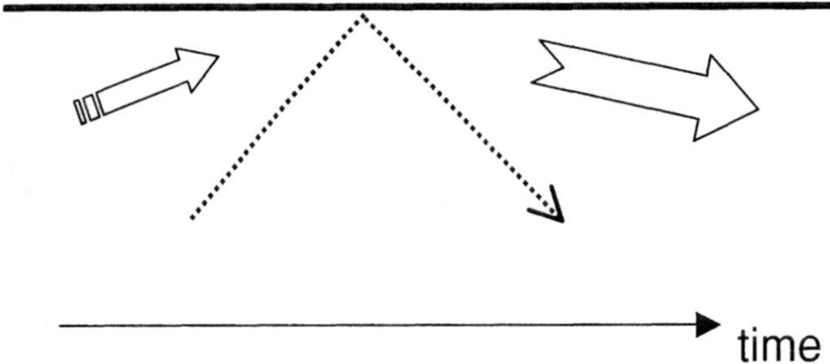

FIG 6.7. Tap production (solid line: passive articulator; dotted line: active articulator; arrows: airflow).

OBSTRUENTS AND SONORANTS

Our categories in this chapter were derived from the hierarchy of articulatory strength, from stops as the strongest through to approximants as the weakest. Another way of grouping consonants refers to their perceived sound quality. Some consonants are more *sonorous* than others (i.e., louder and clearer). The less obstruction there is to the airflow, the more sonorous the resultant sound. This gives us two main groupings: the *sonorants* (sonorous sounds) and the *obstruents* (the sounds with obstructions to the airflow).

Sonorants cover the various approximant types, liquids and glides, and the nasal stops (and, indeed, the vowels). Obstruents are plosive stops, fricatives, and affricates. It is not always clear whether the trills and taps are sonorants (like the other rhotics) or obstruents (like the other stops); for our purposes we will assign them to the obstruents. Nasal stops are sonorants because, although there is a complete closure in the oral cavity, the air flows through the nasal cavity without obstruction.

Such a broad division is sometimes useful phonetically. For example, it may help explain the patterns of voicing we see in the consonants of the world's languages. Obstruents are more commonly voiceless than voiced, because air pressure is expended during voicing that is needed to make obstruent sounds long and clear. On the other hand, sonorant sounds are more commonly found voiced than voiceless, and this is because the laminar (smooth) airflow needs the addition of voice to make the resultant sound loud enough.

The interrelation of the two categorization systems can be seen in the following diagram:

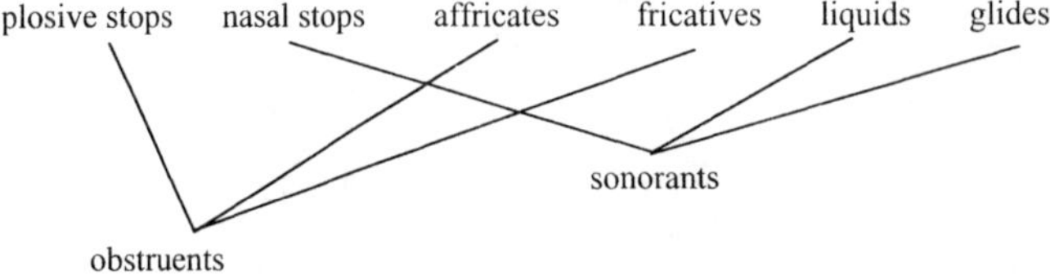

BACKGROUND READING

The standard texts referred to in previous chapters will also provide further reading on this topic. The examples of consonants in various languages are from the sources listed in chapter 5.

EXERCISES

Review Questions

1. Define the terms *stop, fricative*, and *approximant*. What is the main characteristic distinguishing them?
2. Describe the three stages of the production of a plosive.
3. In the speech clinic, we typically find that more children have problems with the production of fricatives than with the production of plosives. Why do you think this is the case?
4. What is the difference between grooved and slit fricatives? Give examples for each category.
5. What is the difference between sibilants and nonsibilants? Give examples for each category.
6. Describe the different categories of approximants.
7. What is the difference between trills and taps?
8. How does the hierarchy of articulatory strength in the classification of consonant types map onto sonorants and obstruents?

Study Topics and Experiments

1. In a textbook on child language acquisition, look up the typical sequence of the acquisition of consonants. What patterns do you find concerning the acquisition of different manners of articulation, and what do you think may cause the pattern in terms of the motor control required for the production of different manners of articulation?
2. Conduct an experiment on voiced phonation in plosives and fricatives. Use the syllables [ɑbɑ], [ɑvɑ], [ɑdɑ], [ɑzɑ]. Record yourself uttering these syllables using a good-quality tape recorder with an external microphone. When you utter each syllable, prolong the consonant as long as possible *while keeping the voicing going* (for [b] and [d] prolong the closure stage of the stop). Measure the duration of the consonants (either with a stopwatch or, preferably, via spectrographic analysis). Comment on your results in light of the discussion above on voicing in plosives.

CD

Listen to the examples of different consonants, and try to imitate as many as possible. Attempt the test items, following the instructions on the CD. Answers to all the exercises are given at the end of the book.

7

Articulation: Consonant Place Types

INTRODUCTION

In the previous chapter we looked at the various manners of articulation that produce consonants. But, as we noted, we also have to be aware of the places of articulation that can be employed. For example, the plosive stops in English can be made with the two lips as articulators ([p, b]), with the tongue tip and/or blade articulating against the alveolar ridge ([t, d]), or with the back of the tongue articulating against the velum ([k, g]). When we describe place of articulation we have to bear in mind that usually, in consonant articulation, there is one active articulator and one passive one. To produce [t, d], the active articulator (the anterior part of the tongue) is placed against the passive one (the alveolar ridge); for [k, g] the back of the tongue is the active, the velum the passive articulator; even for [p, b] we might reckon that the lower lip is the active articulator (say the sounds and feel how much your lower jaw moves), whereas the upper lip moves little if at all.

Because many places of articulation involve tongue movement, we need to have a terminology to cover the main parts of the tongue used in speech. Figure 7.1 is a diagram of the tongue with the main areas shown. Most of these have both English and Latinate names, and we should get to know the adjectives derived from the latter, because they are often used in phonetic description. From apex (tip) we have *apical*; from lamina (blade) we get *laminal*; from dorsum (tongue body) we get *dorsal.*

We also need to know the main divisions for the passive articulators: mainly the roof of the mouth and associated structures, but also extending back into the pharynx and larynx. Figure 7.2 shows many of these. When we describe a place of articulation, we can combine the categories of the active and the passive articulators. For example, [t, d] can be termed *apico-alveolars* (from apex and alveolar), and [k, g] can be called *dorso-velars* (from dorsum and velar). Commonly, however, the active articulator is assumed and only the passive one is named (because there are seldom many options in terms of which active articulator can be coupled with any one passive articulator). Therefore, [t, d] are generally termed *alveolar*, and [k, g] *velar.* In the case of [p, b] we normally use the term *bilabial*, expressing the fact that both lips are involved. *Labial* by itself would be unambiguous in most cases in normal speech, although we need more precise distinctions in disordered speech (see below).

In the next sections we will examine the various places of articulation in turn, grouped into the following categories: labial, anterior lingual, dorsal, and posterior. Some very rare places

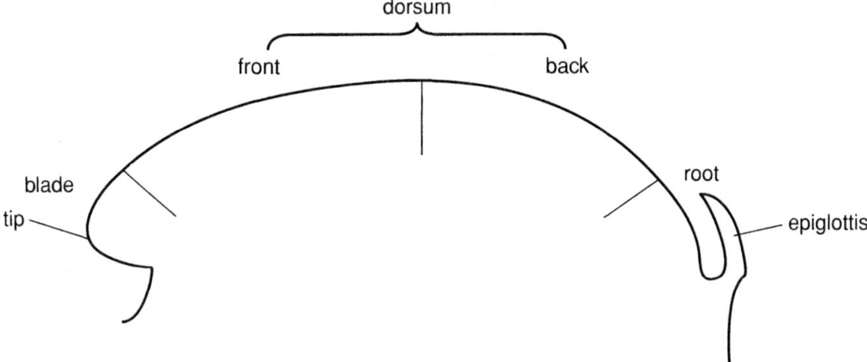

FIG 7.1. Divisions of the tongue.

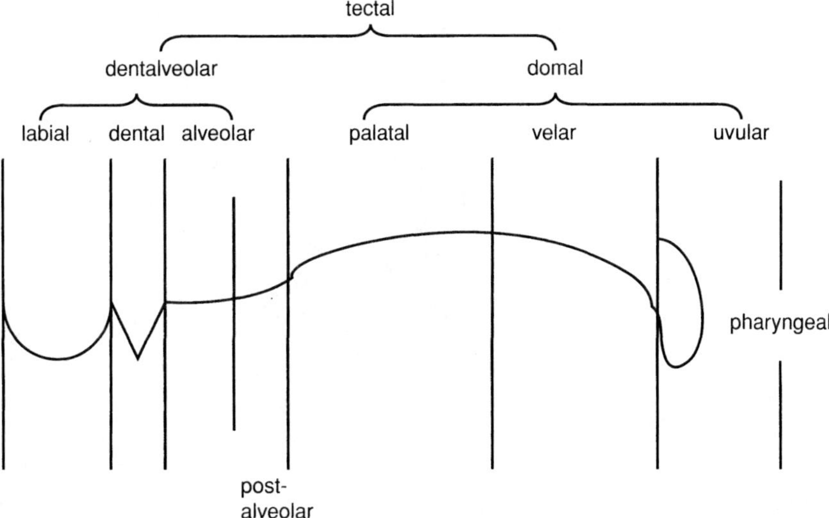

FIG 7.2. The passive articulators.

of articulation are not covered, but readers will find these described in the texts referred to at the end of the chapter.

LABIAL

There are two places of articulation in normal speech that come under this heading: *bilabial* and *labiodental*. These two types are shown in Fig. 7.3. As the name suggests, bilabial consonants are made with the upper and lower lips as the articulators. As we noted above, it is possible to consider the lower lip as the active articulator, though some phoneticians consider both lips as being actively involved to a greater or lesser extent in the production of the sound. Bilabial consonants are commonly found in the languages of the world, and English has bilabial plosives and nasal stops. Bilabial fricatives occur in some languages, and there are even a few instances of the use of a bilabial trill—although we may more often use that sound as an extralinguistic marker of feeling cold!

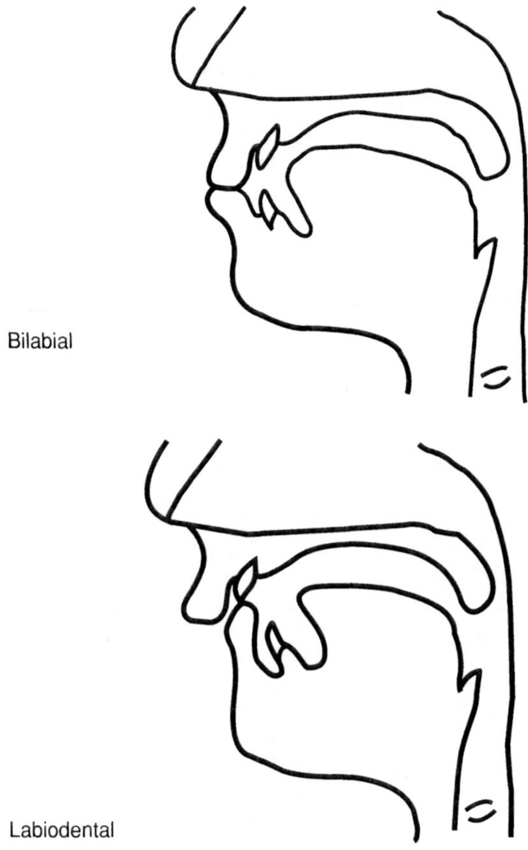

FIG 7.3. Labial articulation types.

> Here are some examples of bilabial consonants in the languages of the world:
>
> | | |
> |---|---|
> | nasal: | [m]—[mat] (Breton) *good* |
> | plosives: | [p], [b]—[pal], [bal] (Hindi) *take care of, hair* |
> | fricatives: | [ɸ], [β]—[ɸu], [βu] (Ewe) *bone, boat* |
> | trill: | [ʙ]—[mbʙuen] (Kele) *its fruit* |

Note that although it is possible to make a purely bilabial approximant, these are not commonly encountered, but a mixed bilabial and velar approximant is found in English ([w]). We discuss these mixed places of articulation in chapter 8.

Labiodental articulations require the lower lip to be brought up to the lower edge of the upper front teeth. Again, the lower lip is generally considered to be the active articulator. For some consonant types (e.g., the fricatives [f] and [v]), it is generally the inner surface of the lower lip that makes contact with the upper teeth; for others (for example, the approximant [ʋ]), the lower lip may be curled inward so that it is its outer surface that is used. However, these different lip postures may also be an individual preference. Labiodental nasals, fricatives, affricates, and approximants are found in natural language, although labiodental plosives are very rare.

Examples of labiodental consonants in the languages of the world are seen as follows:

nasal:	[ɱ]—[kʌɱ̩fi] (English) *comfy (positional variant of English "m")*
fricatives:	[f], [v]—[faka], [vaka] (Portuguese) *knife, cow*
affricates:	[p͡f]—[p͡faɪfən] (German) *to whistle*
approximant:	[ʋ]—[ʋaɻ̩i] (Tamil) *path*

ANTERIOR LINGUAL

There are four main places of articulation made with the anterior part of the tongue (that is, the tip and the blade): *dental, alveolar, postalveolar,* and *retroflex.* These four are illustrated in Fig. 7.4.

In dental articulations, the tip of the tongue is the active articulator and the inside of the upper front teeth is the passive articulator. Dental articulations can be found for all the main consonant types: nasal, plosive, fricative, affricate, and approximant. Whereas English has an alveolar place of articulation for sounds such as [t, d, n, l], many languages use a dental place for these sounds. However, the difference in sound quality between dental and alveolar is slight, and it is comparatively rare to find languages that contrast them (though Malayalam

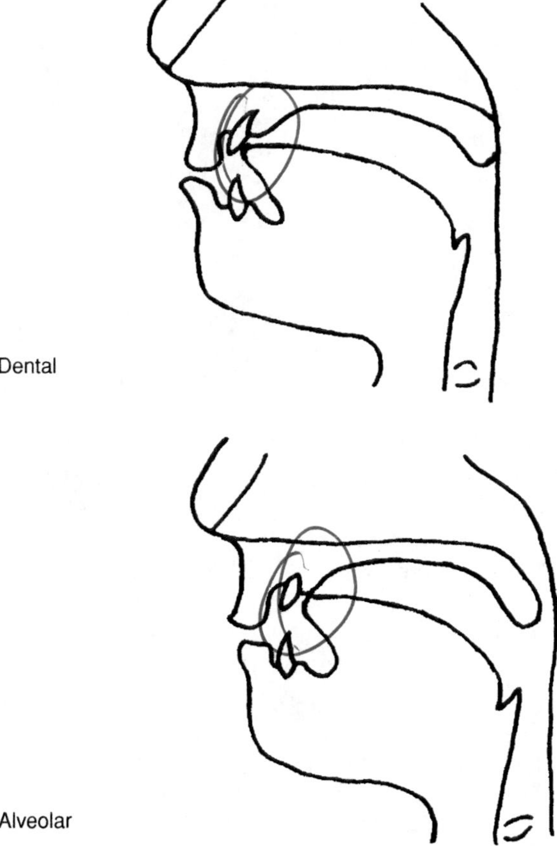

FIG 7.4. Anterior lingual articulation types.

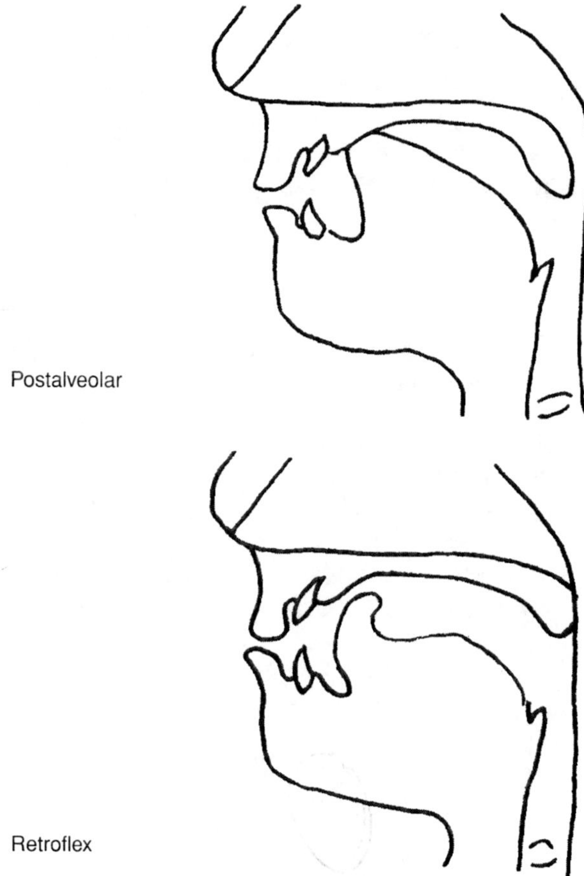

FIG 7.4. (Continued)

in southern India is among the group that do). The IPA, therefore, does not provide separate symbols to distinguish dental from alveolar, and if one wishes to mark the dental place of articulation, then a special diacritic is added beneath the symbol. Dental fricatives normally are slit channel fricatives (though a grooved dental fricative is occasionally found in natural languages). The dental slit fricatives in English (the sounds at the beginning of "thin" and "then") are often pronounced with the tip of tongue placed between the upper and lower teeth. This *interdental* articulation is perceptually very similar to the dental one, and the difference appears to be one of personal preference. You might want to check with colleagues to see whether they have a dental or interdental pronunciation.

Examples of dental consonants in the languages of the world are seen as follows:

nasal:	[n̪]—[n̪u] (French) *we*
plosives:	[t̪], [d̪] — [t̪o], [d̪o] (north Welsh) *roof, yes (past tense)*
fricatives:	[θ], [ð]—[maʊθ], [maʊð] (English) *mouth (noun), mouth (verb)*
lateral approximant:	[l̪]—[l̪iʃu] (Portuguese) *garbage*
trill:	[r̪]—[r̪oː] (Hungarian) *to carve*

Alveolar consonants are made by placing the tip and/or the blade of the tongue up against the alveolar ridge. Some speakers use the tongue tip as the active articulator, some the blade, and some both together; there appears to be no clear sound quality difference here, and it is another example of personal preference. (There are IPA diacritics to mark tip versus blade articulations, however.) All the main manners of consonant articulation are found at the alveolar place. Alveolar fricatives are normally grooved, as in the first sounds of English "sue" and "zoo." However, alveolar slit fricatives can be made, and the so-called "slit-t" of Irish English is just such an example (as in the Irish English pronunciation of final "t" in a word such as "hat").

Examples of alveolar consonants in the languages of the world are seen as follows:

nasals:	[n], [n̥]—[nǎ], [n̥ǎ] (Burmese) *pain, nose*
fricatives:	[s], [z]—[sil], [zil] (English) *seal, zeal*
lateral fricatives:	[ɬ], [ɮ]—[ɬàɬá], [ɮálà] (Zulu) *cut off, play*
affricates:	[t͡s], [d͡z]—[rat͡tsa], [rad͡dza] (Italian) *race, ray (fish)*
lateral approximant:	[l]—[le] (French) *the (plural)*
trill:	[r]—[pɛro] (Spanish) *dog*
tap:	[ɾ]—[pɛɾo] (Spanish) *but*

As the name suggests, postalveolar articulations are made at the rear edge of the alveolar ridge (and often the front edge of the hard palate as well). Although it is possible to produce a wide range of sounds at this position, we generally only find fricatives (with the tongue blade as the active articulator) and a rhotic approximant (using the tongue tip). The postalveolar fricatives are found in English, and have a narrow slit air channel; they are the sounds in the middle of the words "thresher" and "treasure." The postalveolar rhotic approximant is the usual realization of English "r," though in some accents the tongue tip may be bent both up and back. In this case we would refer to the articulation as *retroflex.*

Examples of postalveolar consonants in the languages of the world are seen as follows:

fricatives:	[ʃ], [ʒ]—[ʃu], [ʒu] (French) *cabbage, play (1st pers, sing, present)*
rhotic approximant:	[ɹ]—[ɹɛd] (English) *red*

Retroflex consonants are defined in terms of tongue shape rather than the place of the passive articulator, so in this respect the term differs from the others used in this chapter. These consonants require the tongue tip and blade to be lifted up and bent backward so that, in the case of the stops, for example, the contact is made between the underside of the tongue blade and the border of the alveolar ridge and the hard palate. Retroflex consonants are not found in American English (except for the retroflex version of the rhotic we referred to above that occurs in some varieties), but plosives, nasals, fricatives, and laterals made in this way are common in the languages of India, among others.

Examples of retroflex consonants in the languages of the world are seen as follows:

nasal:	[ɳ]—[ʋaɳɖɪ] (Tamil) *cart*
plosives:	[ʈ], [ɖ]—[ʈal], [ɖal] (Hindi) *postpone, branch*
fricatives:	[ʂ], [ʐ]—[ʂa], [ʐaŋ] (Chinese) *to kill, to assist*
lateral approximant:	[ɭ]—[vaɭ] (Tamil) *sword*
rhotic approximant:	[ɻ]—[báɻà:] (Hausa) *begging*
flap:	[ɽ]—[eɽe] (Gbaya) *hen*

The place *alveolopalatal* is not found often, but two fricatives used, for example, in Polish ([ɕ], [ʑ]) are pronounced with the blade and front of the tongue articulating against the border region of the front of the hard palate and the alveolar ridge.

DORSAL

The dorsal category covers three places of articulation: *palatal, velar,* and *uvular.* These are shown in Fig. 7.5. They all have in common that the body of the tongue is the active articulator: the front of the dorsum for the palatal place, the back of the dorsum for velar and uvular.

The name *palatal* derives from the hard palate, which is the passive articulator for these sounds. English only has one palatal consonant (the glide [j], as at the beginning of "yes"), but palatal nasals, for example, are found in French, Spanish, and Italian (the ñ in "España," for example). Palatal plosives and fricatives are also found, and the voiceless palatal fricative is used in the German word for *I*, "ich." Many English speakers find it difficult to distinguish the difference between palatal, velar, and uvular fricatives, so when you listen to the examples on the CD, note that the palatal fricatives are both higher pitched than the others.

Examples of palatal consonants in the languages of the world are seen as follows:

nasal:	[ɲ]—[aɲo] (Spanish) *year*
plosives:	[c], [ɟ]—[cel], [ɟel] (Turkish) *bald, come*
fricatives:	[ç], [ʝ]—[çon̪i] [ʝàʝàɗə̀] (Greek, Margi) *snow, picked up*
affricates:	[c͡ç], [ɟ͡ʝ]—[c͡ça:n], [ɟ͡ʝa:r] (Sherpa, Hungarian) *north, factory*
lateral approximant:	[ʎ]—[fiʎʎɔ] (Italian) *son*
semivowel:	[j]—[jaɪθ] (Welsh) *language*

Velar consonants require articulation between the back of the tongue body and the soft palate, or velum. Velar sounds are common in the languages of the world. English [k] and [g] (as in "coat" and "goat") are velar stops, and English [ŋ] (as at the end of "sing") is a velar nasal. English lacks velar fricatives, however, and this means that it is typically difficult for monolingual English speakers to make and distinguish these sounds. When listening to the CD, note how much deeper in pitch the velar fricatives are than the palatal ones. Both Spanish and German have velar fricatives, along with other languages you may encounter, such as Dutch, Russian, and Greek.

Examples of velar consonants in the languages of the world are seen as follows:

nasal:	[ŋ]—[ŋă] (Burmese) *a fish*
plosives:	[k], [g]—[kɛʀn], [gɛʀn] (German) *kernel, willingly*
fricatives:	[x], [ɣ]—[exa], [aɣa] (Urhobo) *dance, broom*
lateral approximant:	[ʟ]—[raʟ] (Melpa) *two*
semivowel:	[ɰ]—[ɰiza] (Korean) *doctor*

The uvular place of articulation has the very back of the tongue dorsum as the active articulator. Uvular sounds are not found in English, but are common in many languages, such as Arabic and some Native American languages. The back trilled-r found in standard French and German is often a uvular trill (though it may be a voiced uvular fricative for many speakers), and the back voiceless fricative in languages such as German, Irish, and Welsh may vary between velar and uvular places of articulation. When listening to the uvular fricatives on the CD, you will find that they are low in pitch like the velar ones, but they sound much rougher, because you can hear the vibrations of the uvula itself as the air is forced past it.

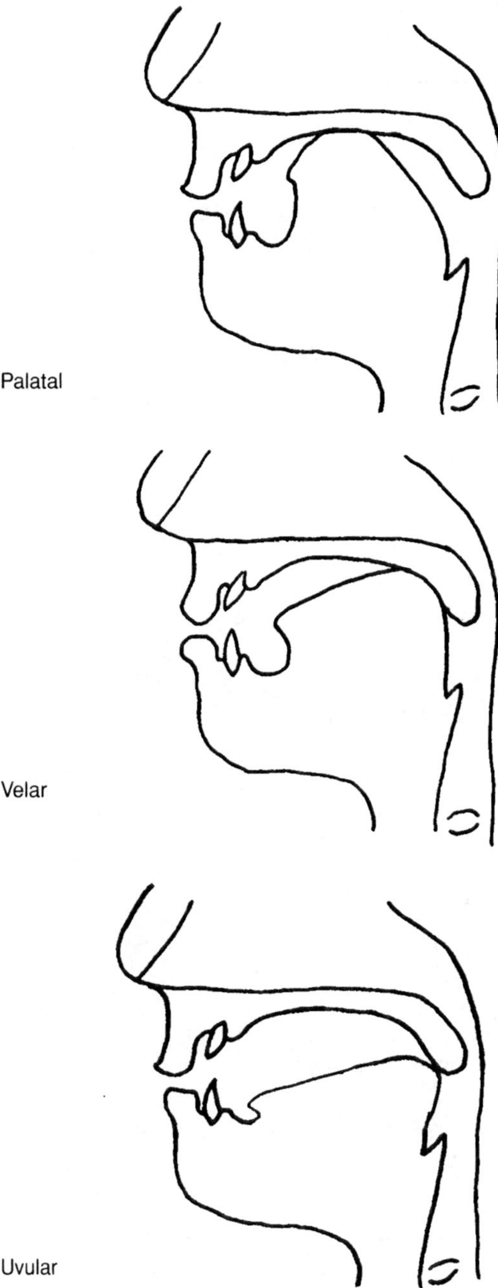

FIG 7.5. Dorsal articulation types.

Examples of uvular consonants in the languages of the world are seen as follows:

nasal:	[ɴ]—[daɴdaɴ] (Japanese) *gradually*
plosives:	[q], [ɢ]—[qaʎu], [ɢar] (Quechua, Farsi) *tongue, cave*
fricatives:	[χ], [ʁ]—[χasa], [ʁatu] (Kwakw'ala, Portuguese) *rotten, mouse*
trill:	[ʀ]—[ʀuʒ] (French) *red*

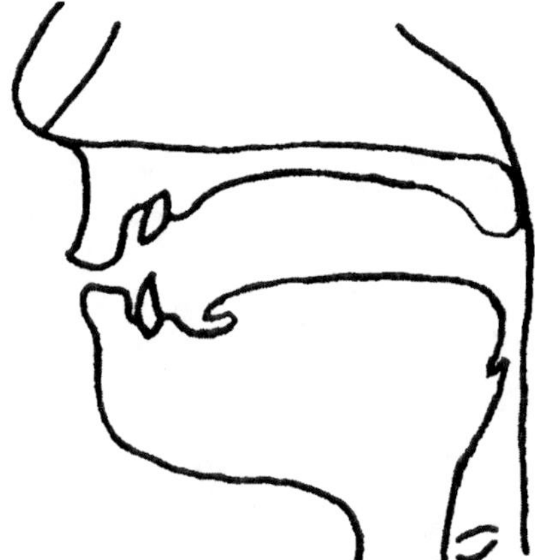

FIG 7.6. Posterior articulation (pharyngeal).

POSTERIOR

This final group of places of articulation includes those where the passive articulator lies outside the oral cavity: the *pharyngeal, epiglottal,* and *glottal* places of articulation. The terminology with these three is not quite consistent. Whereas "pharyngeal" indicates that the pharynx is the passive articulator, at the epiglottal place of articualtion, the epiglottis is the active articulator. "Glottal" means that the articulators are the two vocal folds—both of which count as being active. Figure 7.6 illustrates pharyngeal and epiglottal; diagrams in chapter 3 have provided illustrations of different states of the glottis.

Although pharyngeal articulations are not used in English, they may occur in disordered speech (for example, with cleft palate speakers), so we do need to be aware of them. Pharyngeal sounds are common in Arabic and Hebrew, among others. Pharyngeal fricatives are recorded in natural language, and they are formed by drawing the root of the tongue back into the pharynx. This decreases the air channel through the pharynx for the outflowing lung air, and the airflow becomes turbulent as it is forced through the gap. If the gap is left somewhat wider, the resultant sounds will be approximants. In languages such as Arabic the voiceless pharyngeal is fricative, and the voiced may often be realized as approximant rather than fricative. Apart from these two types, there are no other pharyngeals. The IPA chart in appendix 1 shows some pharyngeal consonants as impossible to make (shaded squares), and others as possible but rarely encountered (blank squares).

Examples of pharyngeal consonants in the languages of the world are as follows:

fricatives: [ħ], [ʕ]—[muħ], [muʕ] (Agul) *barn, bridge*

To show an approximant pronunciation of the voiced pharyngeal, we add the diacritic for lowering to indicate a wider air channel: [ʕ̞].

Epiglottal articulations can be thought of as variants of the pharyngeal type. In these sounds, the epiglottis as well as the tongue root is drawn back into the pharynx. Fricatives and approximants can be made in the same fashion as we saw with pharyngeals. Also, an epiglottal plosive is found in some languages. Here, the epiglottis is pulled right back until it touches the rear wall of the pharynx, to form a closure. This plosive is voiceless, and it seems that it may not be possible to produce a voiced epiglottal plosive, because the pressure differential between sub- and supraglottal air pressure is not sufficient. Although the IPA provides separate symbols for pharyngeal and epiglottal fricatives, it may well be difficult to make pharyngeal sounds without also involving the epiglottis to some extent.

> Examples of epiglottal consonants in the languages of the world are seen as follows:
>
> stop: [ʡ]—[jaʡ] (Agul) *center*
> fricatives: [ʜ], [ʢ]—[ʜor], [ʢor] (Hebrew) *hole, skin (variant pronunciation with pharyngeal)*

The glottal place of articulation really subsumes different states of the glottis. The glottal stop requires closure between the two vocal folds, whereas the voiceless glottal fricative is actually an example of the breath variety of voicelessness. The voiced glottal fricative is the murmur type of phonation. For the sake of convenience, we treat these segments as separate consonants, and we use glottal as their place of articulation. In English we have the voiceless glottal fricative [h], and many varieties also use the glottal stop ([ʔ]). This latter sound may be used, for example, for intervocalic [t], as found in London English, or as a marker of word boundaries, especially before vowel-initial words. We return to this in part II.

> Examples of glottal consonants in the languages of the world are seen as follows:
>
> stop: [ʔ]—[haʔa] (Hawai'ian) *dance*
> fricatives: [h], [ɦ]—[hoː] [ɦut] (Hungarian) *snow*, (Dutch) *hat*

ARTICULATORY DESCRIPTION OF CONSONANTS

We have now introduced the symbols for all the main consonants on the IPA chart. When we describe consonants we can use the full set of parameters that we've looked at in this and the previous chapter. These are:

- airstream
  - location (e.g., pulmonic)
  - direction (e.g., egressive)
- phonation (e.g., voiceless, voiced)
- force of articulation (i.e., fortis or lenis)
- state of the velum (i.e., oral, nasal, nasalized)
- direction of oral airflow (central versus lateral)
- prolongability
- place of articulation
- manner of articulation

Under this system, a sound such as [t] would be described as "pulmonic egressive, voiceless, fortis, oral, central, prolongable, alveolar, plosive stop." Clearly, this is quite a mouthful! In practice, we can take a few of these parameters for granted. So, unless otherwise stated, we assume that the consonant is pulmonic egressive and only add airstream information if we are dealing with ejectives, implosives, or clicks. Because voiceless sounds are nearly always fortis, and voiced ones nearly always are lenis, we can omit the force of articulation category (sometimes it may be more convenient to use the fortis–lenis distinction and omit the phonation one). We usually assume that the consonant is oral, unless it is stated otherwise, and because prolongability is linked to the manner of articulation we normally don't have to include that, either.

This brings us to the so-called "three-term label" of phonation, place, and manner: Our [t] can now be called simply a "voiceless alveolar plosive."

Examples of three-term labels:

[p]—voiceless bilabial plosive
[d]—voiced alveolar plosive
[c]—voiceless palatal plosive
[v]—voiced labiodental fricative
[x]—voiceless velar fricative
[t͡ʃ]—voiceless postalveolar affricate
[ɳ]—voiced retroflex nasal
[ʎ]—voiced palatal lateral approximant
[ɰ]—voiced velar semivowel approximant

ACOUSTIC DESCRIPTION OF CONSONANTS

In chapter 5 we looked at the acoustic analysis of vowel sounds. We can do the same for consonants. In chapters 13 through 15 we will have the opportunity to look in more detail at the acoustic characteristics of English consonants, so in this section we will examine more general features of consonant types.

Because obstruents lack, partly or wholly, a periodic component (see chap. 1), the spectral type analysis of a single moment in time we used for vowels is not appropriate here, because no regular patterns would be observable. Instead we tend to use wideband spectrograms, which show the patterns of frequency across the entire durations of the consonants. Spectrograms are also useful with sonorant consonants, because they can show patterns of voicing and duration, although spectral analyses can usefully be done with these sounds as well.

Obstruents

Plosive stops have an easily recognizable spectrographic signature. Because they involve a short total stoppage of the airflow, the spectrogram displays a short stretch that is almost blank, corresponding to this. For voiceless stops, this stretch is totally blank; for voiced ones, you will be able to see the markings at the base of the spectrogram that denote the voicing buzz. The other easily recognizable feature is the plosive burst (when the air rushes out after the articulators move apart). On a spectrogram we see this as a straight line to the right of the blank stretch that spreads right across the frequency range. Figure 7.7 demonstrates these features for two different plosives: The one to the left of the spectrogram is a voiceless aspirated bilabial plosive taken from the English pronunciation of the word "papa," and the one on the right a voiceless unaspirated bilabial plosive from the French pronunciation of the same word. In each case we see the middle consonant and surrounding vowels. The figure clearly shows the

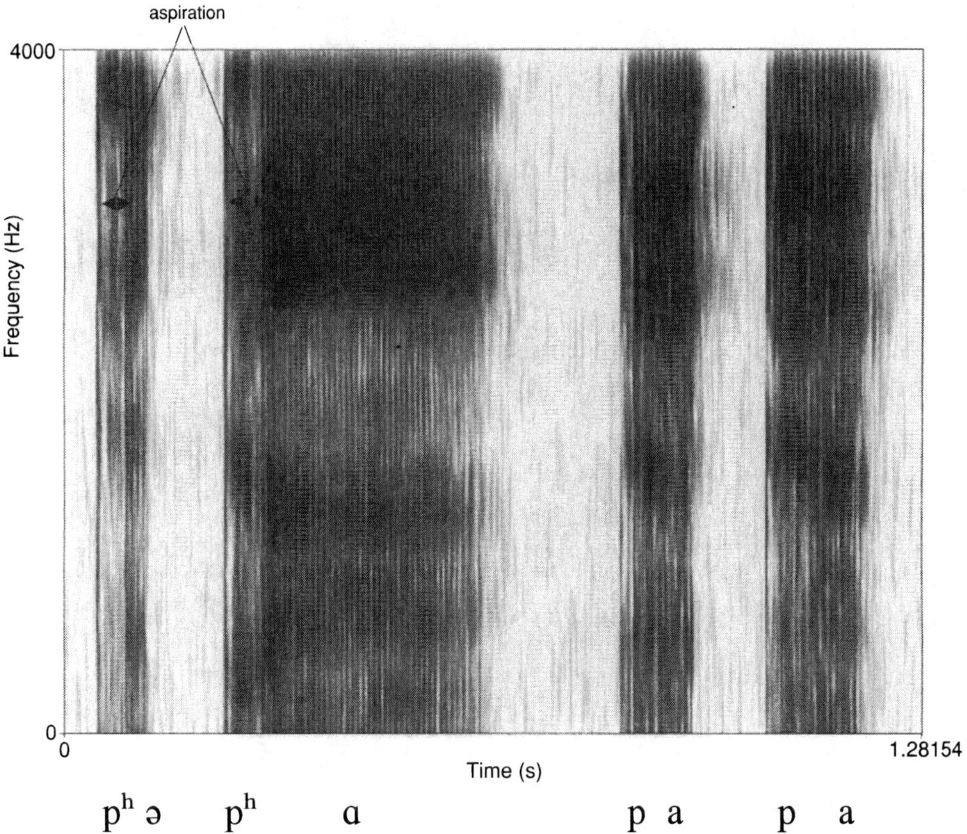

FIG 7.7. Spectrograms of English and French pronunciations of "papa."

closure phase of the stops, the release burst, and for the English example, the voice onset time that corresponds to what we perceive as aspiration.

Differences in place of articulation are not possible to gauge from the closure part of a stop. However, as the articulators move apart on release of the closure and move to the positions to make the following sound, they leave traces in the acoustic record. These *formant transitions*, as they are called (because we can see the formants moving across the frequency range), give information on the place of both the preceding and following sounds. We explore this in more detail in part II.

The spectrogram in Fig. 7.8 shows the characteristics of affricates. As with plosives, we see a blank stretch, corresponding to the closure phase, and a burst of noise on the release of that closure. However, this noise burst has a longer duration, and the markings on the spectrogram show that it is scattered widely across the frequency range. We illustrate affricates with the Italian words "razza" *race* and "razza" *ray-fish*, which have voiceless and voiced alveolar affricates (phonetically [t͡s] and [d͡z]). As well as the affricate release, the spectrogram shows the voicing bar that runs through the closure stage of voiced "razza," and the lack of that bar in voiceless "razza." (Note that although the spellings are identical, standard Italian requires the two different pronunciations dependent on meaning.)

As we noted earlier, obstruents (and fricatives in particular) consist mainly of aperiodic noise. This is clearly seen in Fig. 7.9, which shows a variety of fricatives. The patterns of the front fricatives [f] and [s] can be contrasted with those of the back fricatives [ç] and [x]. You

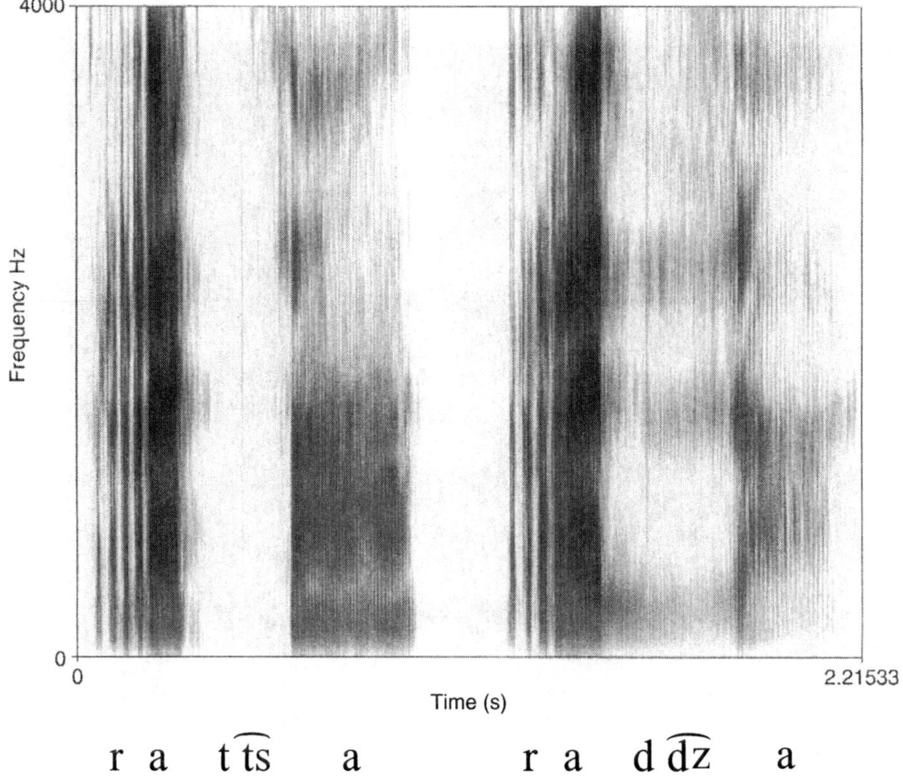

FIG 7.8. Spectrogram of voiceless and voiced affricates in Italian.

can note that the frequency ranges of these sounds differ. So, whereas [s] has its strongest range of frequency between 4000 and about 9000 Hz (and less strong down to about 1500 Hz), [f] has a more compact range of around 8000 to 9000 Hz, with its entire range descending to about 1000 Hz. With the back fricatives, [ç] has its main range from about 4000 to 8000 Hz, whereas [x] starts lower, 1500 to 8000 Hz, with a noticeable formant pattern.

Finally, in this section, we can look at the acoustic characteristics of trills and taps. Figure 7.10 displays the spectrograms of the two Spanish words "perro" *dog* and "pero" *but.* You should be able to recognize the initial plosives now, and the repeated brief contacts of the trill are also clearly noticeable. The tap is similar but, of course, has just the single marking indicating articulator contact.

Sonorants

Nasal stops (and indeed all nasalized sounds) have specific acoustic characteristics that one can look for on a spectrogram. First, they have lower intensity than most other sounds, so the markings on the spectrogram will be fainter during the period that the velum is lowered. Second, the coupling of the nasal to the oral cavity causes certain frequency bands to be suppressed. This is termed *antiresonance*, and an *antiformant* is often said to be in place during nasals at about the 800–2000 Hz level. Finally, the first formant of a nasal sound is generally lower than might be expected for nonnasal sonorants, and this is sometimes called the *nasal formant*. Figure 7.11 shows the nasals in the Spanish words "ano" *after* and "año" *year* (phonetically [n]

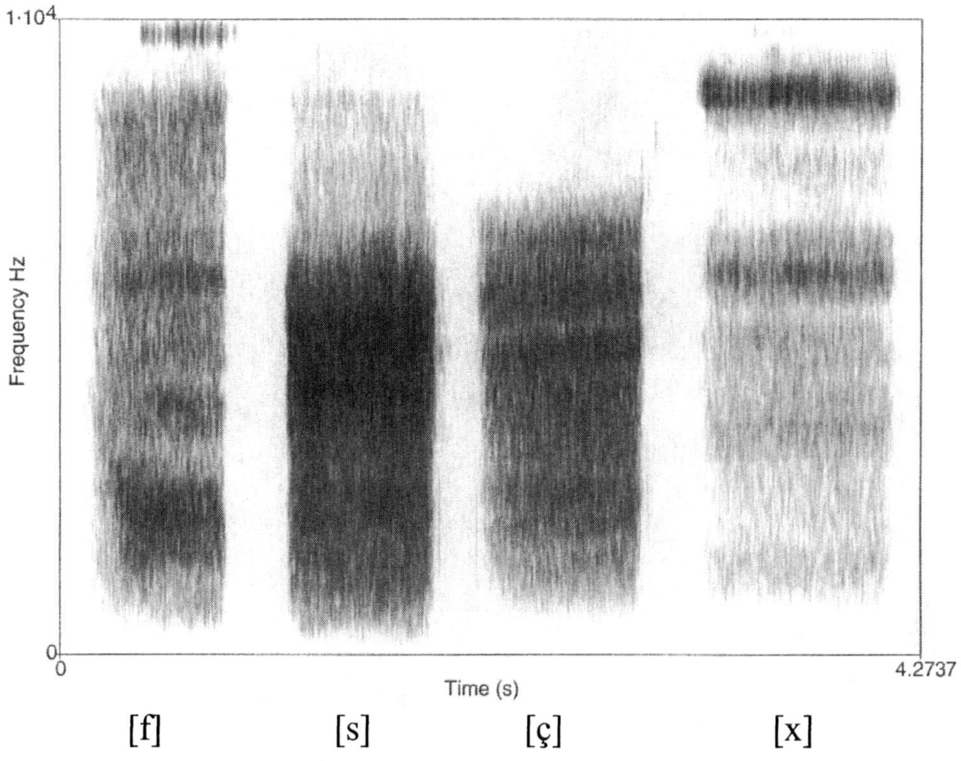

FIG 7.9. Spectrogram of the fricatives [f], [s], [ç], and [x].

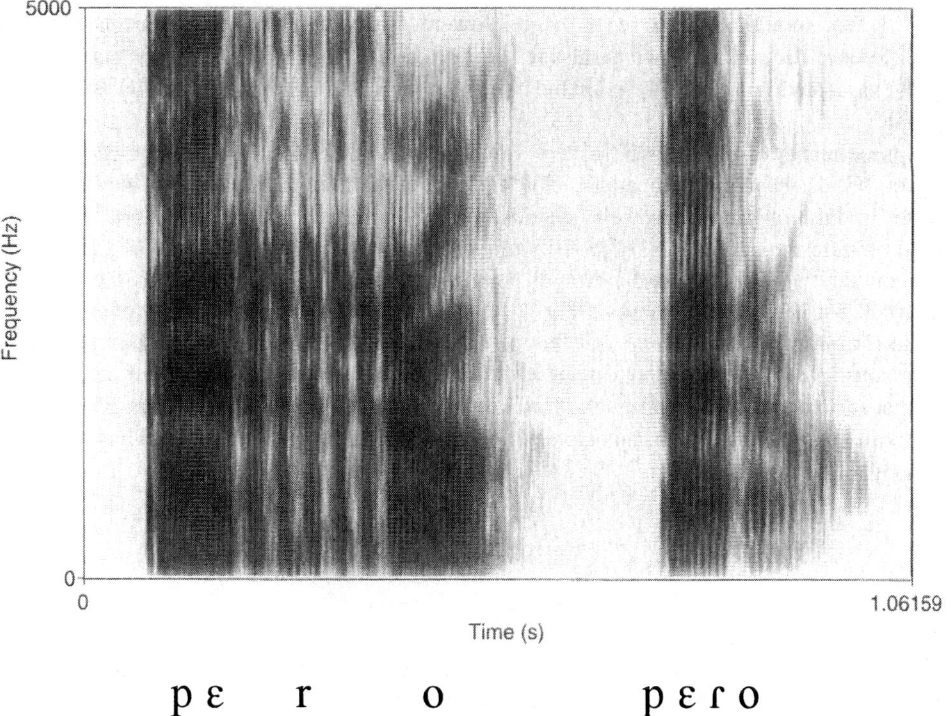

FIG 7.10. Spectrogram of a trill and a tap in Spanish.

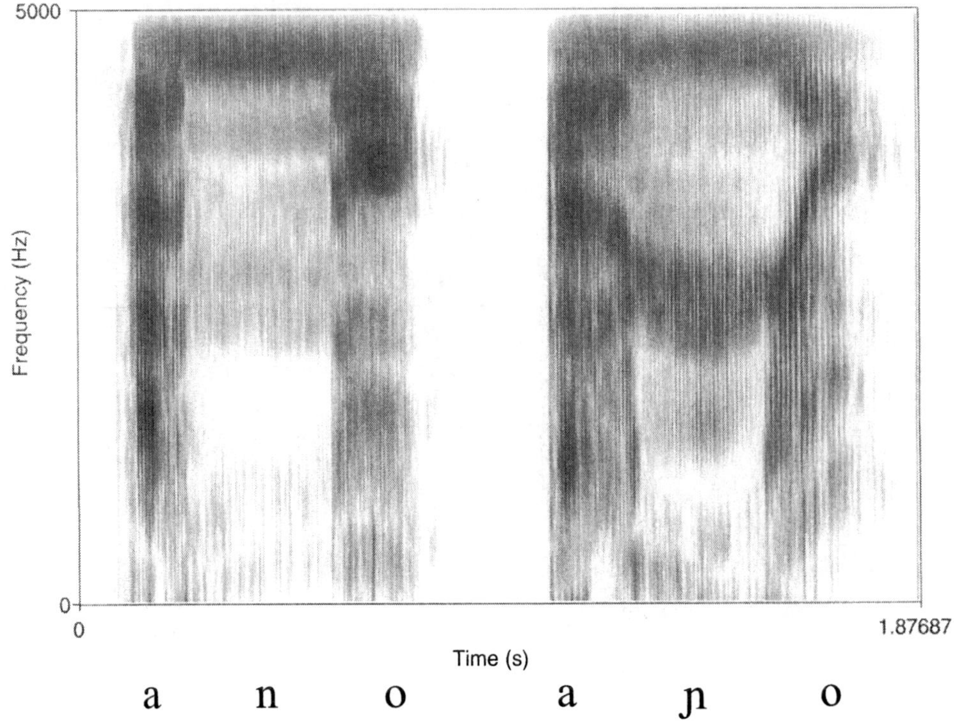

FIG 7.11. Spectrogram of alveolar and palatal nasals in Spanish.

and [ɲ]). You should be able to see the overall lowered intensity of the nasal segments, whereas the differences between the two nasals are manifested mainly in the higher formants, with the palatal nasal having a clear F4, and in the rising and then dipping nature of the formants of the palatal.

Approximants of all types have very vowel-like acoustic structures, with clear formant patterns. Glides have formant patterns close to those of their related vowels, but they are much shorter in duration than the vowels. Liquids, too, have characteristic patterns, and the rhotic liquids demonstrate a lowering of the F1 similar to the one found in rhotic vowels. Liquids are also comparatively short sounds. We will look at the acoustics of the English approximants in part II, but here we can show, in Fig. 7.12, the difference between the European Spanish pronunciation of "llama" *llama* and that of Latin America ([ʎama] versus [jama]). These contrast the palatal lateral approximant with the palatal semivowel approximant, and we can see that differences are found in the formant structure of the initial segments. The palatal approximant has a distinctive gap between formants 2 and 3, whereas the lateral has these two formants close together.

BACKGROUND READING

The examples of consonants from different languages come from various sources: Maddieson (1984), Laver (1994), Ladefoged and Maddieson (1996), the *Handbook of the IPA* (1999), Ball and Rahilly (1999), and the authors' own experience.

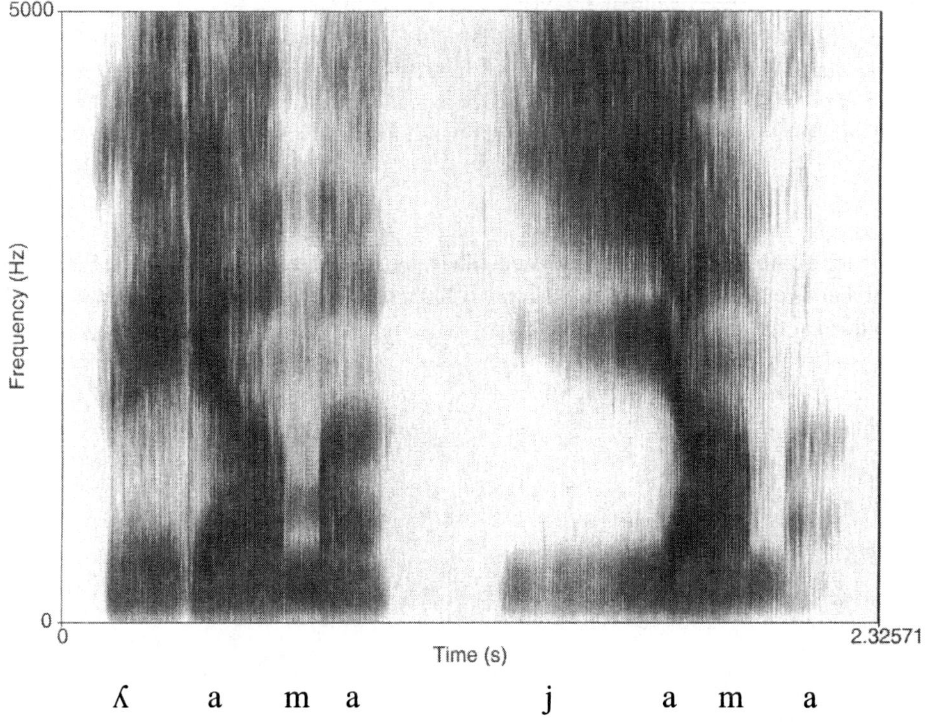

FIG 7.12. Spectrogram of palatal lateral and palatal glide in Spanish.

EXERCISES

Review Questions

1. What is the difference between active and passive articulators?
2. What are the main parts of the tongue that are used in speech?
3. List the main divisions of the oral cavity used to indicate the passive articulator.
4. What places of articulation lie outside the oral cavity, and how do the labels of these differ from labels for other places of articulation?
5. In the articulatory description of consonants, what is the "three-term label"?
6. Give some examples where the three-term label is not sufficient for the articulatory description of a consonant.
7. Describe the main characteristics of the spectrographic signatures of plosives, affricates, and fricatives.
8. Describe the main characteristics of the spectrographic signatures of nasals and approximants.

Study Topics and Experiments

1. In a textbook on child language acquisition, look up the typical sequence of the acquisition of consonants. What patterns do you find concerning the acquisition of different places of articulation, and what do you think may cause the pattern in terms of the motor control required for the production of different places of articulation?

2. Compare spectrographically the acoustic nature of nasal and oral sounds. Record the nasal stops [m] and [n] in the context of preceding and following [ɑ]: [ɑmɑ], [ɑnɑ]. Use a good tape recorder with an external microphone. Input these into a speech analysis program, and print out a wideband spectrogram of each token. Comment on the difference between the oral and nasal segments, paying particular attention to formant structure and intensity.

CD

Listen to the examples of different consonants, and try to imitate as many as possible. Following the instructions on the CD, see if you can identify the test examples. Answers to all the exercises are provided at the end of the book.

8

More on Consonants

INTRODUCTION

In the previous two chapters we have looked at the manners and places of articulation of consonants. There are some aspects of consonant articulation also important for the speech clinician that we have not yet examined, and these are the focus of this chapter. First, we are going to look in more detail at oral stops. There are several ways in which aspects of stop articulation can be modified, and we will investigate each of these. Second, we will look at multiple articulations: double articulations (where both of the articulations are of the same manner) and secondary articulations (where one is weaker than the other). We will also see how these secondary articulations can play a part in the production of distinctive voice qualities.

MODIFICATIONS TO ORAL STOPS

We can consider a stop as having three main stages (as we saw in chap. 6): the *approach* or *closing* phase, when the two articulators are being brought together; the *closure* phase, when they are held together; and the *release* or *opening* phase, when they move apart again. Let us consider the production of [d]. In the approach phase the tongue tip and blade are raised up toward the alveolar ridge until they make a firm contact. During the closure phase the tongue tip is held firmly at the alveolar ridge, and the side rims of the tongue keep an air-tight seal against the inner surface of the upper side teeth. At the onset of the release phase, the tongue tip and blade are pulled sharply down (incidentally also breaking the seal at the tongue rims), and the air that had been compressed behind the closure rushes out. Figure 8.1 shows these stages in diagrammatic form.

Stops—just to be called stops—must, of course, have the middle, closure phase. However, it is possible to modify both phase 1 and phase 3, and in the following sections we will see how this can be done.

Nasal Release of Stops

In the production of an oral, as opposed to a nasal, stop the velum is raised throughout, blocking off the nasal cavity. However, if, instead of moving the articulators apart after the

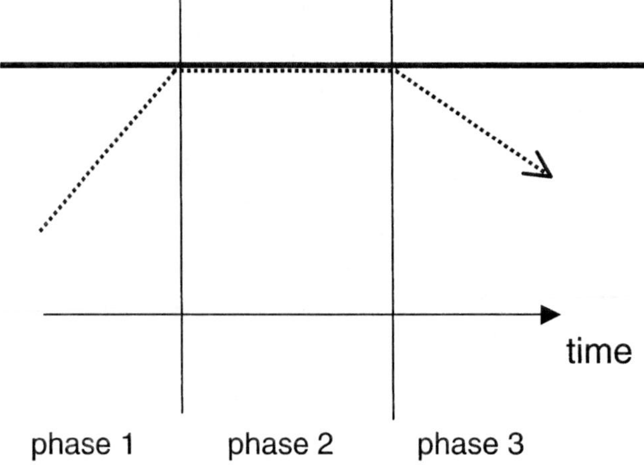

FIG 8.1. Three stages of stop production.

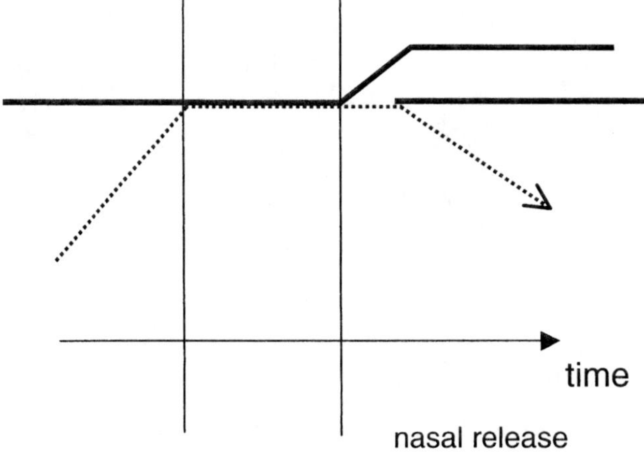

FIG 8.2. Nasal release of stops.

closure phase, the speaker lowers the velum while keeping the articulators in place, then the compressed air will rush out through the nasal cavity (called *nasal plosion*). Only at that point are the articulators moved to make the following sound. This transference of the release phase of the articulators to velic action is called the *nasal release of stops*.

We have to ensure we can tell the difference between a nasal stop and a nasally released (oral) stop. Remember, a nasal stop has the velum lowered all through the production of the sound, but a nasally released stop just has a lowered velum for the release phase.

> In IPA we can symbolize nasal release of a stop by adding a nasal diacritic after the stop concerned, e.g., [t^n], [b^n]. However, because the nasal release normally sounds like a nasal stop homorganic to the oral one (i.e., produced at the same place of articulation), the tendency is simply to write an oral stop followed by a nasal stop: [tn], [bm].

Figure 8.2 shows nasal release diagrammatically.

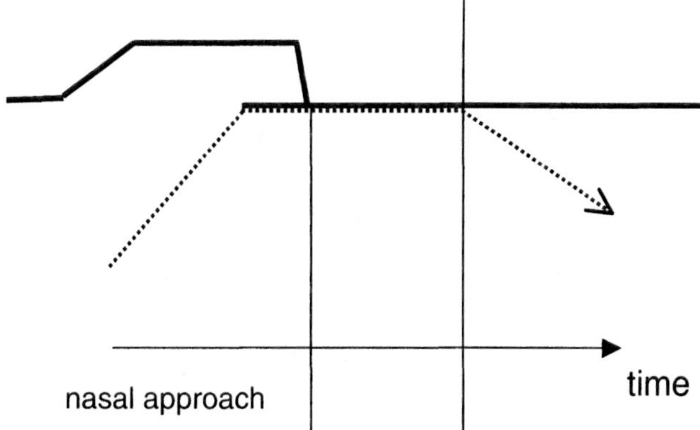

FIG 8.3. Nasal approach to stops.

Most varieties of English have some nasally released stops. If we compare pronunciations of "ribbon" and "ridden" we should note that in the first example the medial [b] is usually released orally, and there is a short schwa vowel between the plosive and the final nasal. On the other hand, the second example normally involves nasal release of the medial [d], with no kind of vowel following it. In IPA, then, "ribbon" is [ɹɪbən], and "ridden" is [ɹɪdn]. (We do have to recognize, though, that in some varieties "ribbon" may well have nasal release as [ɹɪbm]; and in others "ridden" may not have nasal release, as [ɹɪdən].) In examples such as these, the nasal release constitutes the second syllable of the word and it is the nasal part that carries the syllable nucleus (normally this is the task of a vowel). The IPA provides a diacritic to show that the nasal is a *syllabic nasal*: [ɹɪdn̩].

Nasal Approach to Stops

Instead of converting phase 3 of a stop to velic action, we can convert phase 1. In this situation, the articulators come together to form a complete closure in the oral cavity, while the velum is simultaneously lowered. So we have a normal nasal stop at the beginning of this sequence of events. However, instead of the articulators moving off to take up a new position, they are maintained in place, but the velum is lifted so that now the nasal cavity is blocked off. What we have at this point is the closure phase of an oral stop; air pressure builds up and then is let out with plosion at the third phase when the articulators are moved apart. This sequence of events is pictured in Fig. 8.3.

Nasally approached stops sound like a combination of a nasal stop and an oral stop, and are transcribed so in IPA. In English there are many examples such as "hand," "lamp," "thank" ([hænd], [læmp], [θæŋk]). That such combinations are not simply a sequence of two independent sounds is shown by the extreme rarity of nasal–plosive clusters where the nasal and plosive are at different places of articulation. The fact that they are normally homorganic shows how the first phase of the plosive is actually the nasal sound itself.

In just a few words in English we can find a plosive where both the approach phase and the release phase have been transferred to velic action. In a word such as "stampmachine" ([stæmpməʃin]), the velum is lowered while the bilabial articulation is formed, with a resultant [m] sound; then the velum is raised while the articulators remain in place. This causes a period of voiceless silence (heard by us as the [p] part of the combination); then the velum is lowered again so that the compressed air passes through the nasal cavity, which causes us to hear the second [m].

Lateral Release of Stops

Another way of modifying the release phase of an oral plosive is through *lateral release*. In these cases, as the articulators move apart, the compressed air is directed over the side rim of the tongue rather than centrally across the surface of the tongue.

> In IPA this can be shown by a diacritic: [tˡ], [dˡ]. However, because the lateral release normally sounds like a plosive followed by a lateral approximant, we usually transcribe these with two symbols: [tl], [dl].

Laterally released plosives occur in many varieties of English. For example, "middle" [mɪdl] consists of a laterally released [d]; there is no vowel between the [d] part and the [l] part. On the other hand, most speakers' pronunciation of "rubble" [ɹʌbəl] does have a short schwa vowel between the plosive and the lateral, and so is not an example of lateral release. (Of course, there are varieties of English that don't use lateral release, and others where a word such as "rubble" would have lateral release.) In examples such as these, the lateral release constitutes the second syllable of the word and it is the lateral part that carries the syllable nucleus (as we noted earlier, normally this is the task of a vowel). The IPA syllabic diacritic can be used to show that the lateral is a *syllabic lateral*: [mɪdl̩].

Incomplete and Unexploded Stops

The release phase of stops can also be modified by suppressing it altogether. Unreleased stops come about in one of two ways. Incomplete stops are so called because the release phase is not heard. This is because, while the articulators move apart, the compressed air is still stopped because a different articulatory closure has already been put in place elsewhere in the oral cavity. To illustrate this more clearly, let us compare the pronunciation of the English word "apt" with its French cognate "apte." English speakers will bring the two lips together to form the closure for the [p], and hold this for a brief period allowing air pressure to build up. During this closure period, the tongue tip and blade are brought into contact with the alveolar ridge so that, when the lips part at the end of [p], the compressed air cannot flow out because the closure for [t] is already in place. This is shown in the top part of Figure 8.4. French speakers, on the other hand, will move the bilabial closure apart just before they put in place the closure for the [t]. This means we can hear a short period of plosion for [p]. This sequence of events is shown in the lower part of Fig. 8.4. The English [t] is incomplete, therefore; the French [t] is not.

The second way to suppress phase 3 of a stop is not to release the plosion at all. Unreleased stops generally seem to occur utterance-finally and are quite common in many varieties of English. Instead of the articulators parting, the compressed air is released slowly and inaudibly through the nasal cavity, and possibly through the oral cavity after the eventual opening of the closure.

> Both the incomplete stops and the unexploded ones use the same IPA diacritic: "apt" [æp˺t], "map" [mæp˺]. Because these unreleased aspects in English are not used to contrast one sound from another, we usually omit the diacritics when we are undertaking phonemic transcription (see chap. 10).

(a)

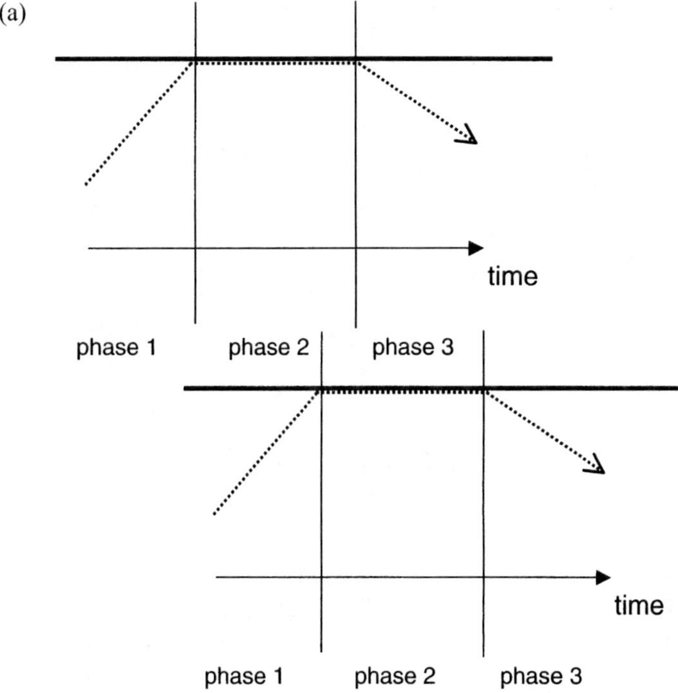

(b)

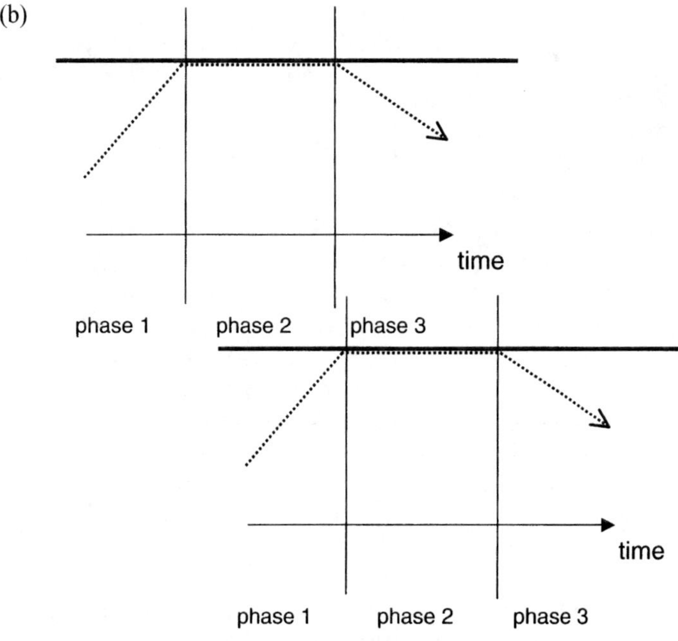

FIG 8.4. (a) Overlapping and (b) nonoverlapping stop sequences.

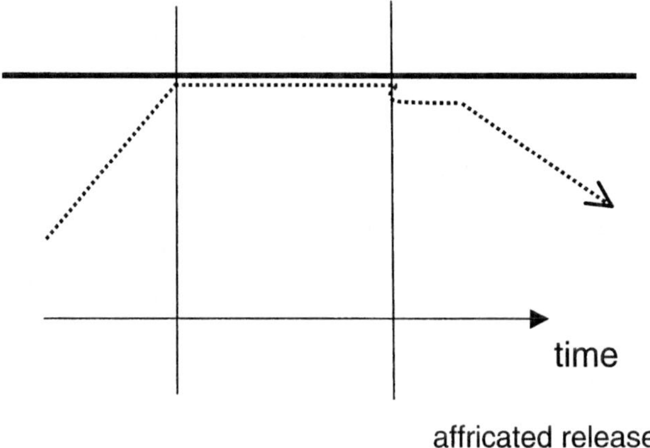

FIG 8.5 Affrication of stops.

Affrication of Stops

In chapter 6 we looked at the affricate manner of articulation and saw that, in effect, this involves a modification to the release phase of an oral stop. It does appear that it is possible to produce a slight amount of affrication on stop release that is normally not deemed sufficient to make the resultant sound a full affricate. For example, in Liverpool English, it is very common to produce voiceless plosives with a slight amount of affrication (turbulent airflow of a fricative nature) on release. This doesn't last long enough to make us consider the sounds affricates, so we call them *affricated stops*. Figure 8.5 shows how the release phase is modified to force the air through a narrow channel and thus produce the turbulence.

> In IPA these affricated stops are shown by adding a small superscript version of the fricative symbol after the plosive. Let's consider some examples from Liverpool, England: "cake" and "tea" may be pronounced [k^{x}eɪk^{x}] and [t^{s}i].

MULTIPLE ARTICULATIONS

As we saw in chapter 7, the main active articulators are the lower lip and various parts of the tongue. The tongue itself is extremely flexible and the tip and blade are able to move independently of the back of the tongue. This, coupled to the fact that the lips are of course separate from the tongue altogether, means it is feasible to produce articulations at two different places at the same time. We will see that such multiple articulations are usually divided into two categories: *double articulations* and *secondary articulations.*

Double Articulations

With double articulations the two strictures (i.e., coming together of articulators) will be in different places, but must be of the same manner. In other words, we can have plosive stops made at the bilabial and velar places of articulation, we can have fricatives made at the postalveolar and velar places of articulation, and we can have approximants made at the bilabial and palatal places of articulation. In each instance we have two of the same manner of articulation: two stops, two fricatives, two approximants. Remember: in these sounds the two articulations occur simultaneously.

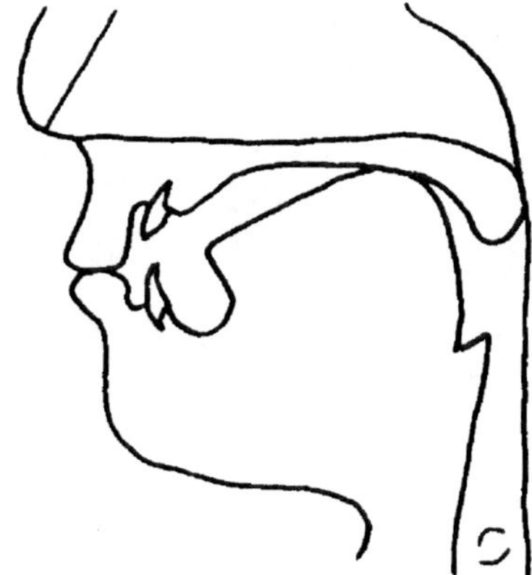

FIG 8.6 Double articulation (labio-velar).

Such double articulations are quite common in natural language. In fact all the examples we quoted in the previous paragraph occur quite frequently. A labio-velar plosive is shown in Fig. 8.6. In English, the semivowel approximant [w] is a double articulation: There is an approximation of the two lips at the same time as there is an approximation of the back of the tongue dorsum to the soft palate.

> The IPA provides some single symbols for commonly occurring double articulations; otherwise two symbols with a tie-bar are used:
>
> double plosives: [k͡p], [g͡b]—[ák͡pá], [g͡be] (Efik, Yoruba) *river, to carry* [labio-velar]
> [p͡ta]—(Bura) *hare* [labio-alveolar]
> double fricatives: [ɧ]—[ɧal] (Swedish) *scarf* [postalveolar-velar]
> [β͡z]—[β͡zose] (Shona) *all* [labio-alveolar)
> double semivowel: [w], [ɥ]—[wi], [ɥi̯t] (French) *yes, eight* [labio-velar; labio-palatal]

Secondary Articulations

A double articulation consists of two simultaneous articulations at different places, where both are of the same manner. When we have a primary and a secondary articulation, on the other hand, the primary articulation is higher on the scale of articulatory strength than the simultaneous secondary one. For example, a bilabial nasal stop [m] can have as a secondary articulation an approximation of the front of the tongue body to the hard palate; an alveolar plosive stop [t] can have an approximation of the back of the tongue body toward the soft palate; and a velar fricative [x] can have a secondary articulation consisting of an approximation of the two lips.

Secondary articulations occur very commonly in speech. For example, in English, when we produce bilabial sounds ([m, p, b]), our tongues get into position early for the following sound; conversely, when we produce consonants with the tongue, our lip shape may be already rounded or spread for a following rounded or spread vowel. When these features are more or less automatic in speech, we rarely need to comment on them. However, in some instances and in some languages, secondary articulations are not simply an automatic reflection of the context of the sound, and they may be used to contrast otherwise identical sounds linguistically.

In such cases we need to note that a secondary articulation is taking place. On these occasions we may need to mark the secondary articulation in any phonetic transcription.

There are four main types of secondary articulations that are used in languages to contrast consonants that are otherwise the same. These secondary articulations are all of an approximant nature, and so can be used with all consonants higher than approximant on the consonant strength hierarchy (for these purposes, lateral approximants count higher than other approximants). The four types are:

- labialization: the addition of bilabial approximation to a primary stricture;
- palatalization: the addition of approximation of the front of the tongue body to the hard palate;
- velarization: the addition of approximation of the back of the tongue body to the soft palate;
- pharyngealization: the addition of approximation of the back of the tongue body and tongue root into the pharynx.

The IPA provides symbols to transcribe secondary articulations:

labialization:	the addition of superscript-w: [gʷ], [sʷ], etc. Consonants that have primary labial articulations are rarely also labialized.
palatalization:	the addition of superscript-j: [dʲ], [fʲ], etc. Consonants that have primary palatal articulations cannot also be palatalized.
velarization:	the addition of superscript–ɣ : [lˠ], [mˠ], etc. Consonants that have primary velar articulations cannot also be velarized.
pharyngealization:	the addition of superscript-ʕ: [tˤ], [ʃˤ], etc. Consonants that have primary pharyngeal articulations cannot also be pharyngealized.

Because velarization and pharyngealization rarely contrast, and are often variants within a language, a common diacritic for both these is the use of the medial tilde ~ : [ɫ].

Labialization is one of the most common secondary articulations, and it is very often found as a context-driven variant. For example, in English the [s] in "soon" differs from the [s] in "seen" in that it has secondary labialization triggered by the following back rounded vowel. Some languages, however, use labialization with a contrastive function that is not context-dependent. So, in the West African language of Twi, we find the words [àkʷá] meaning *a round about way*, and [àká] *(somebody) has bitten*. Labialization is very often found with velar consonants: the Latin letter *Q* reflects a labialized velar stop. It can be found with other places of articulation, even bilabial, because bilabial articulations need not also involve the lip-rounding of labialization.

Palatalization occurs, for example, in Irish. In that language many consonants have a palatalized and a nonpalatalized form. However, these distinctions are not automatic variations caused simply by the context of the consonant. They have a contrastive function, such that the choice of a palatalized sound over a nonpalatalized one will result in a different word or grammatical form (and therefore a different meaning is conveyed). For example, the Irish words "bó" [bo] and "beo" [bʲo] mean *cow* and *alive*, respectively: This meaning difference is carried solely by the choice or otherwise of the palatalized or nonpalatalized initial consonant. Figure 8.7 shows a palatalized and a non-palatalized [t].

Velarization with contrastive function is found in Marshallese (the language of the Marshall Islands in the South Pacific). Here we find pairs of sounds that differ only in the raising of the back of the tongue towards the velum, and this contrast is found with nasals, liquids, and

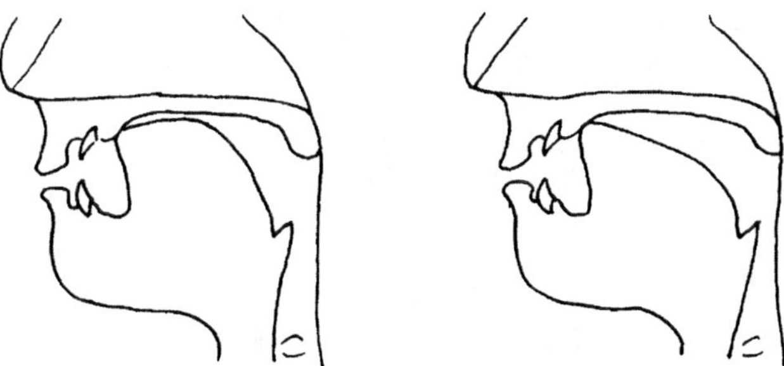

FIG 8.7 Palatalized and non-palatalized [t].

bilabial stops. For example, the words [le] *Ms, Madam* and [lˠe] *Mr., Sir* differ only in the use of velarization.

Arabic is well-known for its contrastive use of pharyngealization. Sounds at many places of articulation exist in so-called emphatic and nonemphatic versions (i.e., pharyngealized and nonpharyngealized), and different letters of the Arabic alphabet are used to write them. For example, the letter س is used to denote [s], whereas the letter ص is the symbol for [sˤ]. The Arabic words [sad] *to prevail* and [sˤad] "letter name" illustrate the contrastive function of this distinction in Arabic.

In English we don't use secondary articulations with a contrastive function. However, there is one instance where the use of a secondary articulation creates a major variant of a consonant, a variant, moreover, that is not simply predictable from context. Although we will look at this in more detail in part II, we can briefly summarize the case here. In many varieties of English there are two major variants of the "l" sound. One of these (called *clear-l*) occurs before vowels and has no important secondary articulation apart from, perhaps, a slight amount of palatalization, especially before high front vowels. The second variant (*dark-l*) occurs after vowels. This variant has a marked degree of velarization, and if you compare your pronunciation of the words "leaf" and "feel" you should be able to hear that difference. (Some English accents have clear-l in both places, and some dark-l in both, however.) This variation is not contrastive in English: the contexts in which we find the two l-varieties are mutually exclusive; therefore no words can ever be contrasted solely by the choice of a clear- or dark-l. Nevertheless, it is not simply an automatic reflex of phonetic context either (as seen by the fact that some accents do not have this usage). We need to remember the distinction because, in disordered speech, there may be different patterns of usage between the clear- and the dark-l. Figures 15.7 and 15.8 show the difference between a clear and dark articulation of [l].

Secondary Articulation and Voice Quality

We saw in chapter 4 how voice quality was affected partly by phonatory activity and partly by supralaryngeal settings. If a speaker adopts any of the four secondary articulations as long-term articulatory settings, then a labialized, palatalized, velarized, or pharyngealized voice quality results. Such a voice quality may be a normal part of the language variety in question (for example, English accents in south Wales are often said to be palatalized), or they may be a personal trait, or even an aspect of a voice quality problem needing intervention.

When we say that someone is using a palatalized voice quality (for example), this means that the speaker is raising the front of the tongue body toward the hard palate during those periods in his or her speech when it is possible to do so. So, when palatal [j] or the high front vowels are being articulated, the tongue is already in that position, and when velar and back vowels are being said, it will be difficult to produce palatalization.

VoQS symbols for the main supralaryngeal voice qualities

$V^{œ}$	labialization (open rounded)	V^{w}	labialization (close rounded)
V^{j}	palatalization	$V^{ɣ}$	velarization
$V^{ʕ}$	pharyngealization	V̶	velarization/pharyngealization

Voice quality settings from various other places of articulation also occur occasionally. The VoQS symbol system (see appendix 1), introduced in chapter 4, provides symbols for a wide range of supralaryngeal settings, from labialization in the front of the mouth, right back to contractions of the faucal pillars at the rear wall of the pharynx.

ACOUSTIC CHARACTERISTICS

In this section we will look at two spectrograms that illustrate some of the features we have discussed in this chapter. We'll return to these features, with specific reference to English, in greater detail in part II of this book. Figure 8.8 is a wideband spectrogram of the word "bidden" spoken in two different ways: to the left is the pronunciation with a schwa vowel between the medial [d] and the final [n]; to the right is the pronunciation with a lateral release of the medial [d] (i.e., [bɪdən] and [bɪdn̩].) The spectrogram shows the short vowel segment in the left-hand version with clearly observable formant structure, followed in turn by the nasal with its less intense characteristics and nasal antiformant; the vowel segment is missing in the right-hand utterance, where the closure of the stop is followed directly by the nasal with its fainter formant markings.

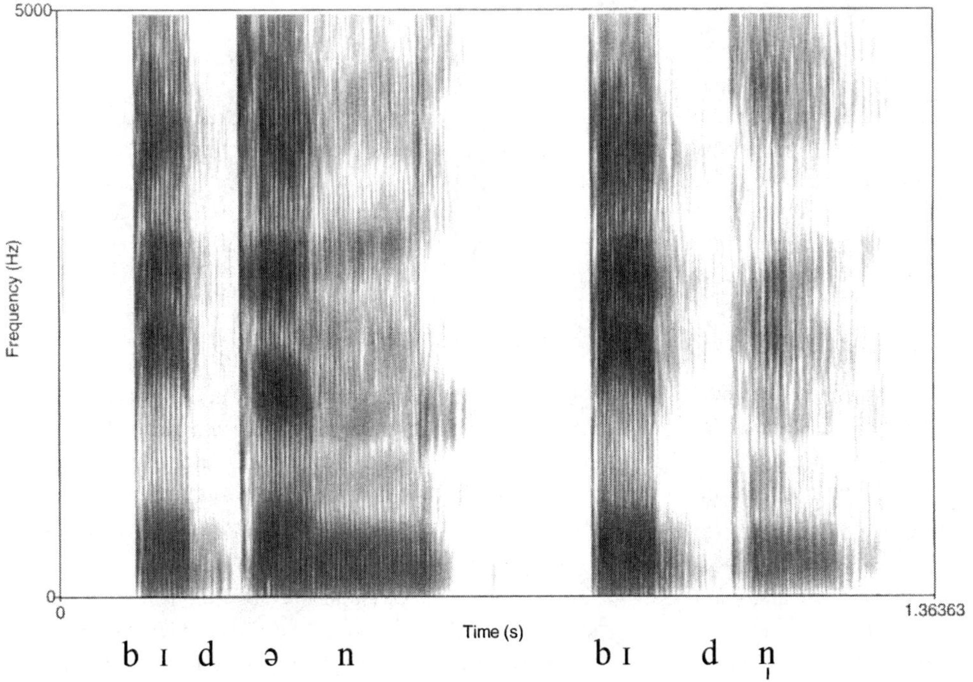

FIG 8.8 Wideband spectrogram of [bɪdən] and [bɪdn̩].

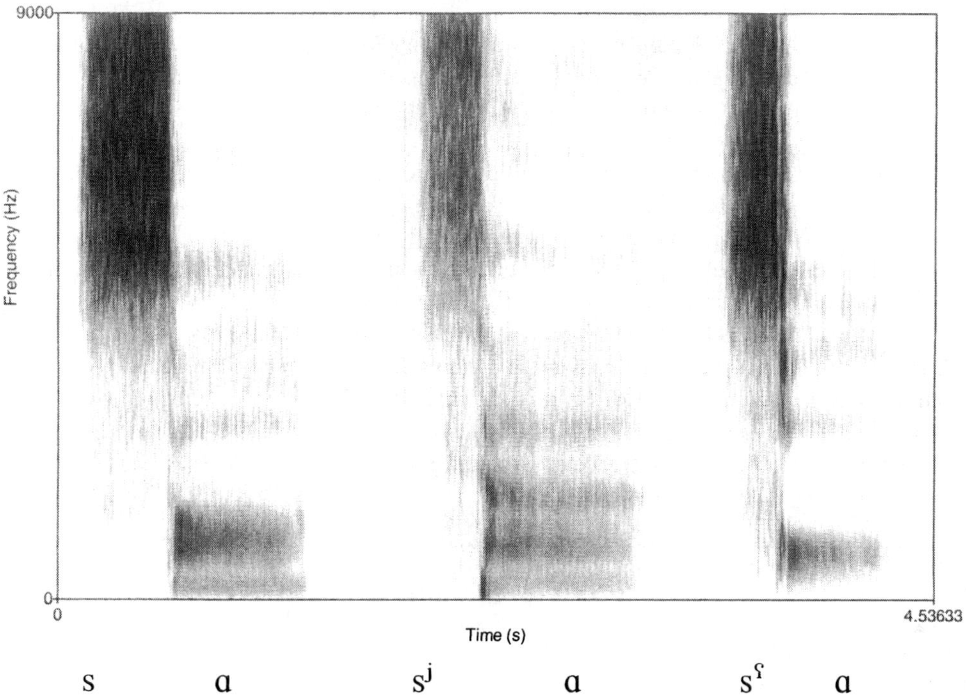

FIG 8.9 Wideband spectrogram of [sɑ], [sʲɑ], and [sˤɑ].

The second spectrogram, shown in Fig. 8.9, demonstrates the acoustic difference between palatalization and pharyngealization. The three syllables shown in the figure are [sɑ], [sʲɑ], and [sˤɑ], that is, a plain, a palatalized, and a pharyngealized version of [s], followed by the vowel [ɑ]. In articulatory terms, the palatalized [s] has the front of the tongue raised toward the hard palate, whereas the pharyngealized [s] has the tongue root drawn back into the pharynx, and all three versions have a main closure between the tongue tip and blade and the alveolar ridge. Figure 8.9 clearly shows the effect of the secondary articulations. Although there is an effect on the fricative component itself (for example, the lower boundary of the frication in the palatalized version is at a higher frequency than the neutral version, whereas it is at a lower frequency for the pharyngealized one), coarticulation effects can also be seen on the following vowels. This can be seen clearly in the lower F1 and F2 in the vowel following the pharyngealized version.

THE IPA CHART

Over the past few chapters we have examined most of the vowels and consonants that are needed to transcribe normal and disordered speech. The IPA arranges all its symbols onto a chart, which is reproduced in appendix 1. This chart is divided into several sections. The grid at the top of the chart illustrates most of the consonants that we have described, and anyone training to be a speech-language pathologist should learn these symbols and know their three-term labels. This grid has place of articulation along the top, and manner of articulation down the side. In each cell the left-hand symbol represents the voiceless sound, and the right-hand its voiced counterpart. For sonorants, no voiceless symbols are provided, because they are so rare, and the voiced symbol is placed to the right of the cell. If we ever do need to transcribe voiceless sonorants, we use the voiced symbol with the addition of the voicelessness diacritic (see chap. 4). Blank cells or parts of cells represent sounds that are possible to produce but for which the IPA has no symbols (because they are rarely if ever encountered in natural language). Shaded cells or parts of cells represent place, manner, and phonation combinations that are considered impossible to produce.

Below to the left is a smaller grid used to display the symbols for clicks, implosives, and ejectives (which we covered in chap. 3). To the right of this grid is the vowel chart that we examined in some detail in chapter 5. Below these at the left is a list of some of the double articulations and rare consonant types, some of which we dealt with in this chapter. In the middle of the chart to the right are lists of special symbols used to mark suprasegmental aspects of speech; we deal with these in chapter 9. At the base of the chart to the left and center is a large grid of diacritics, the little marks that can be added to symbols. Many of these we have already encountered, for example, vowel position diacritics in chapter 5, phonation diacritics in chapter 4, and secondary articulation diacritics in this chapter. These diacritics should also gradually be learned: the extra precision they lend a transcription is often needed when we transcribe severely disordered speech in the clinic.

> IPA place of articulation diacritics:
>
> t̼ linguolabial articulation (tongue-tip to upper lip)
> t̪ dental articulation
> t̺ apical (tongue tip) articulation
> t̻ laminal (tongue blade) articulation
> e̘ advanced tongue root
> e̙ retracted tongue root

BACKGROUND READING

Standard phonetics texts deal with stop articulations and with double and secondary articulations. Laver (1980, 1994) deals in detail with aspects of voice quality. The VoQS symbols are described in Ball et al. (1999). The IPA chart is described in the *Handbook of the IPA* (1999). The examples from various languages were from the same sources listed for chapter 7.

EXERCISES

Review Questions

1. We distinguished between secondary and double articulations. Explain the difference, and give examples for each.
2. How can the approach and closure phases of stops be modified? Give examples.
3. Give examples of the different types of contrastive secondary articulations. What do they all have in common?
4. How do secondary articulation relate to voice quality?
5. Briefly describe the acoustic differences between palatalization, pharyngealization, and a neutral articulatory setting.
6. What is the difference between a *nasal stop* and a *nasally released stop*? Use diagrams to explain the differences in timing of articulatory gestures.
7. What is the difference between an *affricate* and an *affricated stop*?
8. What three basic principles govern the arrangement of the IPA consonant chart?

Study Topics and Experiments

1. Using library and Internet resources, find as many languages that you can that have double articulated plosives. List the languages, where they are spoken, and what language families they belong to. For each language, list the double articulated stops used and, if possible, a sample word plus meaning for each example. Note what the sources say about the precise timing of the two closures.
2. Draw up a list of five words with potential nasal release of stops in English, and five with potential lateral release. Record yourself and at least three other of your colleagues saying these words. Use a good quality tape recorder with an external microphone. Input the tokens into the speech analysis package of a PC. Put wideband spectrograms of the tokens on the screen one by one, and note when a nasal/lateral release is used and when it is a vowel plus nasal/lateral. Print out some of the spectrograms of the different types as examples.

CD

Listen to the examples of different consonants, and try to imitate as many as possible. Identify the test examples, following the instructions on the CD. Answers to all the exercises are given at the end of the book.

9

Suprasegmental Phonetics

INTRODUCTION

In the past few chapters we have been concerned with the segments of speech: that is, the individual vowels and consonants. It is worth noting here that, from a phonetic viewpoint, the idea of individual segments is a convenient fiction. In fact, there are usually no clear-cut boundaries between all the phonetic features of one segment and those of a neighboring segment. However, we *interpret* speech as if it were divided into segments, so we retain this approach out of convenience. We must remember, however, that speech also has aspects that cannot be assigned to individual vowels or consonants, and many of these aspects are very important in conveying meaning. We call the phonetic characteristics of the individual vowels and consonants *segmental*, and phonetic characteristics that stretch over units larger than individual vowels and consonants *suprasegmental*. These suprasegmental aspects of speech are just as likely as the segmental ones to be impaired, so speech clinicians need a detailed knowledge of this area.

> The term *prosody* is often used as a cover term for the suprasegmental aspects of speech. In speech pathology we use the term *dysprosody* when one or more of the prosodic aspects of speech are disrupted.

In this chapter we will examine some of the more important suprasegmental aspects of speech, illustrating them with examples from English and other languages. Probably the three most important of these are stress, length, and pitch, but we will also look at tempo and loudness, and briefly revisit voice quality. As these features stretch over more than one segment, we need to note what their *domain* is, that is to say, what stretch of speech they operate on. As we will see, some have the syllable as their domain; others operate over longer stretches still.

STRESS

We use the term *stress* to describe the fact that certain syllables in speech (of any language) will appear to the listener more prominent (or "stressed") than others. The domain of stress, therefore, is the syllable. We know how this prominence is achieved phonetically. The basic mechanism is to make the stressed syllable louder by increasing the airflow through the vocal tract. This is done by increasing the activity of the muscles of the ribcage. Added to this may be greater muscular activity in the larynx and the articulators, which will be manifested as pitch changes and tenser and longer vowel articulations respectively.

Different languages use stress in different ways. Some languages have predictable stressed syllables: for example, Czech nearly always has stress on the first syllables of words, whereas Polish has stress on the penultimate syllable. (Some small grammatical words will normally not receive stress at all in many languages.) On the other hand, many languages have variable word stress. This means that, although the stress placement is fixed for each individual word, there is usually no way to predict the stressed syllable without hearing the word pronounced by a native speaker. English, German, and Greek are languages with variable stress. Finally, some authorities recognize a third grouping: fixed phrase stress. French, for example, has final syllable stress but, in connected speech, most syllables, except the last one in a phrase, appear to have equal prominence; it is the final syllable in the phrase that appears to carry the stress. Nevertheless, when words are pronounced singly, one can hear the final syllable stress on the word.

Phoneticians recognize various degrees of stress, though for most purposes a simple distinction between stressed and unstressed is sufficient.

Although different dictionaries employ a wide range of devices to mark stress, the IPA only uses marks placed *before* the stressed syllable.

Primary stress: [ˈɪmpɔɹt] "import" (noun); [ɪmˈpɔɹt] "import" (verb)
Secondary stress: [ˌɛksplɔɪˈteɪʃn] "exploitation"

Unstressed syllables remain unmarked.

Speech rhythm in a language derives largely from how stressed and unstressed syllables pattern. In this regard, there appear to be two broad categories: *syllable-timed* languages, and *stress-timed* languages. In syllable-timed languages (for example, Italian and Spanish), there tend to be an equal number of syllables between each two stressed syllables. This produces a comparatively even speech rhythm.

In a stress-timed language, on the other hand, stressed syllables tend to occur with fairly regular time-intervals between them; they are said to be *isochronous*. (This term means "identical in time," though actually the timing units only tend toward this.) English is a stress-timed language and we can see that there can be a variable number of syllables between each two stressed syllables, but a roughly equal amount of time (this, of course, implies that some syllables will take longer to say than others). The units that stretch from one stressed syllable to just before the next stressed syllable (which may consist of one, two, or more syllables) are termed *feet*. As an example, we can look at the following phrase, where there are both one and two syllables between stressed syllables, and where the single-syllable feet will take longer to say than each syllable in the double-syllable feet (stressed syllables are shown in italics; the upright line shows the division between feet):

"*Pat* has | *got* a | *bright* | *red* | *coat*"

Stress-timed languages tend to have a less even rhythm than syllable-timed ones, and often the strong rhythmic alternation between stressed and unstressed syllables in these languages results in a weakening of the unstressed syllables. This is a notable feature of English, where unstressed syllables may undergo simplification of consonants and reduction of vowel qualities toward lax vowels such as schwa. Compare, for example, the emphatic pronunciation of "and" with its normal reduced form in the following phrases:

"I want cookies *and* coffee" versus "I want cookies and coffee"
['ænd] [əŋ]

LENGTH

The duration of segments is also considered to be one of the prosodic aspects of speech. At first sight, this may seem odd, because we talk about long and short vowels and long and short consonants. However, length really operates over the domain of the syllable because, when we have a long vowel (for example), the rest of the syllable (any surrounding consonants) tends to be shorter, and when we have a short vowel, the surrounding consonants tend to be longer. This is only a tendency; we don't mean to say that all syllables have the same length (as we saw in the previous section for stress-timed languages, this is not the case). Nevertheless, because of this adjustment to the length of syllables between the vowel and consonant durations, we consider length to be suprasegmental. Further, the fact we noted earlier about syllable length in stress-timed languages being controlled to some extent by the patterns of feet is also indicative of the suprasegmental characteristic of length.

> The IPA marks long vowels with a special diacritic that looks somewhat like a colon [oː].
> Half-long if needed is shown with just the upper dot of this diacritic [oˑ].
> Short is denoted by a "breve" mark, placed above the vowel symbol [ŏ].
> Long consonants can also have the length diacritic added, but it is common practice to show these by simply doubling the consonant symbol [-nn-]. Doubling is also occasionally used with vowels instead of the diacritic.

In some languages (such as English), vowel length (or quantity) is a noncontrastive aspect of the sound system. So, although the vowel [i] (as in "see") is longer than the vowel [ɪ] (in "sit"), this difference in length is subsidiary to the difference in tongue position (or vowel quality). However, in other languages, vowel quantity may be the only (or main) difference between vowels. Languages as different as Korean, Finnish, Arabic, and Japanese all distinguish pairs of vowels by their length (although this may be restricted to certain varieties of these languages). We can take the following examples:

Korean: [il] "day"—[iːl] "work"
Finnish: [tuleː] "comes"—[tuːleː] "blows"
Arabic: [qaːla] "he said"—[qaːlaː] "they (masc. dual) said"
Japanese: [kiro] "wear (imperative)"—[kiroː] "cut (tentative)"

Although it is unusual for languages to contrast more than two degrees of length, Estonian uses three degrees of consonant length and of vowel length, short, half-long, and long, although some of these are restricted to certain word types. The Mexican language Mixe does clearly contrast three degrees of length (Laver, 1994):

Mixe: [poʃ] "guava"—[poˑʃ] "spider"— [poːʃ] "knot"

As we noted earlier, some languages may also contrast short and long consonants, often called single and double (or geminate) consonants. Italian regularly does this, and shows it clearly in its orthography by doubling the consonant letters that represent the long consonant.

In the IPA transcriptions we'll also use the double symbol convention to show the geminate consonants.

Italian: [nonɔ] "ninth"—[nonnɔ] "grandfather"

English does not have many words with double consonants; but there are a few examples where they have come about due to compounding, or the addition of a prefix or a suffix. So, for example, the words "bookcase," "guileless," and "unknown" all have double consonants at their syllable boundaries (although the spellings wouldn't suggest this): [bʊkkeɪs], [gaɪlləs], [ʌnnoʊn].

PITCH

The pitch of the voice is adjusted through the tension of the vocal folds. If their tension is increased (through movements of the arytenoid cartilages), the vocal folds will vibrate more quickly. We perceive an increased rate of vibration as a rise in the pitch of the voice; conversely, our perception of lower pitch derives from a slowing in vocal fold vibration. (It is worth remembering that terms such as *high pitch* and *low pitch* are only metaphors we use to refer to our perception of different vocal fold vibration rates: There is nothing inherently "high" or "low" about these pitch differences.)

Linguistically, languages can use pitch in two different ways: through *tone* and through *intonation*. We will examine these two features in turn.

Tone

The domain of tone is the syllable (or, to be more precise, all the voiced segments of the syllable: Pitch changes cannot be marked by voiceless segments, because they have no vocal fold vibrations). Tone is a contrastive use of syllable pitch used to distinguish one word from another. In other words, languages that use tone may have sets of words that have the same strings of consonants and vowels but different pitch patterns. In English, if we alter the pitch pattern of any word the meaning stays the same (though we may sound more or less certain or emphatic). In tone languages, on the other hand, altering the tone of the syllable typically alters the word itself. We can exemplify this from Mandarin Chinese, one of a large number of tone languages in the Far East:

high level	meaning "mother"	[mā]	妈
high rising	meaning "hemp"	[má]	麻
low dipping	meaning "horse"	[mǎ]	马
high falling	meaning "scold"	[mà]	骂

The IPA provides two different systems to mark tones: diacritics above the vowel nucleus of the syllable, and tone letters placed after the syllable. We can illustrate both systems with data from Thai:

[k^hâ:]	[k^ha:˧˨] 32	"to dangle"
[k^hȁ:]	[k^ha:˨˩] 21	"spice"
[k^hā:]	[h^ha:˥˩] 51	"price"
[k^hắ:]	[k^ha:˦˥] 45	"to trade"
[k^hã:]	[k^ha:˨˩˥] 215	"leg"

A variety of other systems are also often found, such as numerical marking of tone levels (1 lowest pitch level, 5 highest; so 32 means fall from level 3 to level 2).

Tone languages include Thai, Chinese, Burmese, Tibetan, and Vietnamese. These languages are sometimes termed *contour tone* languages, because most of the contrastive pitch types involve a movement from high to low, mid to high, etc. Tone languages are also widespread in Africa, and most of these are *register tone* languages, where the pitches tend to be level: high level, mid-level, low level, and so forth. Zulu in South Africa distinguishes just high and low tones, whereas Yoruba in West Africa uses high, mid, and low. Some Native American languages are register tone languages and others are contour tone or mixed languages. We can illustrate register tone with the following example from Igbo (a language spoken in southeastern Nigeria), where the tone change shows the relationship between the two nouns:

[àg͡bà] "jaw" [èŋwè] "monkey"
[àg͡bá èŋwè] "the jaw of the monkey"

> Diacritics and tone letters can also be used with register tones.
> The following Igbo example has low tone—high tone—low tone—low tone:
>
> [àg͡bá èŋwè] [a˩g͡ba˥ e˩ŋwe˩]

Intonation

Intonation is the linguistic use of pitch over groups of syllables, and signals syntactic and semantic information. Although intonation, like tone, also exploits pitch changes, its domain is the intonation phrase. The intonation phrase varies in length, depending upon what the speaker decides to say, and the way in which he or she wishes to say it. For example, a specific intonation pattern will be placed on a simple utterance such as "yes," or on a much longer utterance, such as "what time are you going out today?" We will examine the intonation of English in detail in chapter 17; here, we will look at the basic units of intonation only. Interestingly, whereas only some languages use tone, all languages have intonation systems. This means that in a tone language, the precise pitch movements for a specific tone may be modified depending on the overall intonation pattern of the phrase being spoken.

One of the main purposes of intonation is to highlight new information over given information. Consider the different ways you would say the phrase "Pat's going to town" in the following contexts:

1. Who's going to town? — Pat's going to town.
2. Where's Pat going? — Pat's going to town.

In sentence 1 "town" is given information; therefore we need to highlight "Pat" in the reply. In sentence 2, "Pat" is given, and "town" is new. To highlight the most important piece or pieces of information through intonation, we employ pitch changes on the stressed syllable of the relevant word. So, for example, in the reply to sentence 1, we might well produce quite a large fall of pitch on the syllable "Pat," whereas in the reply to sentence 2 we'd be likely to locate a pitch fall on the syllable "town." Phoneticians term the syllable with this major pitch change the *nucleus* of the intonation pattern (*tune*), or the *tonic* syllable.

All languages will have a set number of different possible *nuclear* patterns, and these are also likely to differ from dialect to dialect. These patterns often involve change in pitch direction (e.g., fall, rise, rise–fall), but level pitches can also be found (for example, a mid-level pitch is often used in English when counting specific items). The heart of an intonation pattern, then, involves partly the location of the nucleus, and partly the choice of the nuclear pattern.

However, as soon as we have an intonation phrase that is longer than one or two syllables, we also have to examine the pitch patterns over the nonnuclear parts. These are normally divided into pre- and postnuclear (or pre- and post-tonic) sections. Although in languages such as English the nuclear syllable tends to be toward the end of the intonation phrase, there are exceptions to this. Prenuclear patterns will extend over all the syllables before the nucleus and, in English, these tend to be either a level high or a level low pitch (although sometimes a stepping up or down from syllable to syllable is used). Postnuclear patterns in English are determined by the nucleus: If the nucleus involves a fall, postnuclear syllables remain low in pitch, but if the nucleus involves a rise, then postnuclear syllables continue to rise.

The various possible combinations of prenuclear, nuclear, and postnuclear patterns constitute a set of intonation tunes for the language or dialect. These tunes, together with the syntax of the utterance (e.g., the use of a declarative, interrogative, or imperative sentence pattern), are responsible for part of the overall meaning of the utterance. Intonation may be responsible for distinguishing major utterance functions (such as question versus statement), precise aspects of meaning, or the attitude of the speaker. Because intonation can be disordered in some clients in the speech-language pathology clinic, we will need to examine English intonation in more detail later in this book.

A wide variety of different methods have been employed to try and capture intonation in transcription. Perhaps the easiest to read is the musical-score approach, where the upper and lower lines represent the top and bottom pitch levels; the large and small dots represent stressed and unstressed syllables, and the tails to the dots show pitch movement during a syllable. The following shows an example of the use of this method.

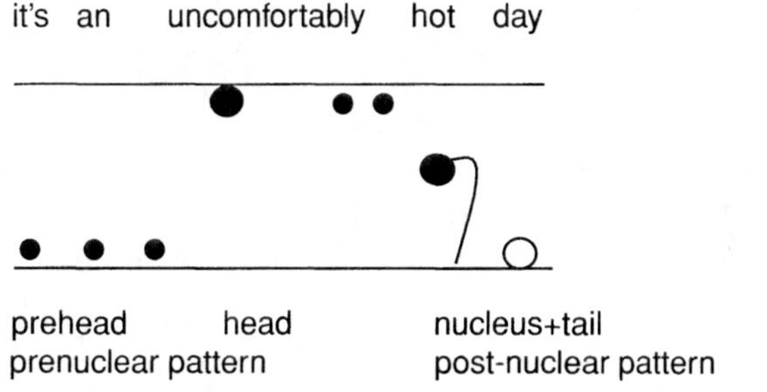

BOUNDARY EFFECTS

Effects related to speech boundaries can be found at various points: between words, between syllables, and between segments.

Word boundary phenomena are concerned with effects holding between the final sounds of a preceding word and the initial sounds of a following word. In rapid speech, changes may occur at word boundaries that would not be evident if the words were pronounced slowly or in isolation. For example, we find *assimilation*, where one sound becomes more like (sometimes even identical to) another. When the sound affected is the first sound of the following word, we talk of progressive assimilation; regressive assimilation affects the final sound of the preceding word. English demonstrates regressive assimilation of place of articulation when the affected sound is an alveolar, and full details of these changes are given in chapter 16.

Other word boundary phenomena include *elision* (the loss of a sound), which in English often occurs in word final consonant clusters where one consonant is elided; *compression* (the loss of unstressed syllables) is also common in some varieties of English. *Liaison* (the adding of a sound at the end of a word) is common in French, for example, to avoid a word ending in a vowel being followed immediately by a word beginning with a vowel.

Assimilation in English:	[tɛn] + [mɛn] → [tɛm mɛn] "ten men"
Elision in English:	[nɛkst] + [wik] → [nɛks wik] "next week"
Compression in English:	[laɪbɹəɹi] → [laɪbɹi] "library"
Liaison in French:	[e] + [il] → [et il] "est il" (is he)

Our main concern with syllable boundaries is where the division occurs between one syllable and the next. Sometimes this is clear. In some languages, syllables within words always start with an onset consonant; therefore, in a word that has the structure CVCV (C = consonant, V = vowel), the syllable boundary must be after the first V, and before the second C. In English, syllable division isn't always so clear, and this has led some phoneticians to posit that medial consonants in English may sometimes be both the end of one syllable and the beginning of the next (this is called *ambisyllabicity*). There are also some occasions where the choice of the syllable boundary can actually change the meaning. Consider these examples from English: "an aim"—"a name," "ice cream"—"I scream," "that's tough"—"that stuff." In the latter two cases, the [t] of "tough" and the [k] of "cream" are slightly different from the [t] of "stuff" and the [k] of "scream" (see chap. 13), but in the first instance we can only make the difference through manipulating very small durational and pausing differences between the two phrases. Examples within words can also be found: "lightening" has three syllables, while "lightning" has only two.

The IPA marks syllable boundaries with a small dot, although normally we do not need to show these. Between words we can simply use a gap to show the difference.

"an aim"—"a name"	[ən eɪm]—[ə neɪm] or [ən.eɪm]—[ə.neɪm]
"I scream"—"ice cream"	[aɪ skɹim]—[aɪs kɹim] or [aɪ.skɹim]—[aɪs.kɹim]
"lightening"—"lightning"	[laɪt.n̩.ɪŋ]—[laɪt.nɪŋ]

Effects at segmental boundaries are often called *coarticulations*. As we noted at the beginning of the chapter, consonants and vowels do not have neat boundaries where all phonetic features change at the same time. In fact, we find instances where phonation and articulation are slightly out of step: In English, for example, we often turn off voicing somewhat before the end of a word-final voiced consonant; we find instances where velic lowering is a little early for a following nasal stop, or velic raising a little late after a preceding nasal stop, leading to nasalization of surrounding vowels; where lip-rounding is started in advance of a rounded vowel and the preceding consonant is also lip-rounded; and where the need to move the tongue forward for a front vowel causes the preceding consonant to be made further forward in the mouth than usual. All these are coarticulatory effects. We have not the space to go into these in detail here, but major coarticulatory characteristics of English sounds will be described in part II of this book.

Finally, we can briefly consider pausing. Pauses can occur at almost any point in natural speech (even sometimes in the middle of a word). For speech-language pathologists, it can be important to record pauses accurately (for example, in people with stuttering). Pauses can be measured from the acoustic record, but it is also usually possible to do this via impressionistic transcription. Various different methods have been suggested to mark pauses, but the *Extensions to the IPA* for disordered speech recommend the use of periods within parentheses for short pauses, and actual durations in seconds for longer ones. In this way, (.) would stand for a pause equivalent to one beat of the speaker's current rhythm, with (..) and (. . .) as longer pauses; a notation such as (4 sec) would mark really long pauses.

OTHER PROSODIC FEATURES

There are several other suprasegmental aspects of speech that are important for the speech-language pathologist. These all have the utterance (or part of the utterance) as their domain, and have less of a linguistic impact than those prosodic features we have discussed previously. Nevertheless, impairment to any of these may seriously affect a speaker's intelligibility. The first of these is *voice quality*. We have examined both the phonatory and supralaryngeal aspects of voice quality already (chaps. 4 and 8, respectively), so we will not revisit this topic here. We will, however, return to specifically disordered aspects of voice quality in chapters 19 and 20.

The second of these aspects is *tempo*. This refers to the speed of speech and, of course, speakers may speed up and slow down at any point during an utterance. Unless one is doing very fine-grained analyses of conversation, transcriptions of normal speech often ignore tempo. However, in a variety of speech disorders (including fluency disorders, acquired neurogenic disorders, and hearing impairment), we may well be interested in whether a client is using normal tempo, excessive speed, or excessive slowness in speech, and whether the tempo has altered after therapy. Naturally, we can use acoustic instrumentation to find precise measures of tempo, but normally an impressionistic measure will suffice. Because tempo is very important in music, a range of terms has been developed for musicians, and some of these have been adopted into phonetic terminology and symbolization. For fast speech the term *allegro* is used, whereas for slow speech the term is *lento*. If the tempo is unmarked, it is assumed to be neither fast nor slow. It is rarely necessary to use any further degrees of speed.

Finally, we can consider loudness. As with tempo, loudness may be affected by disorders such as hearing impairment or neurological damage and, also as with tempo, terms from music have been adopted to describe different levels of loudness. Loud and soft are termed *forte* and *piano*, respectively (abbreviated *f* and *p*), and very loud and very soft are *fortissimo* and *pianissimo* (*ff* and *pp*). Again, unmarked sections of speech are deemed to be of normal loudness.

These musical terms can be included in phonetic transcriptions through the use of the brace convention. In this approach, a stretch of transcription into IPA of the speech of an individual is bracketed off using braces, and the braces are labeled with a suprasegmental symbol (e.g., voice quality, tempo, or loudness).

> The following examples show the use of labeled braces for marking suprasegmental aspects of speech. The example utterance is "the rainbow is a division of white light into many beautiful colors."
>
> Voice quality (creak at end):
> [ðə ˈɹeɪnbou ɪz ə dɪˈvɪʒn əv ˈwaɪt ˈlaɪt ɪntʊ ˈme{C ni ˈbjutɪfʊl ˈkʌlɚz C}]
> Tempo (slow at the start):
> [{$_{lento}$ ðə ˈɹeɪnbou ɪz ə dɪˈvɪʒn $_{lento}$} əv ˈwaɪt ˈlaɪt ɪntʊ ˈmeni ˈbjutɪfʊl ˈkʌlɚz]
> Loudness (loud in middle):
> [ðə ˈɹeɪnbou ɪz ə dɪˈvɪʒn əv {$_{f}$ ˈwaɪt ˈlaɪt $_{f}$} ɪntʊ ˈmeni ˈbjutɪfʊl ˈkʌlɚz]
> Tempo and loudness (throughout):
> [{$_{pp,allegro}$ ðə ˈɹeɪnbou ɪz ə dɪˈvɪʒn əv ˈwaɪt ˈlaɪt ɪntʊ ˈmeni ˈbjutɪfʊl ˈkʌlɚz $_{pp,allegro}$}]

ACOUSTIC ANALYSIS OF SUPRASEGMENTALS

As we have done with the vowels and the consonants, we can look at how the main prosodic features discussed in this chapter can be displayed through acoustic analysis. First, we can consider stressed and unstressed syllables. Figure 9.1 shows an intensity trace of the two words "import" (noun) and "import" (verb) discussed earlier. The intensity trace clearly shows that in the noun the first syllable is more intense than the second, and in that in the case of the verb, the opposite is the case.

To illustrate length, we can compare the two Italian words *nono* "ninth" and *nonno* "grandfather" in the phrase *il nono nonno* "the ninth grandfather." The spectrogram in Fig. 9.2 shows the medial nasal stops in each word, and we can clearly see the longer duration in the word *nonno*. (In fact, in this example, the durations were 41 ms and 25 ms, respectively.)

Finally, we can look at pitch changes. Fig. 9.3 shows a pitch trace superimposed over a spectrogram containing the four Chinese words we noted earlier: 妈 [ma˥] "mother," 麻 [ma˧˥] "hemp," 马 [ma˨˩˦] "horse," and 骂 [ma˥˩] "scold," which have a high level tone, a high rising tone, a low falling–rising tone, and a high falling tone, respectively, in the Putonghua (Mandarin) dialect of Chinese. The pitch trace shows the pitch movement on these syllables clearly.

Finally, we can plot a pitch trace over an entire intonation phrase. In Fig. 9.4 we have the utterance noted earlier, "it's an uncomfortably hot day," said with the same intonation pattern we diagrammed above. The pitch trace shows the movement of the pitch from low for the first few syllables, to high for the middle syllables, with a fall at the end.

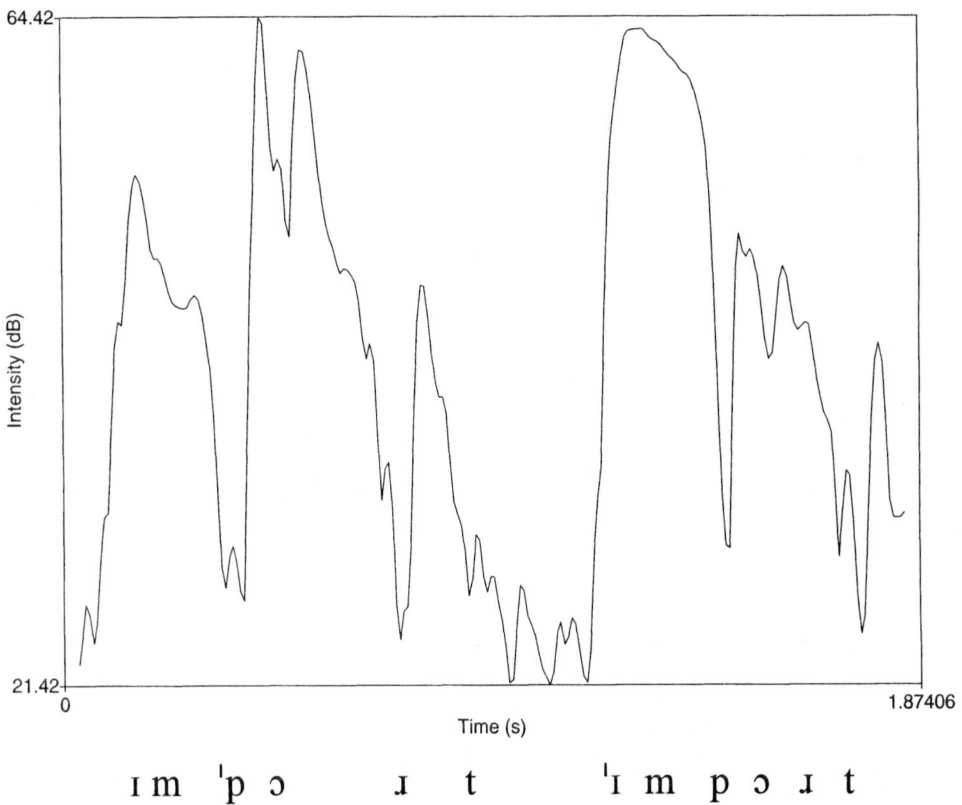

FIG 9.1. Intensity trace of "import" (verb) and "import" (noun).

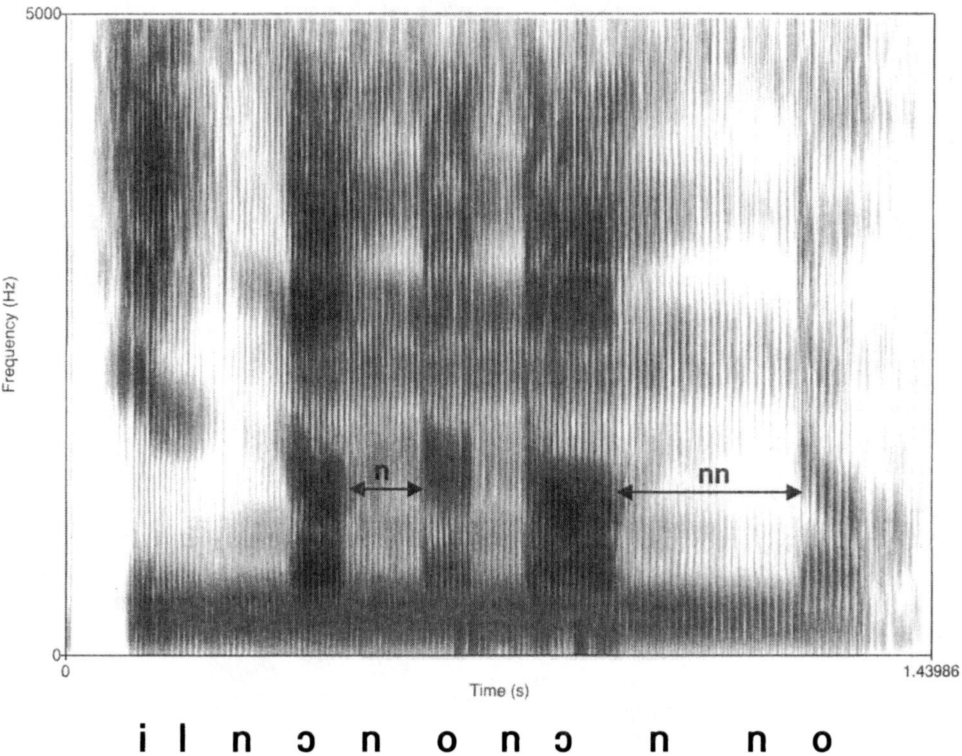

FIG 9.2. Wideband spectrogram of *il nono nonno*.

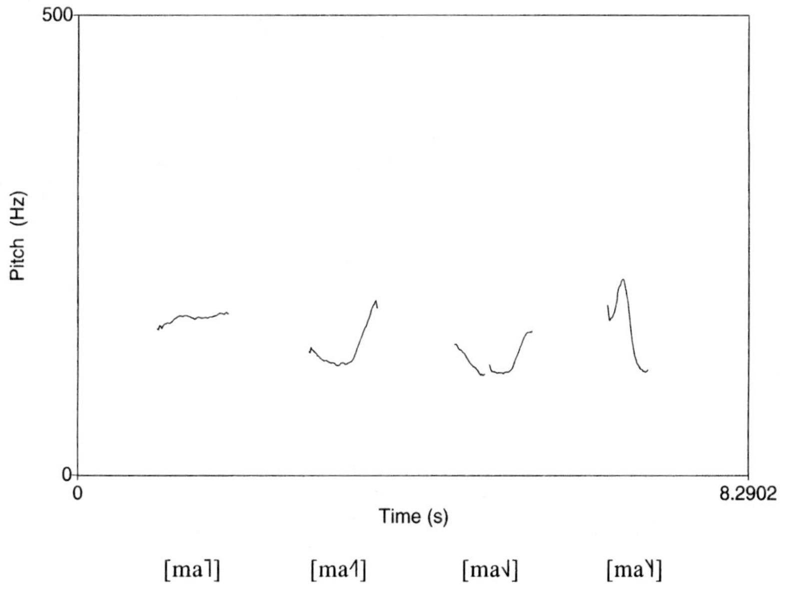

FIG 9.3. Pitch trace of 妈 [ma˥] "mother," 麻 [ma˧˥] "hemp," 马 [ma˨˩˦] "horse," and 妈 [ma˥˩] "scold."

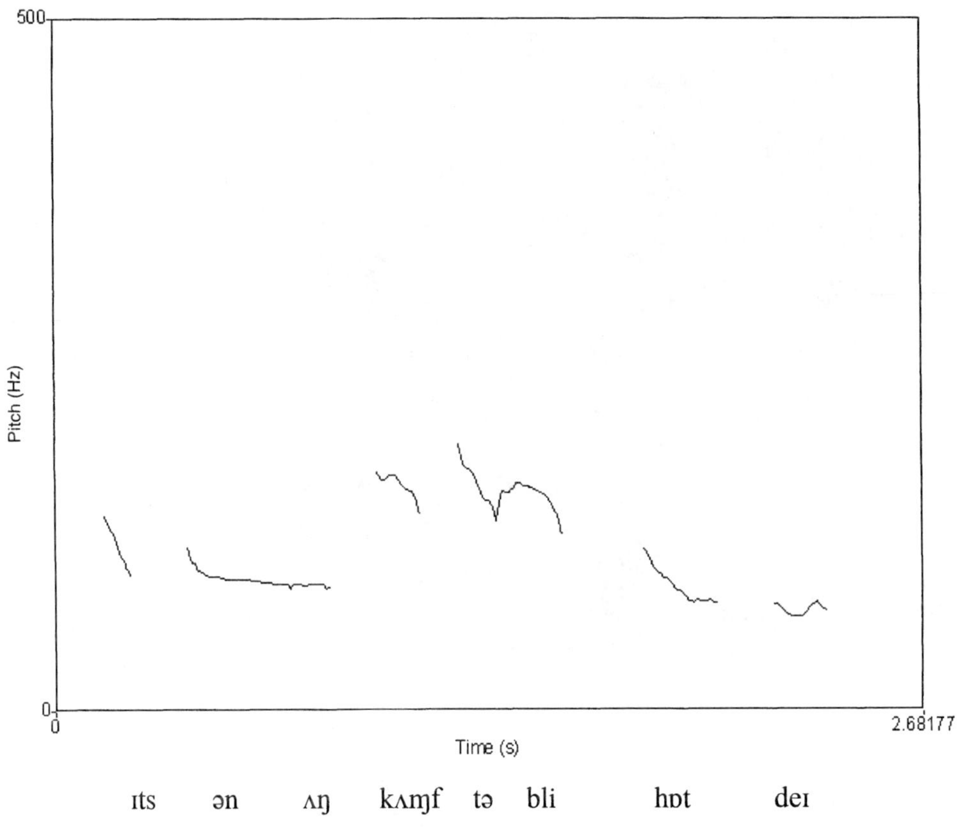

FIG 9.4. Pitch trace of "it's an uncomfortably hot day."

BACKGROUND READING

Standard phonetics texts all deal with suprasegmentals, though some give more detail than others. The Igbo tone example can be found in Ladefoged's *A Course in Phonetics* (1993); the Thai example is from Ball, Rahilly, and Tench (1996). Other examples are from the sources noted in chapter 7. Thanks to Liang Chen for providing the chinese characters for the Mandarin examples.

EXERCISES

Review Questions

1. What are segmental and suprasegmental aspects of speech?
2. What is stress, what is its domain, and how is stress achieved?
3. What is the difference between stress-timed and syllable-timed?
4. What is the difference between tone and intonation?
5. What are register and contour tones?
6. What does intonation contribute to utterance meaning?
7. What are the main types of word boundary phenomena? Give examples.
8. What are coarticulations? Give examples.

Study Topics and Experiments

1. Using library and Internet resources, find descriptions of at least four tone languages, two from Asia and two from Africa. How many different tones do these languages use, and what are they?
2. Using library and Internet resources, find descriptions of the intonation systems of at least two languages other than English. What is the meaning potential of the intonation systems?

CD

Listen to the examples of different prosodic features of speech, and try to imitate as many as possible. Try to identify the test examples following the instructions on the CD. Answers to all the exercises are given at the end of the book.

II

English Phonetics

10

Phonetic and Phonological Description

THE DIFFERENCE BETWEEN PHONETICS AND PHONOLOGY

Part I of this book was concerned with the phonetic description of the production and transmission of speech sounds. We did not comment on how any of these sounds patterned in particular languages (although, of course, we did provide examples of the use of many of the sounds). In other words, our phonetic approach was independent of specific language use. When we do examine the *function* of sounds within a particular language, as opposed to just looking at their *form*, we discover a different—though related—area of study. To demonstrate why this is so, let us consider two languages that may share some of the same speech sounds, where their form is identical, but their function (in terms of their distribution in word structure) differs.

Both English and Zulu have a voiced velar nasal: [ŋ]. However, in English this sound can only appear at the end of syllables (e.g., "sing," "sang," "sung," and "song"), whereas in Zulu it can occur at the beginning (e.g., "ngakho" *therefore,* "ngapha" *on this side*, "ngempela" *really*). Both English and Spanish allow a sequence of the sounds [s] and [p], but whereas in English these can come at the beginning of a syllable, in Spanish they can only occur across a syllable boundary; compare English "Spain" with Spanish "España." Both English and Hindi have voiceless aspirated and voiceless unaspirated plosives. However, in English the choice between these two types is strictly governed by context: In syllable-initial position all plosives are aspirated unless they follow [s], in which case they are unaspirated (compare "pill" [pʰɪl] and "spill" [sp⁼ɪl]). In Hindi, on the other hand, these sounds can both be used in the same syllable positions, and the use of one rather than the other will determine the meaning of the word (in other words they are *contrastive* sounds): /p⁼al/ *take care of*, /pʰal/ *knife blade*. Conversely, whereas Spanish and English both have a voiced dental fricative ([ð]), only in English is this contrastive with [d] (e.g., "then"–"den" /ðɛn/–/dɛn/). In Spanish, [ð] is a positional variant linked with [d]: [d] is used word-initially ("dos" *two* [dos]), with [ð] used word-medially and -finally ("Madrid" [maðrið]).

These, and many other examples, demonstrate the need to consider how sounds are used, or distributed, in languages separately from how they are produced. This area of study is sometimes called *linguistic phonetics*; the term we normally use is *phonology*. The examples we gave above illustrate two main areas of interest within phonology. First, the phonological description of a language will include a list of the contrastive sounds used in the language (that is, sounds capable of distinguishing between two words, with different meanings), together with the ranges of variants each sound has and where these variants are found. This is the phonological *system* of a language. Second, the phonological description will specify where in a syllable a sound can occur, and into what combinations of sounds each sound can enter. This is the phonological *structure* of a language. We will look at these two areas in more detail in the following section.

We need to understand this distinction well, because clients in the speech clinic may present with phonetic problems, phonological problems, or both. Treatment may well differ depending on this difference, so it is vital that the clinician can tell apart phonetic and phonological aspects of speech.

PHONOLOGICAL SYSTEM AND STRUCTURE

System

The phonological system is the set of consonant and vowel units that make up the words of a specific language or language variety. However, we don't want to list every tiny shade of sound difference at the phonological system level, because we are only interested in sound differences that are *contrastive*: that is, differences that can be used to contrast one word with another word. Once we have established these contrastive units of sound, then we can see what variants each of these units has (the noncontrastive nuances), and when one uses each of these variants. How can we tell whether the difference between two sounds is contrastive, or whether it is noncontrastive and the two sounds are simply variants of a single phonological unit? A relatively simple test is to look for *minimal pairs.* A minimal pair is a pair of words from the language that you are investigating that differ in only one sound (the sound has to be at the same place in each word). So, to take examples from English, we can easily think up many such pairs: "pit"–"bit"; "cap"– "cab"; "lopping"–"lobbing" would be three such pairs. In these three examples we find that the word pairs differ only in the choice of [p] or [b]. In other words, it is the use of the [p] or the [b] that contrasts the meanings of the word pairs. Therefore, for English at any rate, [p] and [b] must belong to separate phonological units. We call these units *phonemes*, and we write the phoneme symbols in slant brackets: /p/, /b/, and so forth.

Through examining hundreds of minimal pairs, with the relevant sounds (as in our three examples) at the beginning, end, and in the middle of words, we can draw up a list of all the contrastive consonants and vowels for the language we're studying. Of course, different dialects of a language may differ in this respect. For example, although most dialects of English have the same number of consonant phonemes (24), the number of vowel phonemes (including diphthongs) may vary from 17 to 20. (There are also dialects that have two or three consonants less than the standard 24.)

But what do we do about the sound differences that clearly are not contrastive, because we cannot find any minimal pair words? For example, in English we can find a voiceless alveolar plosive, a voiceless postalveolar plosive, and a voiceless dental plosive, but none of these can be found contrastively in minimal pairs of words. We may well suspect that these are all variants of a basic voiceless anterior (front) plosive—but how do we prove this? To examine whether sounds are variants (we term these *allophones*) of a phoneme we can use the *complementary distribution* test. Complementary distribution means that we find one allophone in a particular phonetic context (e.g., word-initial; after a rounded vowel; before a nasal consonant), where we never find the other allophone(s). In other words, each allophone has its particular context, and other allophones cannot occur there. Let's return to our example from English. The three sounds we noted are written in IPA as [t], [t̠], and [t̪] (note that allophones go into square

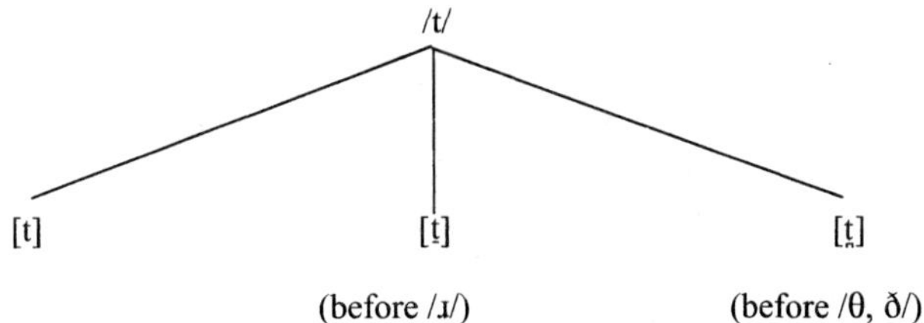

FIG 10.1. Some allophones of /t/ in English.

brackets). Taking the last one first, we find the dental variant only before dental fricatives (e.g., in words such as "eighth") and nowhere else; we find the postalveolar variant only before /ɹ/, and nowhere else (e.g., "attract"); the alveolar variant we find in most other contexts (there are other allophones of /t/ which we will ignore for the moment). It is clear that these allophones arose due to articulatory pressures: because words such as "eighth" have a dental fricative, it is easier to produce the /t/ in front of that fricative as a dental, because this avoids moving the tongue tip from the alveolar to the dental position. Likewise, in words such as "attract," because the /ɹ/ is postalveolar, it saves effort if the tongue goes straight to the postalveolar position and doesn't have to be moved from alveolar back to postalveolar. We can draw up a tree diagram for each phoneme, showing its allophones and the contexts where they occur. Part of such a tree for English /t/ would look like the one given in Fig. 10.1 (this is simplified, because we have omitted several other allophones).

It is not sufficient to group allophones as members of a phoneme solely based on the fact that their contexts of use are mutually exclusive, however. The allophones concerned must also be *phonetically similar*. In the example we've been using the three allophones were all anterior voiceless plosives. This is important to bear in mind, because it is possible to find examples of sounds that are in mutually exclusive contexts, but cannot be allophones of a single phoneme because they are not phonetically similar. Looking again at English, we can find an example with the sounds [h] and [ŋ] (note that square brackets are used also to denote sounds irrespective of any later phonemic analysis). [h] in English can only occur at the beginnings of syllables, immediately in front of a vowel: "happy," "behave" (final "h" in spellings such as "oh" is silent). On the other hand, [ŋ] is only found at the ends of syllables: "wrong," "singing." So, technically, [h] and [ŋ] are in complementary distribution, because they occur in mutually exclusive environments. However, we would not want to claim that they are allophones of the same phoneme, as the two have very little in common phonetically, other than that they are both consonants. [h] is a voiceless glottal fricative, whereas [ŋ] is a voiced velar nasal: the three-term labels do not overlap at all.

Finally, we can note that some phonemes may have allophones that are not in complementary distribution. These cases often involve a stylistic option: There may be a choice of two (or sometimes more) pronunciations for a particular phoneme in a particular context. Whether you use one or the other won't result in a change of meaning (there are no minimal pairs, and the sounds concerned cannot be phonemically contrastive), but it may result in a pronunciation that sounds more formal, more regional, more middle class, and so forth. Looking at English, we can consider the allophones available for /p/ in word-final position. One option is to use a weakly aspirated, yet fully released plosive [p^h], whereas another is to use an unreleased stop [p˺]. There is no difference at all to the meaning of, for example, "cap" when pronounced with final [p^h] or with [p˺]. Therefore, these two sounds are both allophones of /p/, but allophones in *free variation* rather than complementary distribution. Some speakers may use from time to time all free variation allophones, usually with a stylistic motive; other speakers may stick to just one of the free variants most or all of the time.

The notions of phonemes and allophones are important in phonetic transcription. In a *broad* transcription we usually only transcribe the phoneme values used by the speaker (and we show this by putting the symbols into slant brackets). *Narrow* transcription aims to record as much detail as possible and so should include as many of the allophonic distinctions used by the speaker as can be detected. In the clinic, broad phonemic transcription may not be much help, because many clients' speech cannot be adequately described by relying on the phoneme system of the target language.

Structure

As we noted earlier, the phonological structure of a language determines which combinations of units (consonants and vowels) from the system can occur where. The domain of interest here is the syllable. Syllables all have nuclei, and these are usually vowels, which we can represent with V. (Certain sonorant consonants can also be syllable nuclei, and we describe those found in English in later chapters.) The nucleus may be preceded by an onset consonant (C) and may also be followed by a coda consonant. To take some examples from English, a simple V syllable is found in "O!" or in "I" or "eye"; a CV syllable is seen in "show"; a VC syllable in "owed"; and a CVC syllable in "showed."

This way of writing syllable shapes suggests that the onset, nucleus, and coda are all equally independent units of the syllable. However, this is not the case, as we can appreciate when we consider how rhyming works. When we rhyme syllables together ("cat," "sat," "mat," and so on), we rhyme the nucleus and the coda together. On the other hand, when we use alliteration, we alliterate only the onset consonant: "Peter Piper picked a peck of pickled peppers." So syllables really consist of a hierarchy of the units, as seen in Fig. 10.2.

Not all languages allow the full range of V, CV, VC, and CVC syllable shapes we've described for English. Japanese, Italian, and Spanish, for example, have comparatively few syllables with a final coda consonant, and some languages have restrictions on syllables with empty onsets.

Apart from simply listing syllable shapes, the structure of a phonology describes which particular Cs and Vs from the complete system of Cs and Vs can go into these slots, and which combinations of Cs and Vs are allowed. For example, in English [ŋ] cannot go into the onset C slot, only into the coda C slot. Further, even when it is in the coda slot, only a few Vs from the full set of English Vs can precede it in the nucleus. To show this we can list the following four words: "sing," "sang," "song," and "sung." The vowels in these words are the only ones that can go into a V slot before [ŋ]. (If we allow "oink" as a word, then that adds a fifth—but in this word only!) Interestingly, if /ŋ/ is followed by /kθ/, as in "length," then one more vowel is found.

Finally, we can consider clusters of consonants. Many (but not all) languages allow consonant clusters. The phonological structure determines which clusters are found and in which position (onset or coda). It will also determine any patterns in these clusters, and whether these patterns alter in multisyllable words as opposed to single syllable words. English is particularly rich in such clusters. We allow up to three consonants in the onset position, and up to four in the coda position, and we can show this by the code $C^{0\text{–}3}$ $VC^{0\text{–}4}$. There are, however, patterns to these clusters. So, if we have three consonants in onset position, the first is always /s/, the second is always a voiceless plosive, and the third is one of the approximants (consider "splash," "string," "squeamish"). Other languages are much more parsimonious in their cluster use. Some may allow no clusters at all (for example, Chinese). Some may allow certain

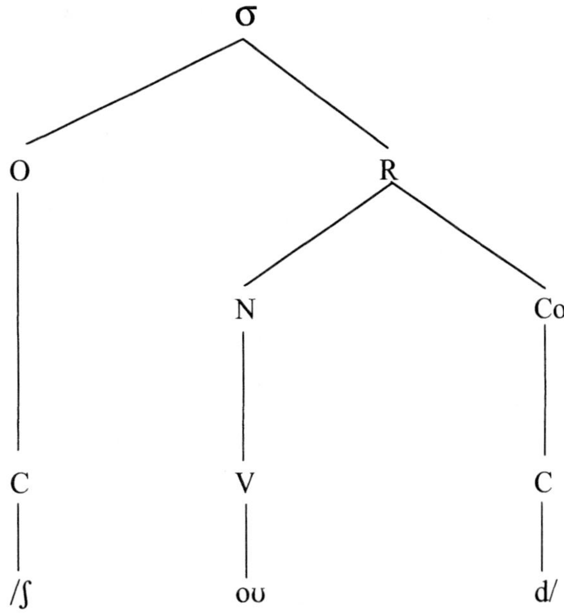

FIG 10.2. Syllable diagram for "showed." σ: syllable; O: onset; R: rime; N: nucleus; Co: coda; C: consonant; V: vowel.

clusters but not necessarily all those found in English. For example, Spanish only allows /s/ plus plosive to occur across a syllable boundary (which technically means they don't count as clusters), so where English has "*Sp*ain," Spanish has "E*s*.*p*aña" (where the period marks the syllable boundary). There are also languages that have clusters not found in English. Hebrew, for example, has initial /bn–/ clusters, and Georgian has /d͡zl–/ and /t͡ʃrd–/.

CLINICAL PHONOLOGY

The concept of the phoneme has of course been applied to the phonological analysis of disordered as well as normal speech. Early attempts at classifying speech disorders used a four-point scale: addition of a phoneme; loss of a phoneme; substitution of one phoneme for another phoneme; distortion of a phoneme through a nonphonemic change (though this last type does not distinguish between using the wrong allophone of the target phoneme and using a sound from outside the phonological system of the language altogether).

> To gauge the severity of disordered speech it was suggested that the error types be graded, with distortion the least severe and deletion the most. However, such a metric often doesn't equate with the degree of intelligibility, and won't account for the underlying source of patterns of similar errors.

However, it soon became clear that using these categories often obscured patterns of speech error that speakers might be displaying. For example, if a client used [b] instead of /p/, [d] instead of /t/, and [g] instead of /k/, it would appear from the strictly phonemic approach to analysis that he or she had three substitution errors. This, however, would not show the obvious pattern behind these errors: that they all involve the change from a target voiceless consonant to a voiced one, and that all other aspects of the target sound other than voicing are in fact accurate. Clinical phonologists therefore turned from strictly phoneme-by-phoneme analysis to descriptions based on phonological *distinctive features* that had long been in use by those working on the sound systems of normal speech.

Under a distinctive features (DF) approach, the error noted above would be one involving a single feature ([voice]), and could be expressed in the form of the following *rule*:

$$[-\text{voice}] \rightarrow [+\text{voice}] \ / \ [+\text{cons}, -\text{cont}]$$

This represents a statement such as: "the feature minus voice (i.e., voicelessness) is changed to plus voice (i.e., voiced) in the context of a plus consonantal sound (i.e., a consonant) that is also minus continuant (i.e., a noncontinuing, or stop, sound)."

> To gauge severity with DFs it was suggested that the number of feature changes could be counted. However, because features are often not directly related to phonetic characteristics, this was not always helpful.

Because this is not a book on clinical phonology, we will not here go into the debate concerning the nature of phonological features, which specific features one needs, or whether features should be only +/− (like the example above), be multivalued, or be single-valued. We do include, however, in appendix 2, a full list of the binary features normally encountered in clinical work and a full list of the unary primes (i.e., single-valued features) recommended by some researchers for work with clinical data.

Before leaving this topic we need to mention briefly one other approach to characterizing the speech error patterns commonly encountered in the clinic. The proponents of *natural phonology* have proposed that a series of *natural processes* exist in phonology. These processes are natural because they occur time after time in the studies of the languages of the world. Specifically, they occur in the acquisition of phonology by children learning to speak, and they occur when languages change over time. It seems that in both these cases there are many patterns that turn up irrespective of the language being studied. (Not all patterns in historical change or in language acquisition fit into the concept of natural processes, however; some idiosyncratic patterns are also observed.) When we turn to speech errors, it seems that many of these (though certainly not all) are also examples of such processes. Among the commonly occurring processes are *context-sensitive voicing* (initial consonants become voiced, final ones become voiceless); *fricative stopping* (fricatives become stops at the same place of articulation); *velar fronting* (velar sounds are realized as alveolars); and *weak syllable deletion* (unstressed syllables are deleted).

> Some phonological processes act to simplify the phonological system (e.g., velar fronting removes all velars from the system); others simplify the structure (e.g., weak syllable deletion removes unstressed syllables only). See appendix 2 for a list of common processes.

Many of the processes, when they occur during the period of normal phonological acquisition, have specific ages attached to them (i.e., we know when the normally developing child would stop using the process and acquire the correct pronunciation). This allows us to rate, approximately, the delay in a child's phonological acquisition. However, not all authors promoting the use of processes for clinical analysis have realized that these processes should be *natural*; that is to say, they should be tied to naturally occurring patterns. When idiosyncratic patterns do emerge in the data there is a tendency just to make up another process name and to lump this pattern in with all the others. Another problem is that process approaches do not make explicit whether the error is at the phonemic level or the allophonic level, whether it involves sounds from within the target system only, or whether the client is using sounds from outside that system.

In fact, with all analyses of speech error data, we need to distinguish between the phonological and the phonetic levels, between changes within the system and outside it, and between what the speaker intends and what the listener perceives. We return to these points in more detail in chapter 19.

THE SYSTEM AND STRUCTURE OF ENGLISH

The following chapters in this part of the book deal with the consonants, vowels, and suprasegmental aspects of the General American accent of English (GA) and of the Received Pronunciation (i.e., standard) of British English (RP); other varieties of English are dealt with in a later chapter. We need first to introduce the system of phonemes of the variety, and note briefly some of the structural possibilities allowed. If we know the various norms of English pronunciations we will be better able to distinguish disordered speech from differences due to dialect.

General American English

This variety (also called Standard American) is often considered to be the variety of pronunciation in North America that is least marked by region. Wells (1982) defines General American as the variety that "do[es] not show marked eastern or southern characteristics" (p. 470). Cruttenden (2001) notes further that it is this variety that serves as a second language model for learners of English in parts of Asia (e.g., the Philippines) and in Latin America. The variety does have a number of accents that differ in precisely how the phonemes are realized. However, the basic system and structure are the same across this range, as described in the following subsections.

Phonological System

GA has six plosive stops, three voiceless and three voiced. The pairs are found at the bilabial, alveolar, and velar places of articulation: /p, b, t, d, k, g/. There is also a pair of affricates, at the postalveolar place: /tʃ, dʒ/.

There are three nasal stops, all voiced, at the same places of articulation as the plosive stops: /m, n, ŋ/.

The accent has nine fricatives; voiceless and voiced pairs at the labiodental, dental, alveolar, and postalveolar places, and a single voiceless fricative at the glottal place of articulation: /f, v, θ, ð, s, z, ʃ, ʒ, h/.

The remaining four consonants are all approximants. GA has one lateral approximant (alveolar), /l/; one central approximant (postalveolar), /ɹ/; and two semivowel approximants (labiovelar and palatal), /w, j/. All these are voiced.

Note the symmetry in the plosive and nasal stop systems,

p b	t d	k g
m	n	ŋ

but the lack of symmetry with the fricative system,

f v	θ ð	s z	ʃ ʒ	h

There are four front unrounded monophthongal vowels: high front tense /i/, high front lax /ɪ/, mid front /ɛ/, and low front /æ/.

There are four central vowels, two nonrhotic and two rhotic: lower central /ʌ/ and higher central schwa /ə/ are nonrhotic, whereas unstressed shwar /ɚ/ and stressed /ɝ/ are rhotic.

There are four back monophthongal vowels: unrounded low back /ɑ/, rounded mid back /ɔ/, lax high back /ʊ/, and tense high back /u/.

Note the symmetry in the monophthong system (the rhotic vowels are omitted for clarity):

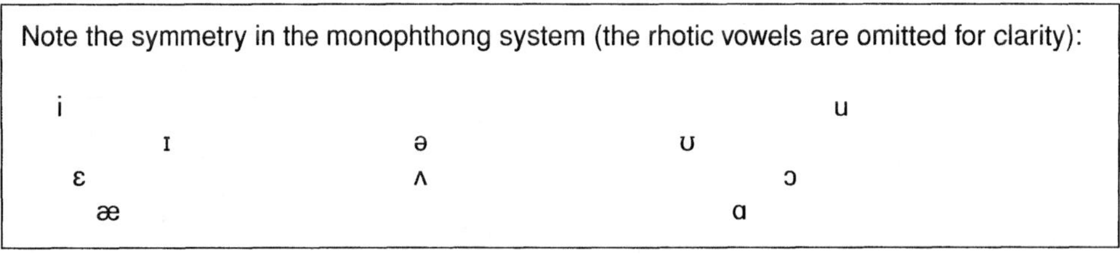

Finally, GA has five diphthongs: mid front rising /eɪ/, low front rising /aɪ/, mid back rising /oʊ/, low back rising /aʊ/, and mid back fronting /ɔɪ/.

Note the symmetry in the diphthong system, with the exception of /ɔɪ/:

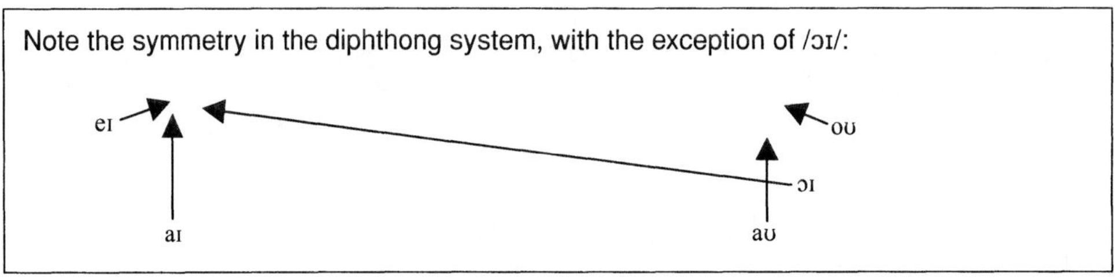

The relative frequency of GA English vowels and consonants has been worked out by several researchers using a variety of representative spoken texts. Table 10.1 shows frequencies adapted from the work of Edwards (2003) and Delattre (1965).

RP British English

This variety is also a nonregional variety, but in British terms. The accent was originally associated with those who had been educated at prestigious private schools, and was eventually adopted as the standard of pronunciation in the broadcast media. Even though it has undergone many changes, and although it is threatened by the emergence of competing forms based around London pronunciations, RP still has an undoubted prestige, and is the target accent for second language learners of English in many parts of the world.

Phonological System

The consonant system of RP is the same as that for GA. The vowel systems differ, however. There are four front unrounded monophthongal vowels: high front tense /i/, high front lax /ɪ/, mid front /ɛ/, and low front /æ/. The mid front vowel is often transcribed with /e/ in British phonetics texts, but we retain /ɛ/ here to enable direct comparison with the GA system.

There are two central vowels: lower central /ʌ/ and higher central schwa /ə/.

There are five back monophthongal vowels: unrounded low back /ɑ/, and rounded low back /ɑ/, rounded mid back /ɔ/, lax high back /ʊ/, and tense high back /u/.

Note the near symmetry in the monophthong system:

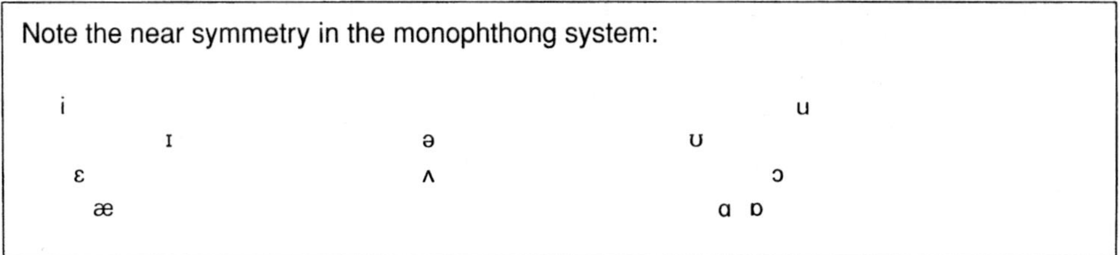

TABLE 10.1
Frequency of GA English Consonants and Vowels

Sound	*Percentage of Consonants*	*Percentage of Vowels*	*Percentage of Consonants and Vowels*
/t/	12.77	——	7.85
/ə/	——	20.12	7.76
/n/	11.46	——	7.04
/ɪ/	——	14.44	5.57
/ɹ/	8.32	——	5.11
/l/	7.69	——	4.72
/s/	7.47	——	4.59
/æ/	——	9.44	3.64
/d/	5.65	——	3.47
/i/	——	8.49	3.28
/z/	4.90	——	3.01
/m/	4.74	——	2.91
/ð/	4.61	——	2.83
/ɑ/	——	6.99	2.70
/k/	4.30	——	2.64
/ɛ/	——	6.85	2.64
/w/	3.67	——	2.26
/u/	——	5.60	2.16
/b/	3.48	——	2.14
/aɪ/	——	5.50	2.12
/h/	3.26	——	2.01
/v/	3.17	——	1.95
/oʊ/	——	4.95	1.91
/f/	2.86	——	1.75
/eɪ/	——	3.95	1.52
/p/	2.35	——	1.45
/ŋ/	2.20	——	1.35
/j/	2.01	——	1.23
/ɚ/	——	2.90	1.13
/ʌ/	——	2.87	1.11
/g/	1.57	——	0.96
/aʊ/	——	2.20	0.84
/ɔ/	——	2.00	0.77
/ʊ/	——	2.00	0.77
/θ/	0.97	——	0.60
/ɝ/	——	1.50	0.57
/ʃ/	0.88	——	0.54
/dʒ/	0.88	——	0.54
/tʃ/	0.63	——	0.39
/ʒ/	0.16	——	0.10
/ɔɪ/	——	0.20	0.08

RP has five rising diphthongs: mid front rising /eɪ/, low front rising /aɪ/, mid back rising /əʊ/, low back rising /aʊ/, and mid back fronting /ɔɪ/. Because it is a nonrhotic accent (i.e., post-vocalic -r is not found), RP replaces certain vowel+/ɹ/ sequences with centering diphthongs. Three of these are still found in RP, /ɪə/, /ɛə/, and /ʊə/, while /ɔə/ may still be used by older speakers and some regional accents.

Note the symmetry in the centering diphthong system:

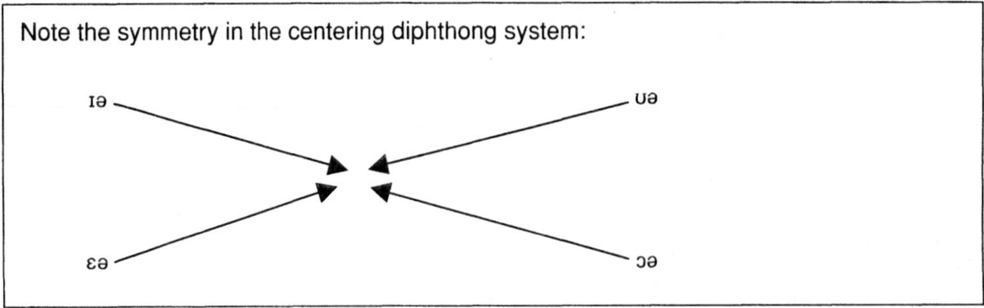

Table 10.2 shows frequencies of RP English vowels and consonants adapted from the work of Fry (1947).

Clearly some of the differences between Tables 10.1 and 10.2 are due to the dialect differences. Other slight differences in ordering will be due to the choice of texts used to establish these frequencies.

TABLE 10.2
Frequency of RP English Consonants and Vowels

Consonants	%	*Vowels*	%
/n/	7.58	/ə/	10.74
/t/	6.42	/ɪ/	8.33
/d/	5.14	/ɛ/	2.97
/s/	4.81	/aɪ/	1.83
/l/	3.66	/ʌ/	1.75
/ð/	3.56	/eɪ/	1.71
/ɹ/	3.51	/i/	1.65
/m/	3.22	/əʊ/	1.51
/k/	3.09	/æ/	1.45
/w/	2.81	/ɒ/	1.37
/z/	2.46	/ɔ/	1.24
/v/	2.00	/u/	1.13
/b/	1.97	/ʊ/	0.86
/f	1.79	/ɑ/	0.79
/p/	1.78	/aʊ/	0.61
/h/	1.46	/ɜ/	0.52
/ŋ/	1.15	/ɛə/	0.34
/g/	1.05	/ɪə/	0.21
/ʃ/	0.96	/ɔɪ/	0.14
/j/	0.88	/ʊə/	0.06
/dʒ/	0.60		
/tʃ/	0.41		
/θ/	0.37		
/ʒ/	0.10		
Total	60.78%	Total	39.21%

Phonological Structure

As noted earlier, English allows syllable shapes V, CV, VC, CVC. We also noted that consonant clusters were allowed in onset and coda positions, and the number of consonants in these clusters could be abbreviated as $C^{0-3}VC^{0-4}$. We do not have the space here to list all the Cs and Vs allowed in their various combinations. We can, however, pick out some of the important patterns, especially the initial and final consonant clusters. We will do this in terms of the various syllable patterns available to English. A listing of possible combinations of segments is often called *phonotactics*.

V. There are a few words that consist of a vowel only. Among these are “a” /ə/, /eɪ/; “I,” “eye” /aɪ/; “owe,” “O!,” “oh” /oʊ ~ əʊ /; “ah” /ɑ/; “oy” /ɔɪ/.

V-. All the vowels can occur in syllable-initial position except /ʊ/.

CV-. /ŋ/ does not occur initially; /ʒ/ occurs initially only in loan words, and then only before the vowels /i/ or /ɪ/. Other consonants can mostly occur with any vowel following them, though there are some gaps (especially before /ʊ/ and /ɔɪ/).

CCV-. Initial two-consonant clusters are as follows (brackets show clusters used in only some varieties; most British varieties use these forms):

p + l, ɹ, j
t + ɹ, (j), w
k + l, ɹ, (j), w
b + l, ɹ, j
d + ɹ,, (j) , w
g + l, ɹ, j, w
f + l, ɹ, j
θ + ɹ, (j) , w
ʃ + ɹ,

s + l, w, p, t, k, m, n

m, (n), v, h + j

It should be noted that C+j clusters only occur before /u/ or /ʊ/; and /tw–, dw–, gw–/ occur before a restricted set of vowels.

CCCV-. Initial three-consonant clusters are as follows (brackets show clusters used only by some speakers):

s + p + l, ɹ, (j)
s + t + ɹ, (j)
s + k + l, ɹ, j, w

-V. All vowels can occur finally except /ɪ, ɛ, æ, ʌ, ʊ/. Final /ʊ/ may be found in the word “to” before a word beginning with a vowel.

-VC. The following consonants do not occur finally: /h, j, w/. /ʒ/ occurs only after /ɪ, ɑ, u, eɪ/ in loan words; /ŋ/ occurs only after /ɪ, æ, ɑ, ʌ/; /ð/ occurs only after /ɪ, i, u, eɪ, aɪ, oʊ, aʊ/; /g/ occurs only after /ɪ, ɛ, æ, ʌ, ɑ, i, ɝ, eɪ, oʊ/. Only /d/ occurs after all the vowels, and no vowel occurs before all the consonants.

-VCC. Final two-consonant clusters are as follows:

p + t, θ, s
t + θ, s

k + t, s
b + d, z
d + z
g + d, z
tʃ + t
dʒ + d
m + p, d, f, θ, z
n + t, d, tʃ, dʒ, θ, s, z
ŋ + k, d, z
l + p, t, k, b, d, tʃ, dʒ, m, n, f, v, θ, s, z
f + t, θ, s
v + d, z
θ + t, s
ð + d, z
s + p, t, k
z + d
ʃ + t
ʒ + d
ɹ + p, t, k, b, d, g, tʃ, dʒ, m, n, l, f, v, θ, s, z, ʃ

The final set of /ɹ/ clusters do not occur in RP or other nonrhotic accents (i.e., accents that do not have a postvocalic-r). Some of these clusters arise due to the addition of suffix morphemes (for example, plural, past tense, possessive).

-VCCC. Final three-consonant clusters are as follows:

p + s + t
t + s + t
k + s + t
d + s + t
m + p + t
n + s, tʃ + t
ŋ + s, k + t
l + s, p, k, tʃ + t
s + p, k + t
ɹ + p, k, tʃ, f, s, ʃ + t

n + dʒ, z + d
l + dʒ, m, v + d
ɹ + b, g, dʒ, m, n, l, v, z + d

p + t, θ + s
t + θ, + s
k + t, + s
m + p, f + s
n + t, θ + s
ŋ + k + s
l + p, t, k, θ + s
f + t + s
s + p, t, k + s
ɹ + p, t, k, f, v + s

n	+	d	+	z
l	+	b, d, n, m, v	+	z
ɹ	+	b, d, g, m, n, l, v	+	z
k	+	s	+	θ
n	+	t	+	θ
ŋ	+	k	+	θ
l	+	f	+	θ

Again, /ɹ/+consonant clusters do not occur in RP.

-VCCCC. Final four-consonant clusters occur in only a handful of words, and all arise from the addition of a morphological suffix to an existing three-consonant cluster. Examples include:

/−mpts/ "prompts"
/−mpst/ "glimpsed"
/−lkts/ "mulcts"
/−lpts/ "sculpts"
/−lfθs/ "twelfths"
/−ksts/ "texts"
/−ksθs/ "sixths"
/−ntθs/ "thousandths"

Both these clusters and three-consonant final clusters are subject to simplification in rapid speech, usually through the deletion of any alveolar plosive; e.g., "facts" pronounced as /fæks/; "prompts" pronounced as /pɹɑmps/.

BACKGROUND READING

There are many books on phonology and on clinical phonology that will expand on the materials presented here. At an introductory level, readers may wish to refer to Bauman-Waengler (2004); more advanced readers could consult Ball and Kent (1997). The account of the phonotactics of English is adapted from Cruttenden (2001).

EXERCISES

Review Questions

1. What are the two main concerns of phonological description, and why does phonology always deal with a specific language, or specific languages?
2. What are minimal pairs, and how are they used in phonological analysis?
3. What are allophones, and how can we determine whether two sounds are allophones, or two different phonemes?
4. Find as many examples as you can of consonant clusters in English (make sure you don't get misled by spellings!), and describe the patterns you find.
5. What are distinctive features?
6. What are some advantages and disadvantages of a process approach to clinical phonology?
7. Using any language you know other than English, list four differences between the systems, and four between the structures.

Study Topics and Experiments

1. In a published source or from your instructor, find a data sample of transcribed child speech, or speech from someone with a phonological disorder. It should contain at least fifty utterances. Attempt to work out the contrastive segments contained in the sample. How does the person's contrastive system differ from that of an adult speaker (or someone without a phonological disorder)?
2. Using a speech sample from a child below the age of 3;6 (= 3 years, 6 months), analyze the syllable structures you find. How do they differ from those you would expect in adult language?

CD

It is important that you listen to, and do the exercises in, part 10 of the accompanying CD. These exercises provide a revision of all the sounds covered in part I of the book.

11

Monophthongs of English

INTRODUCTION

As we saw in chapter 5, vowels—unlike consonants—are not easily described in terms of strictures between the active and passive articulators. We also noted that, although it is possible to use articulatory descriptions of vowels, these are not as precise as articulatory descriptions of consonants. This was because just a slight movement of the tongue in terms of tongue height or tongue anteriority (how far front or back the highest part of the tongue is) causes perceptible differences in the quality of the vowel. We described how, for these reasons, some phoneticians prefer to use a perceptual rating system (the cardinal vowel system) and to describe vowels in terms of how close they sound to one of the cardinal vowel values.

In this chapter and in chapter 12 we will use both systems to describe the vowels of English. We will provide a description of tongue position and lip shape for the English vowels, and we will also plot the vowels onto a vowel diagram (derived from the cardinal vowel system) to show their perceptual values.

We also suggest names for the phonetic symbols, both in this chapter and in the following four for the remaining vowels and the consonants. It is clearly easier to use a short name for a symbol as an alternative to describing the sound with the full articulatory label (though we should be able to do that as well). For most of the consonants, symbol names present little difficulty, because we can adopt the usual name of the letter of the alphabet from which the symbol is derived. However, many of the vowel symbols differ in shape from orthographic letters, and others that are the same often have different values in the International Phonetic Alphabet (IPA) than they do in English orthographic usage. For vowels, therefore, we recommend that we name the symbol using the IPA value (unless the symbol has an acceptable other name).

The entry for each vowel and consonant of English in this and the following chapters includes a section on common spellings of the relevant sounds. It should be noted that we do not attempt to include every possible spelling (some are restricted to just one or two words). It should also be noted that spellings listed for one vowel or consonant may well also represent others, and we do not have the space to cross-reference all these usages. In referring to orthographic usage, spellings used in English are shown in angled brackets (e.g., <th>) to distinguish them from phonetic symbols. The order of vowels in this chapter follows the vowel diagram, starting at high front and working our way around to high back.

We also provide illustrations of the acoustic characteristics of each vowel in this chapter and in chapter 12 by providing a spectrogram of the vowel in a sample word, and also a spectral analysis of a point halfway through the vowel (to avoid the influence of surrounding sounds). In each case, the dark bands on the spectrogram and the peaks on the spectrum clearly show the formant structure of the vowel. We also give typical measurements of the fundamental frequency and the first three formants of the vowels for men, women, and children (mostly based on Peterson and Barney, 1952, and Hillenbrand, Getty, Clark, and Wheeler, 1995).

The vowels of English share certain phonetic features: they are all voiced (in all contexts), and they all involve a free flow of laminar (smooth) air over the tongue. Naturally, there are other features that help us distinguish groups of vowels and individual vowel phonemes. First, we can divide the vowels into monophthongs (vowels where the main allophones do not involve any major movement of the tongue) and diphthongs (where the main allophones do have a gliding movement of the tongue from one position to another). The monophthongs of English are often divided into three groups: four each of front vowels, central vowels, and back vowels (though some varieties have an extra back vowel). The central vowels in turn can be grouped into rhotic and nonrhotic examples. Another way of grouping these vowels is into the *tense* group (vowels where the tongue is tense, usually peripheral to the vowel area, and long in duration) and the *lax* group (the tongue is not tense and the vowels are usually not peripheral and are generally shorter in duration than the tense ones).

The diphthongs are normally classed into those that move to a high front position and those that glide to a high back position, or in terms of their starting points. In this chapter we examine the front and back monophthongs, and we turn to the remainder in chapter 12. Although there are many similarities between the vowel systems of General American and British Received Pronunciation, there are some differences. We show these differences through the initials "GA" and "RP" in the text.

For all the vowel variants described in this chapter, the vocal folds vibrate throughout the production of the vowel, producing voiced phonation; the soft palate is raised so that it blocks off the nasal cavity, resulting in purely oral airflow; and the tongue adopts a convex shape unless otherwise stated.

THE HIGH FRONT VOWELS

The English monophthongs constitute a symmetrical system, with two high front vowels, two lower front vowels, two high back vowels, and two lower back vowels. The high front pair consists of one tense and one lax vowel.

The High Front Tense Vowel

/i/

This vowel is usually described as being a high front tense unrounded vowel. /i/ can occur word-initially, before and after consonants, and word-finally in open syllables. Because the IPA symbol does not represent the same sound as the traditional name of the letter of the alphabet <i>, we suggest calling the symbol "ee" /i/, or "dotted-i."

Spelling

There are many different ways of spelling /i/. The most common are:

<e> (often with silent <e> after the consonant) be these
<ee> see been
<ea> sea bean

Other, less common, spellings also occur:

<ie> believe
<ei> deceive
<ey> key
<i> (with silent <e>) police
<y> pretty

Some spellings are found in only very few words:

<eo> people
<ay> quay

Note: Many of the spellings noted above can represent other vowels, and so may be listed in other entries.

The most usual allophone of this phoneme is produced in the following way. The highest point of the tongue arch is raised to a position slightly behind and below the highest frontest position possible for a vowel. The side rims of the tongue may make light contact with the inner surfaces of the upper side teeth. The tongue is tense during the production of this vowel, which belongs to the group of long vowels. The lip shape for the vowel is spread. In terms of the cardinal vowel system, English /i/ would be plotted onto the vowel chart as seen in Fig. 11.1, and with the symbolization [i̞-].

The following are the main allophones of /i/:

- [iː] full length vowel, found in open syllables and before voiced consonants (e.g., "see," "seed").
- [iˑ] reduced length vowel, found before voiceless consonants (e.g., "seat").
- [ɪi] or [ɪi] vowel with diphthongal quality, variant realization in open syllables.
- [i^ə] slight centralizing glide, found before dark-l (e.g., "seal").
- [i̠] retracted vowel found in unstressed open syllables (e.g., "pretty").
- [ĩ] nasalized allophone found before nasal consonants (e.g., "seen"). Less nasalization occurs after a nasal consonant ("neat").

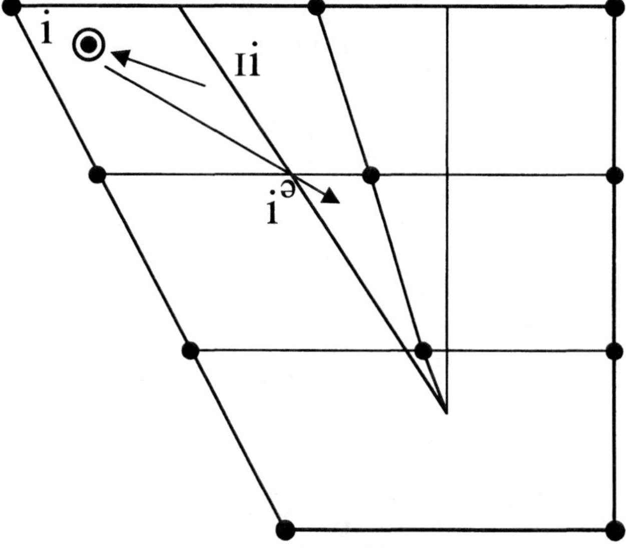

FIG 11.1. Cardinal vowel values of the main allophones of /i/.

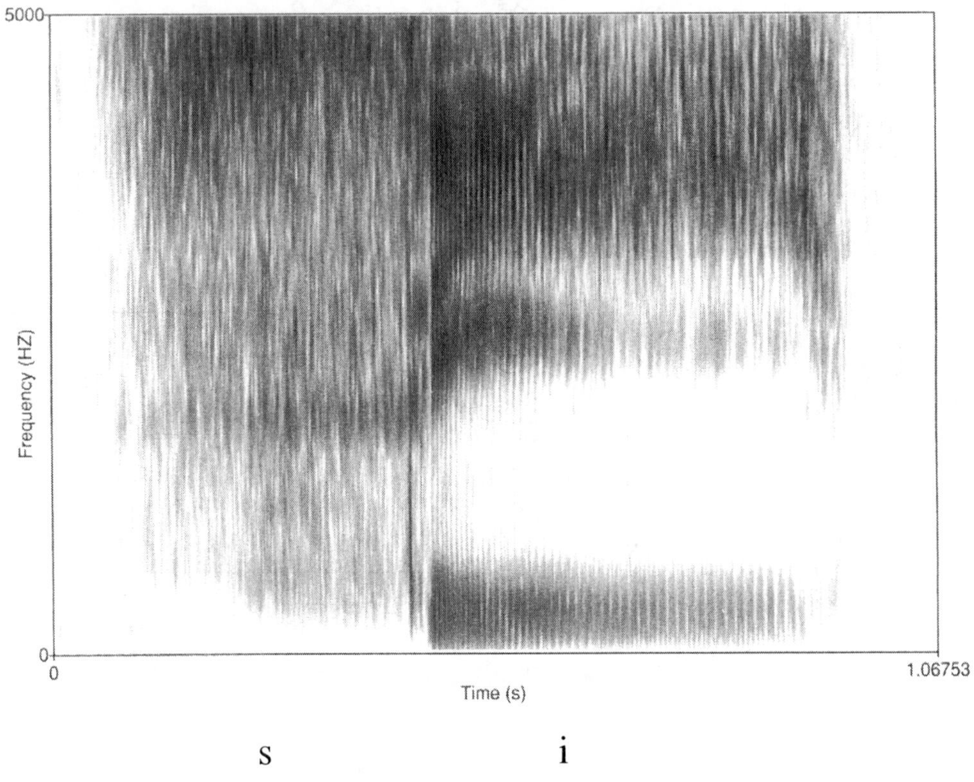

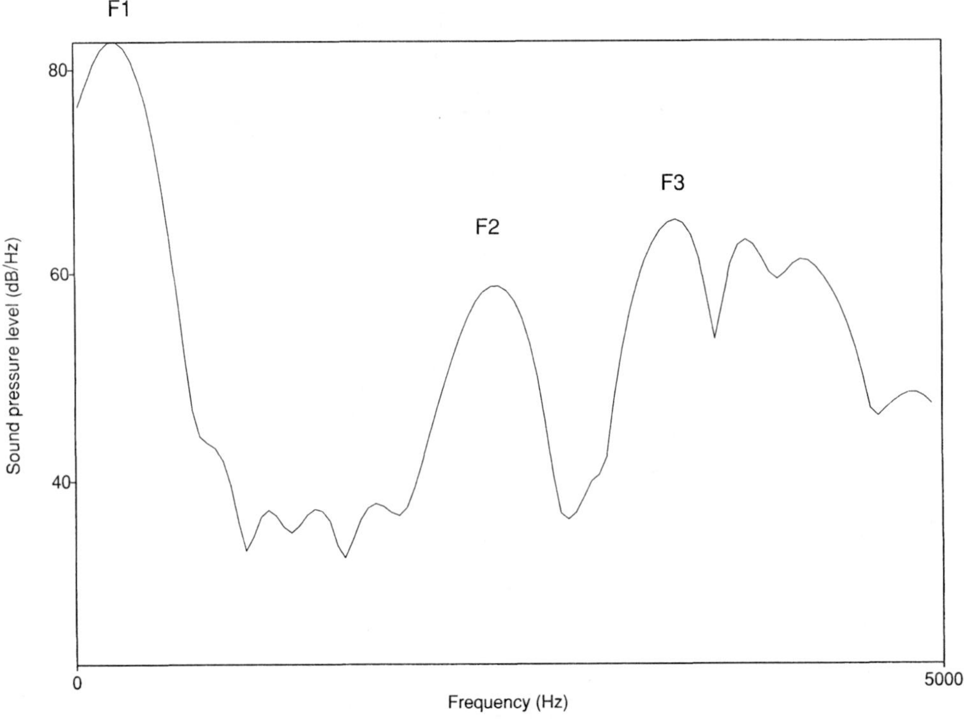

FIG 11.2. Wideband spectrogram and spectrum of the vowel in "see."

TABLE 11.1
Typical Formant Values for /i/

	F0	*F1*	*F2*	*F3*
Men	138	342	2322	3000
Women	227	437	2761	3372
Children	246	452	3081	3702

Figure 11.2 shows a spectrogram of the vowel /i/ in the word "see," together with a spectrum of the vowel taken halfway through the duration of the vowel. Table 11.1 gives typical values for the F0 and F1–F3 of /i/ in men, women, and children.

The High Front Lax Vowel

/ɪ/

This vowel is usually described as being a high front lax unrounded vowel. /ɪ/ can occur word-initially, before and after consonants, but not word-finally in open syllables. The symbol for this sound can be called "ih" /ɪ/, or "cap(ital)-i," or "small-cap-i."

Spelling

There are several different ways of spelling /ɪ/, the most common are:

<i> pit this in
<y> symbol gym

Other, less common, spellings also occur:

<e> pretty houses
<a> (with silent <e>) image private

Some spellings are found in only very few words:

<ui> built building
<u> busy business minute
<o> women
<ei> forfeit

Note: many of the spellings noted above can represent other vowels, and so may be listed in other entries.

The commonest allophone of this phoneme is produced with the highest point of the tongue arch raised to a position substantially behind and below the highest frontest position possible for a vowel. The side rims of the tongue may make light contact with the inner surfaces of the upper side teeth. The tongue is lax during the production of this vowel, which belongs to the group of short vowels. The lip shape for the vowel is slightly spread. In terms of the

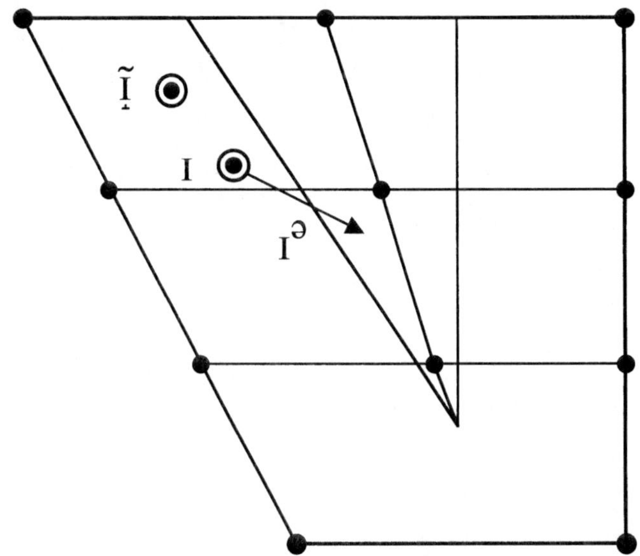

FIG 11.3. Cardinal vowel values of the main allophones of /ɪ/.

cardinal vowel system, English /ɪ/ would be plotted onto the vowel chart as seen in Fig. 11.3, and with the symbolization [ï].

The following are the main allophones of /ɪ/:

- [ɪ] full length vowel, found before voiced consonants (e.g., "hid").
- [ɪ̆] reduced length vowel, found before voiceless consonants (e.g., "hit").
- [ɪᵊ] slight centralizing glide, found before dark-l (e.g., "hill").
- [ɪ̃] nasalized allophone found before nasal consonants (e.g., "win"). Less nasalization occurs after a nasal consonant ("nib").
- GA; not RP [ɪ̝̃] raised and nasalized allophone found before velar nasal consonants (e.g., "wing"), although this is not raised as far as the vowel /i/. Interestingly, in some southern US dialects the opposite occurs, with a lower vowel before the velar nasal.

Figure 11.4 shows a spectrogram of the vowel /ɪ/ in the word "sit," together with a spectrum of the vowel taken halfway through the duration of the vowel. Table 11.2 gives typical values for the F0 and F1–F3 of /ɪ/ in men, women, and children.

In unstressed final open syllables (words such as "city," "economy," and "university"), there is often confusion as to whether /i/ or /ɪ/ is being used. The vowel heard most often in General American and RP English is longer than /ɪ/, but shorter than /i/ in stressed syllables. It is usually more retracted than /i/, but not as low as /ɪ/. It is not clear, therefore, whether this vowel should be thought of as an allophone of /i/ or of /ɪ/ (there is never any contrast

TABLE 11.2
Typical Formant Values for /ɪ/

	F0	*F1*	*F2*	*F3*
Men	135	427	2034	2684
Women	224	483	2365	3053
Children	241	571	2552	3403

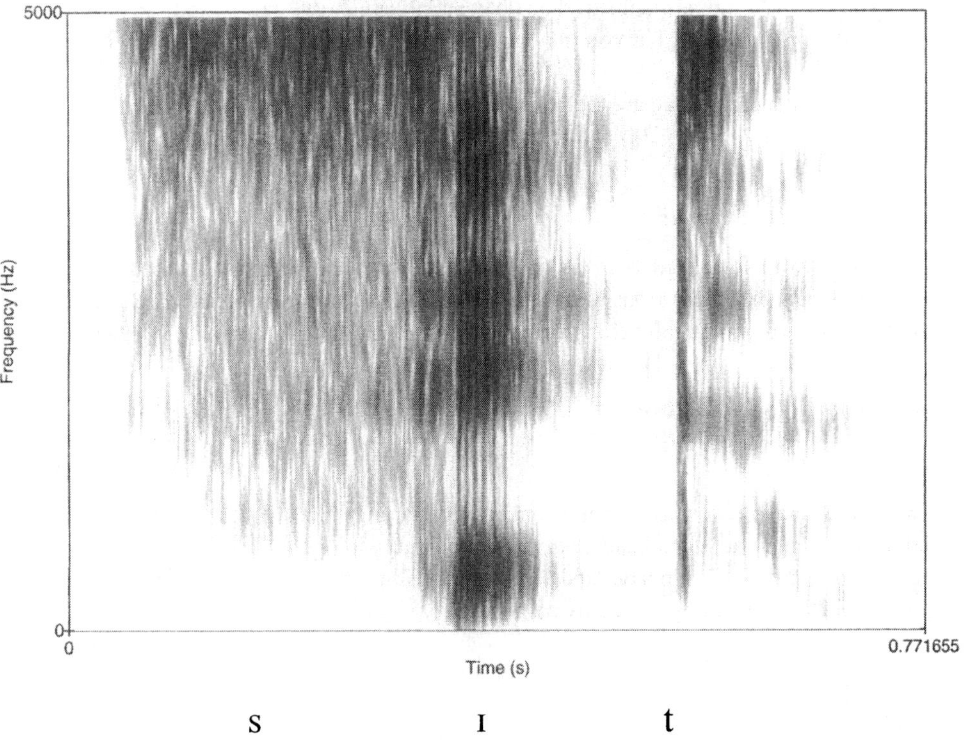

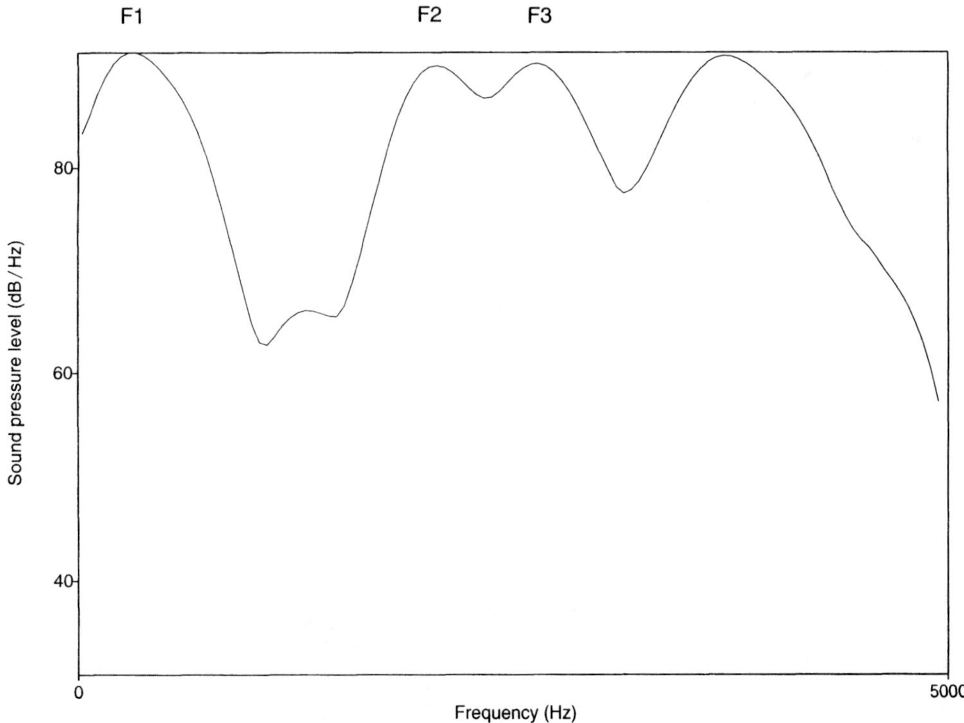

FIG 11.4. Wideband spectrogram and spectrum of the vowel in "sit."

between these two phonemes in unstressed open syllables). As we saw earlier, we classify this vowel as an allophone of /i/, but you may encounter other authors treating it as an allophone of /ɪ/.

Finally, we can note that we use the vowel symbol /ɪ/ followed by /ɹ/ in rhotic contexts such as "ear" /ɪɹ/.

The Lower Front Vowels

The two lower front vowels are both lax and unrounded. It should be noted that the vowel that some authors treat as a tense front vowel ([e]) is considered in this book as a diphthong ([eɪ]) because its most common realizations are diphthongal.

The Mid Front Lax Vowel

/ɛ/

This vowel is usually described as being a mid front lax unrounded vowel. /ɛ/ can occur word-initially, before and after consonants, but not word-finally in open syllables. This IPA symbol is derived from the Greek alphabet and we suggest calling the symbol "eh" /ɛ/, or "epsilon," or "Greek-e." In transcribing RP, many authorities prefer the symbol /e/ for this vowel.

Spelling

The most common spelling of /ɛ/ is

<e> bed extra went

Other, less common, spellings also occur:

<ea> head breath
<ei> deceive
<a> many

Some spellings are found in only very few words:

<ai> said
<ay> says
<ie> friend
<ei> heifer
<eo> Geoffrey
<ue> guess

Note: many of the spellings noted above can represent other vowels, and so may be listed in other entries.

The primary allophone of this phoneme is produced by raising the highest point of the tongue arch to a position about halfway between the highest frontest position possible for a vowel and the low front position. The side rims of the tongue may make light contact with the inner surfaces of the upper side teeth. The tongue is lax during the production of this vowel (but not as lax as for /ɪ/), which belongs to the group of short vowels. The lip shape for the vowel is loosely spread. In terms of the cardinal vowel system, English /ɛ/ would be plotted onto the vowel chart as seen in Fig. 11.5, and with the symbolization [ɛ̝] or [e̞].

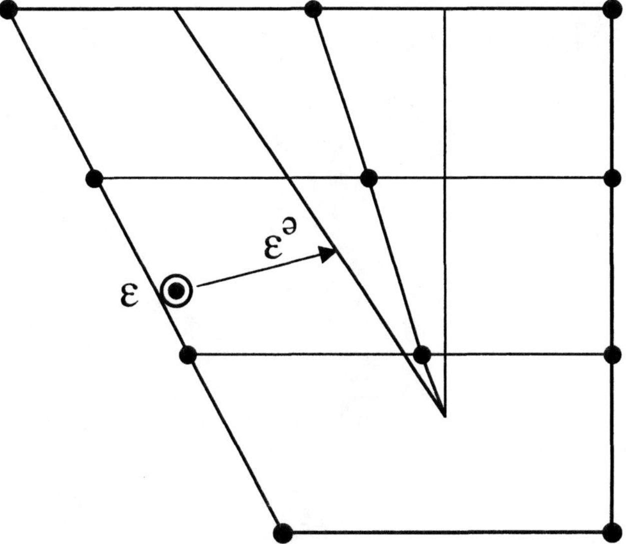

FIG 11.5. Cardinal vowel values of the main allophones of /ɛ/.

The following are the main allophones of /ɛ/:

- [ɛ] full length vowel, found before voiced consonants (e.g., "dead").
- [ɛ̆] reduced length vowel, found before voiceless consonants (e.g., "debt").
- [ɛ^{ə}] slight centralizing glide, found before dark-l (e.g., "bell").
- [ɛ̃] nasalized allophone found before nasal consonants (e.g., "hen"). Less nasalization occurs after a nasal consonant ("net").

Note that we use the vowel symbol /ɛ/ followed by /ɹ/ in rhotic contexts such as "air" /ɛɹ/.

Figure 11.6 shows a spectrogram of the vowel /ɛ/ in the word "set," together with a spectrum of the vowel taken halfway through the duration of the vowel. Table 11.3 provides typical values for the F0 and F1–F3 of /ɛ/ in men, women, and children.

The Low Front Lax Vowel

/æ/

This vowel is usually described as being a low front lax unrounded vowel. /æ/ can occur word-initially, before and after consonants, but not word-finally in open syllables. This IPA symbol is derived from the Early English alphabet usage and we suggest calling the symbol by the Early English name "ash" (which also contains the vowel sound, of course).

TABLE 11.3
Typical Formant Values for /ɛ/

	F0	*F1*	*F2*	*F3*
Men	127	580	1799	2605
Women	214	731	2058	2979
Children	230	749	2267	3310

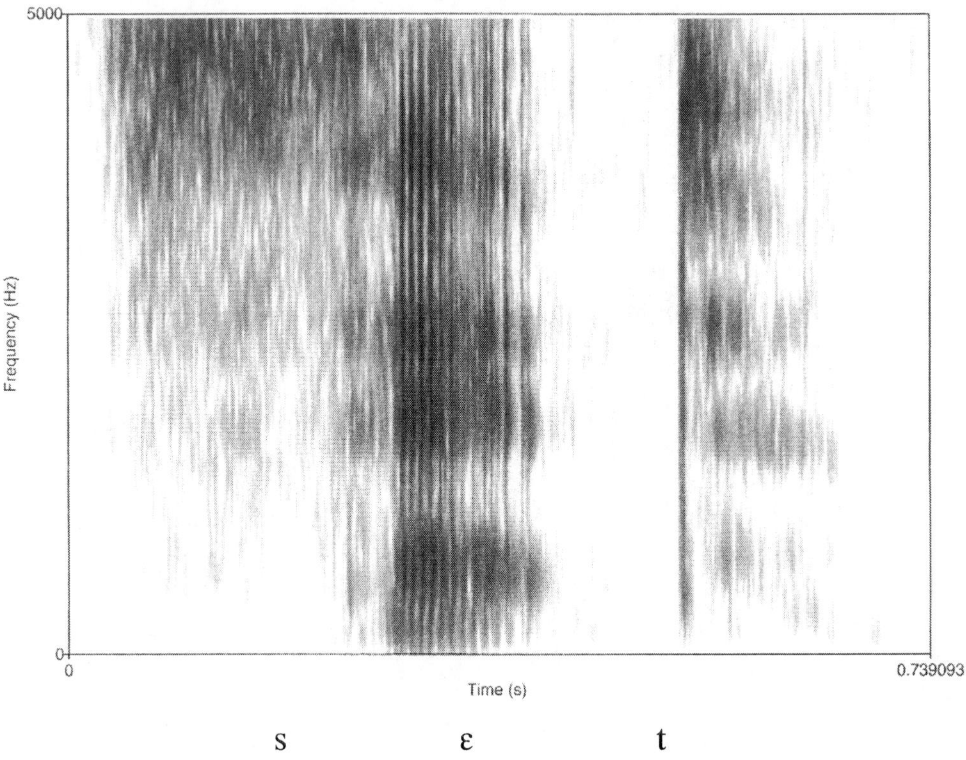

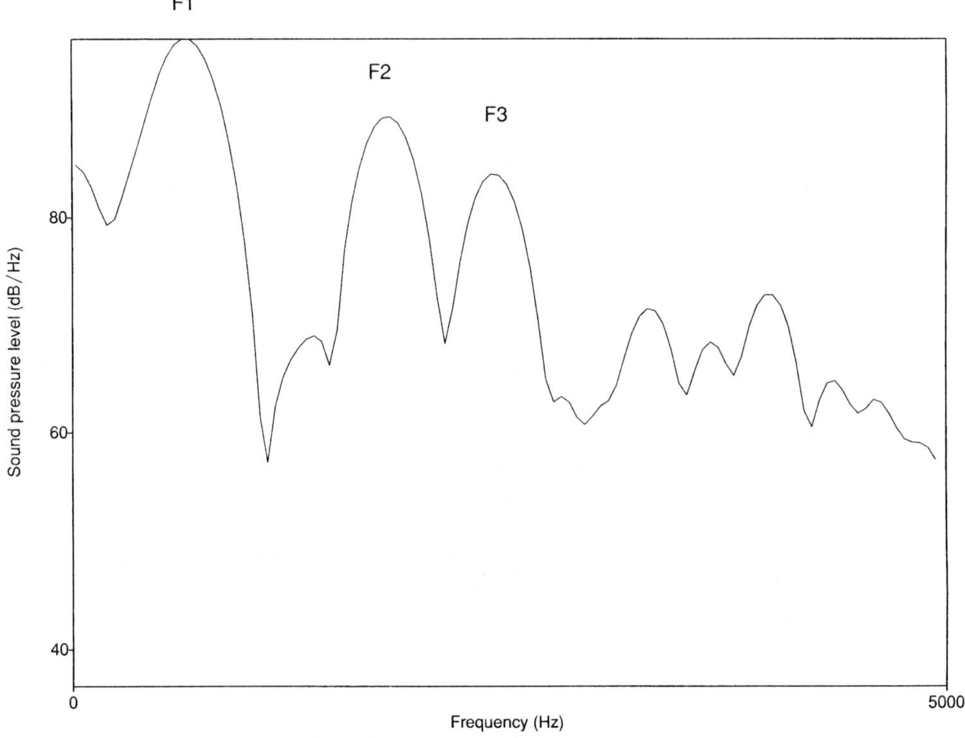

FIG 11.6. Wideband spectrogram and spectrum of the vowel in "set."

Spelling

The most common spelling of /æ/ is

<a> bad lamp apple

Other, less common, spellings also occur:

<ai> plaid
<ua> guarantee
<i> meringue timbre

Some spellings are found in only very few words:

<ei> reveille

Note: Some of the spellings noted above can represent other vowels, and so may be listed in other entries.

For the usual allophone of this phoneme the highest point of the tongue arch is lowered to the lowest frontest position possible for a vowel. The rear side rims of the tongue may make light contact with the inner surfaces of the upper side teeth. The tongue is lax during the production of this vowel (but tenser than for /ɪ/ or /ɛ/), which belongs to the group of short vowels (although it is noticeably longer than the other lax vowels). The lip shape for the vowel is neutrally open. In terms of the cardinal vowel system, English /æ/ would be plotted onto the vowel chart as seen in Fig. 11.7, and with the symbolization [a̝] or [ɛ̞]; in current RP the vowel is nearer to cardinal vowel 4.

The following are the main allophones of /æ/:

- [æ] full length vowel, found before voiced consonants (e.g., "had").
- [æ̆] reduced length vowel, found before voiceless consonants (e.g., "hat").
- [æᵊ] slight centralizing glide, found before dark-l (e.g., "scalp").
- GA not RP [æ̝̃] raised and nasalized allophone found before nasal consonants (e.g., "hand"), although note that the vowel does not become as raised as /ɛ/ (compare "man" and "men"). Less nasalization and no raising occurs after a nasal consonant ("gnat").

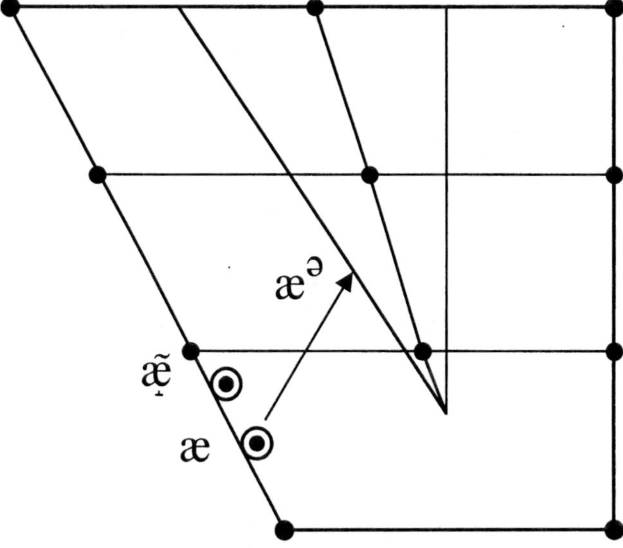

FIG 11.7. Cardinal vowel values of the main allophones of /æ/.

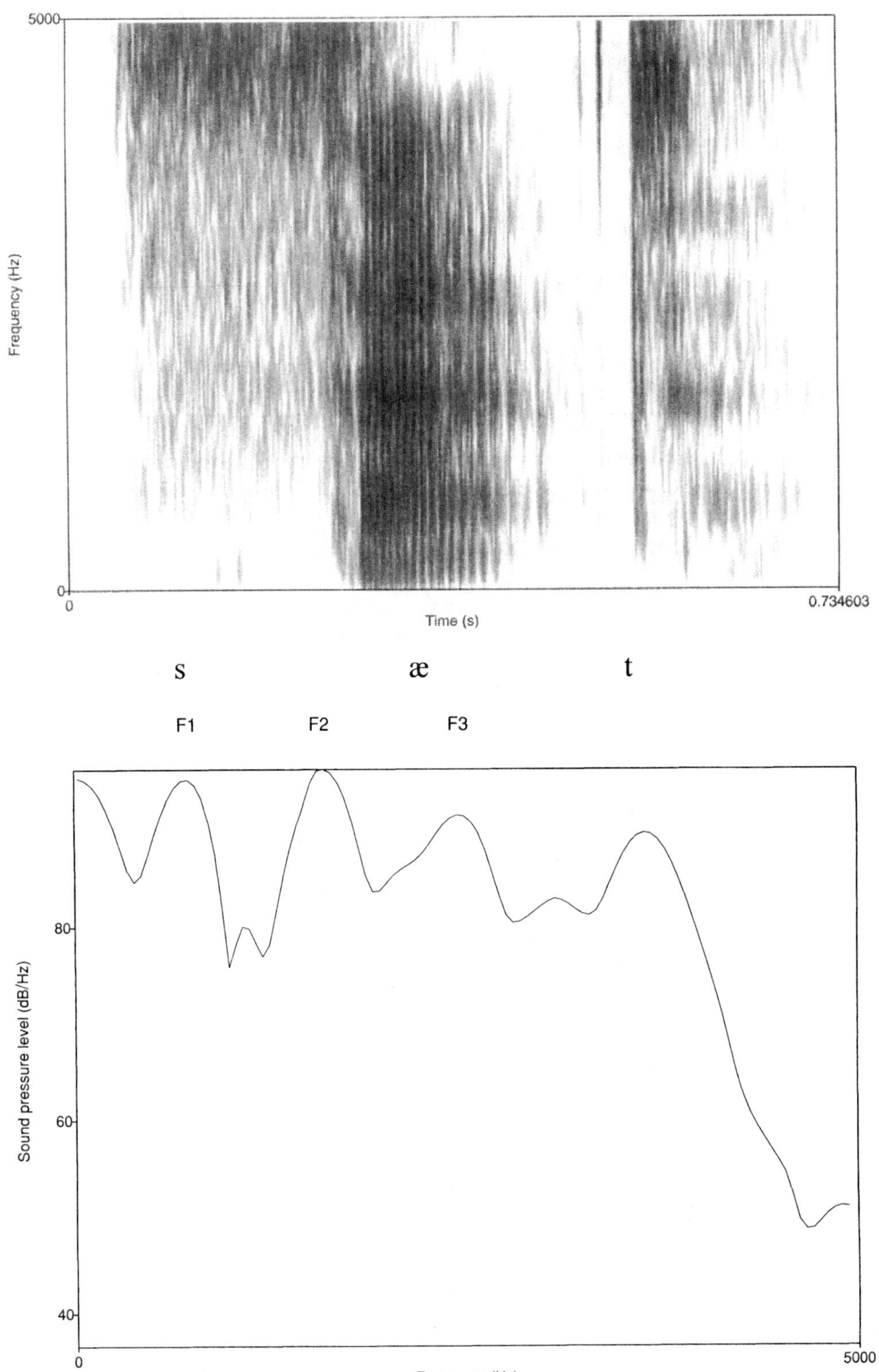

FIG 11.8. Wideband spectrogram and spectrum of the vowel in "sat."

TABLE 11.4
Typical Formant Values for /æ/

	F0	*F1*	*F2*	*F3*
Men	123	588	1952	2601
Women	215	669	2349	2972
Children	228	717	2501	3289

Figure 11.8 shows a spectrogram of the vowel /æ/ in the word "sat," together with a spectrum of the vowel taken halfway through the duration of the vowel. Table 11.4 gives typical values for the F0 and F1–F3 of /æ/ in men, women and children.

THE LOWER BACK VOWELS

The two lower back vowels differ in both lip shape and tenseness. Whereas /ɑ/ is unrounded and tense, /ɔ/ is rounded and more lax. It should be noted that the vowel that some authors treat as a tense back rounded vowel ([o]) is considered in this book as a diphthong ([oʊ]) because its most common realizations are diphthongal. We also include a third low back vowel (/ɒ/) out of strict sequence in terms of the vowel diagram. This vowel is found in RP and some US accents, but not in GA.

The Low Back Tense Vowel

/ɑ/

This vowel is usually described as being a back low tense unrounded vowel. /ɑ/ can occur word-initially, before and after consonants, and word-finally in open syllables. Because the IPA symbol does not represent the same sound as the traditional name of the letter of the alphabet <a>, we suggest calling the symbol "aah" /ɑ/, or "script-a."

Spelling

There are many different ways of spelling /ɑ/; the most common are:

<o> top not (GA)
<a(r)> father car

Other, less common, spellings also occur:

<aa> aardvark
<ua> guardian
<ea> hearth

Some spellings are found in only very few words:

<e> sergeant
<a> spa

Note: /ɑ/ may be used to represent other spellings; see note in spelling box of the next subsection. Also, many of the spellings noted above can represent other vowels, and so may be listed in other entries.

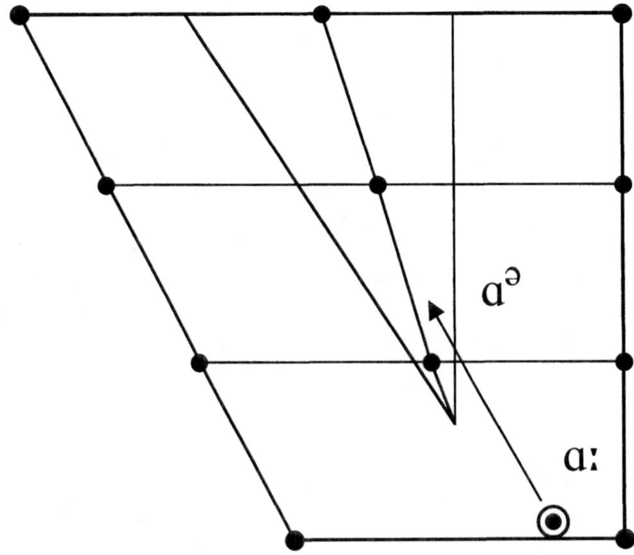

FIG 11.9. Cardinal vowel values of the main allophones of /ɑ/.

The highest point of the tongue arch is lowered to a position slightly in front of the lowest, backest position possible for a vowel to make the most common allophone of this phoneme. The side rims of the tongue make no contact with the inner surfaces of the upper side teeth. The tongue is tense during the production of this vowel, which belongs to the group of long vowels. The lip shape for the vowel is neutrally open. In terms of the cardinal vowel system, English /ɑ/ would be plotted onto the vowel chart as seen in Fig. 11.9, and with the symbolization [ɑ+]

The following are the main allophones of /ɑ/:

- [ɑː] full length vowel, found in open syllables and before voiced consonants (e.g., "spa," "pod" GA).
- [ɑˑ] reduced length vowel, found before voiceless consonants (e.g., "pot" GA; "part" RP).
- [ɑᵊ] very slight centralizing glide, found before dark-l (e.g., "Paul" GA; "marl" RP).
- [ɑ̃] nasalized allophone found before nasal consonants (e.g., "sawn" GA; "carn" RP). Less nasalization occurs after a nasal consonant ("mark").

Figure 11.10 shows a spectrogram of the vowel /ɑ/ in the word "shah," together with a spectrum of the vowel taken halfway through the duration of the vowel. Table 11.5 shows typical values for the F0 and F1–F3 of /ɑ/ in men, women, and children.

There is considerable variation in the use of /ɑ/ and /ɔ/ in many words; see the discussion at the end of the following subsection.

TABLE 11.5
Typical Formant Values for /ɑ/

	F0	*F1*	*F2*	*F3*
Men	123	768	1333	2522
Women	215	936	1551	2815
Children	229	1002	1688	2950

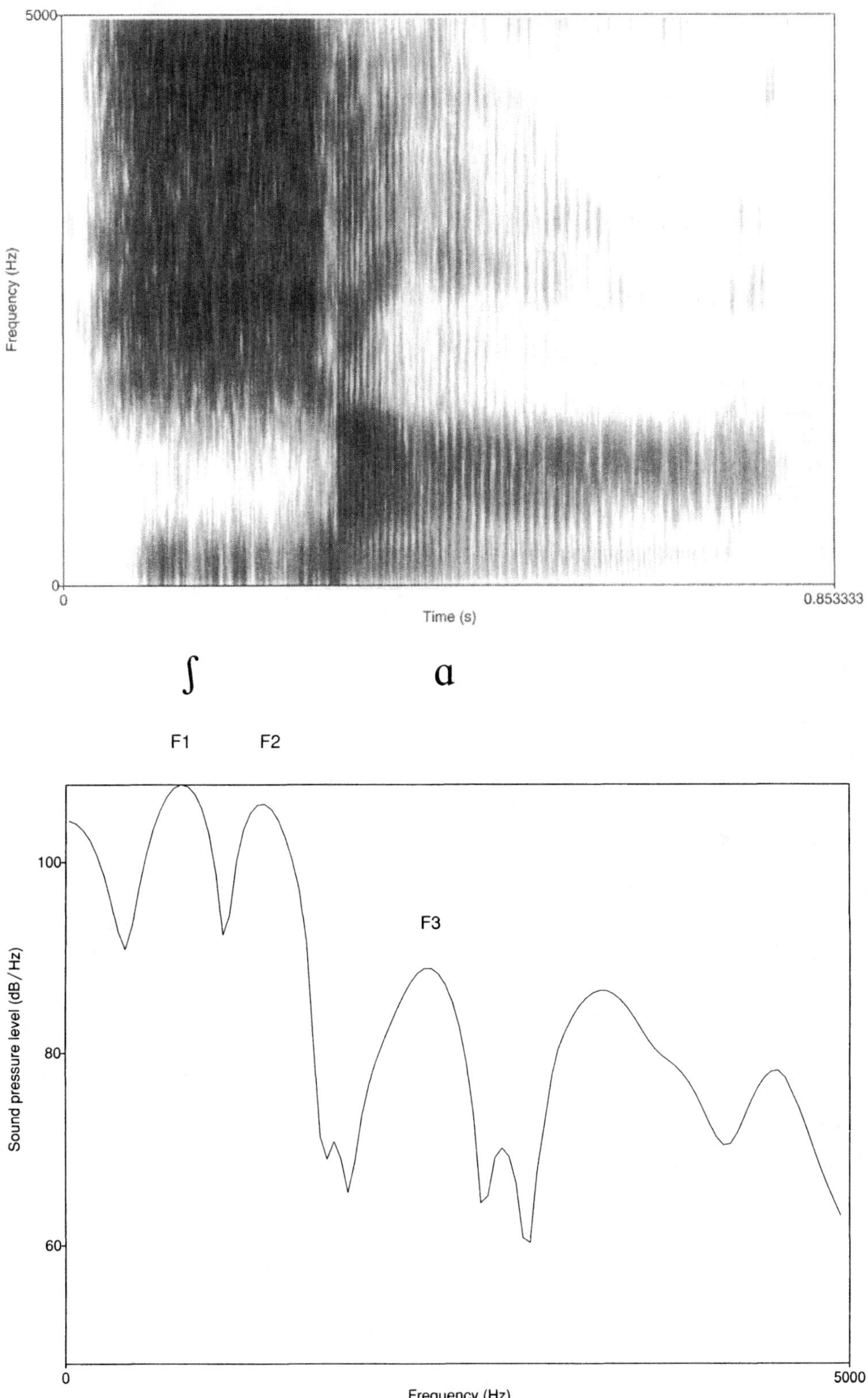

FIG 11.10. Wideband spectrogram and spectrum of the vowel in "shah."

The Mid Back Vowel

/ɔ/

This vowel is usually described as being a half-low back rounded vowel. /ɔ/ can occur word-initially, before and after consonants, and word-finally in open syllables. Although some authorities class the vowel as lax, it is tenser and longer than most other lax vowels. We suggest calling the symbol "aw" /ɔ/, or "open-o."

Spelling

The most common spellings of /ɔ/ are:

<o>	cloth	off (not-RP)
<au>	cause	author
<augh>	daughter	taught
<aw>	saw	yawn
<a>	tall	talk
<ough>	thought	ought

Other spellings with following <r> also occur:

<ar>	war
<or>	torn more
<our>	court
<oar>	boar
<oor>	door

Note: This vowel is subject to much variation, and so some speakers of GA may use different vowels for these examples. Also, many of the spellings noted above can represent other vowels, and so may be listed in other entries.

The primary allophone of this phoneme is produced as follows: The highest point of the tongue arch is raised to a position about a quarter of the way up from the lowest backest position possible for a vowel. The side rims of the tongue make no contact with the inner surfaces of the upper side teeth. The tongue is probably more tense than lax during the production of this vowel, which belongs to the group of long vowels. The lip shape for the vowel is open rounded. In terms of the cardinal vowel system, English /ɔ/ would be plotted onto the vowel chart as seen in Fig. 11.11, and, being very close to cardinal vowel 6, can be symbolized as [ɔ]. The most common allophone of this vowel in RP is higher, being about halfway between cardinal vowels 6 and 7.

The following are the main allophones of /ɔ/:

- [ɔː] full length vowel, found before voiced consonants and in open syllables (e.g., "cawed," "caw").
- [ɔˑ] reduced length vowel, found before voiceless consonants (e.g., "caught").
- [ɔᵊ] slight centralizing glide, found before dark-l (e.g., "ball"), imperceptible in many speakers.
- [ɔ̃] nasalized allophone found before nasal consonants (e.g., "pawn"). Less nasalization occurs after a nasal consonant ("nor").

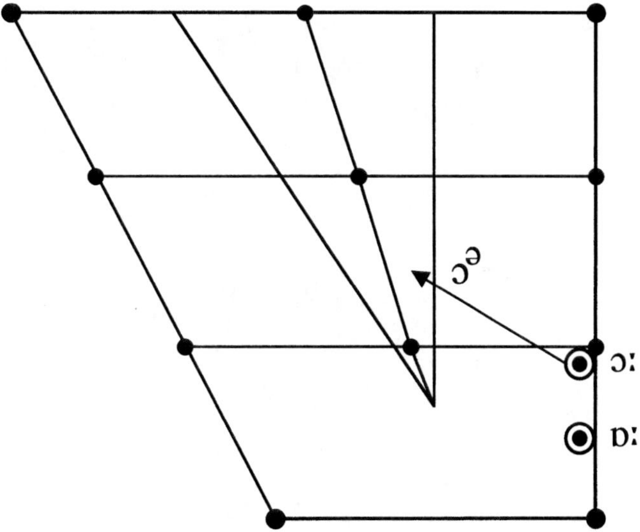

FIG 11.11. Cardinal vowel values of the main allophones of /ɔ/.

Figure 11.12 shows a spectrogram of the vowel /ɔ/ in the word "saw," together with a spectrum of the vowel taken halfway through the duration of the vowel. Table 11.6 gives typical values for the F0 and F1–F3 of /ɔ/ in men, women, and children.

As we noted earlier, the usage of this vowel is subject to variation in American English. While most of the spellings with following <r> use the /ɔ/ vowel, the majority of the other spellings can be pronounced with /ɑ/. In some areas, a laxer, lower, rounded realization ([ɒ]) may be used for some of the non-<r> spellings. This last vowel is phonemically distinct in British and some southern and eastern accents of American English (e.g., "cot" ~ "caught" /kɒt/ ~ /kɔt/); see the next subsection. Finally, we can note that some words with following <r> (e.g., "four") have a variant pronunciation with [o], an allophone of /oʊ/ (see chap. 12). We return to regional differences with this vowel in chapter 18.

The Low Back Rounded Vowel (RP)

/ɒ/

This vowel is usually described as being a low back rounded vowel. /ɒ/ can occur word-initially, before and after consonants, but not word-finally in open syllables. This is a lax vowel. We suggest calling the symbol "ɒ" /ɒ/, or "turned-a."

TABLE 11.6
Typical Formant Values for /ɔ/

	F0	*F1*	*F2*	*F3*
Men	121	652	997	2538
Women	210	781	1136	2824
Children	225	803	1210	2982

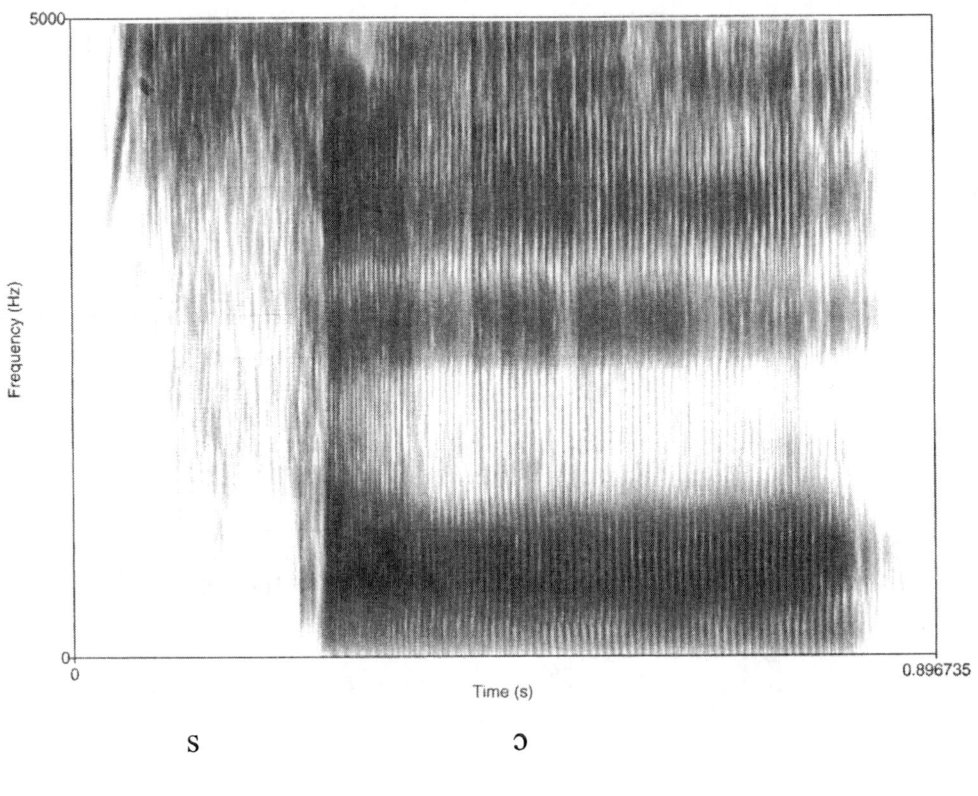

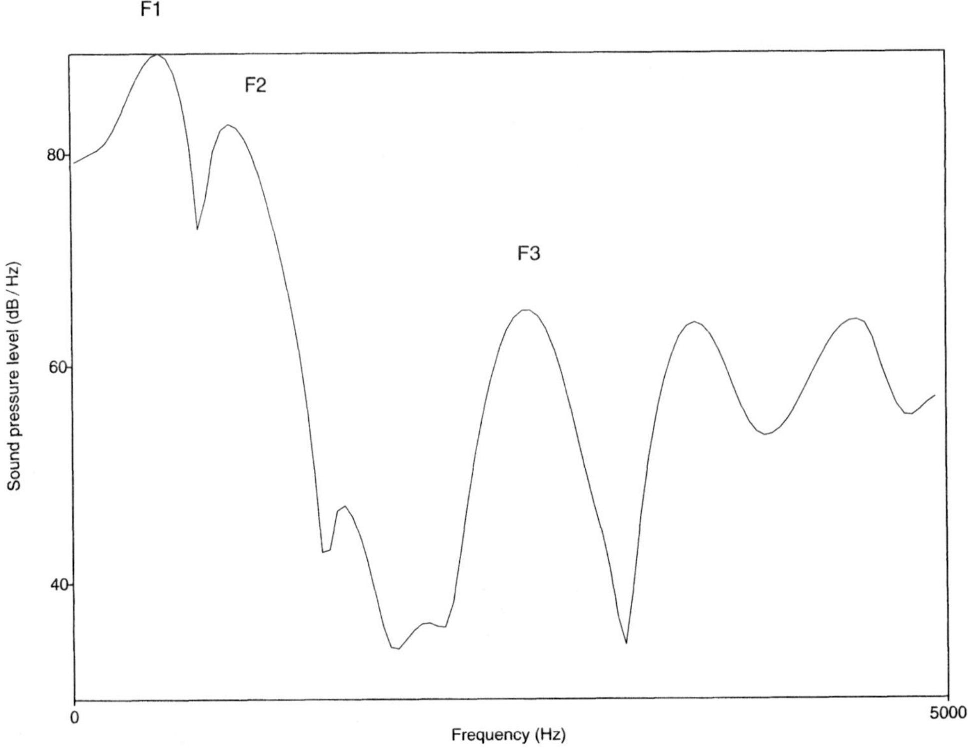

FIG 11.12. Wideband spectrogram and spectrum of the vowel in "saw."

Spelling

The most common spellings of /ɒ/ are:

<o> cloth off dog gone
<a> was what swan
<ou> cough
<ow> knowledge
<au> because laurel
<a> yacht

Note: Also, many of the spellings noted above can represent other vowels, and so may be listed in other entries.

For the commonest allophone of this phoneme the highest point of the tongue arch is lowered to a position close to the lowest, backest position possible for a vowel. The side rims of the tongue make no contact with the inner surfaces of the upper side teeth. The tongue is lax during the production of this vowel, which belongs to the group of short vowels. The lip shape for the vowel is open rounded. In terms of the cardinal vowel system, English /ɒ/ would be plotted onto the vowel chart as seen in Fig. 11.13, and with the symbolization [ɒ].

The following are the main allophones of /ɒ/:

- [ɒ] full length vowel, found before voiced consonants (e.g., "dog").
- [ɒ̆] reduced length vowel, found before voiceless consonants (e.g., "dock").
- [ɒ^{ə}] slight centralizing glide, found before dark-l (e.g., "doll"), imperceptible in many speakers.
- [ɒ̃] nasalized allophone found before nasal consonants (e.g., "Don"). Less nasalization occurs after a nasal consonant ("nod").

Figure 11.14 shows a spectrogram of the vowel /ɒ/ in the word "sot," together with a spectrum of the vowel taken halfway through the duration of the vowel. Studies on American

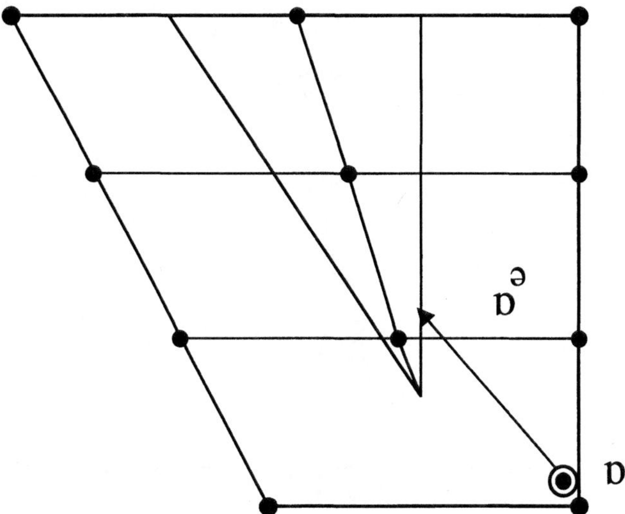

FIG 11.13. Cardinal vowel values of the main allophones of /ɒ/.

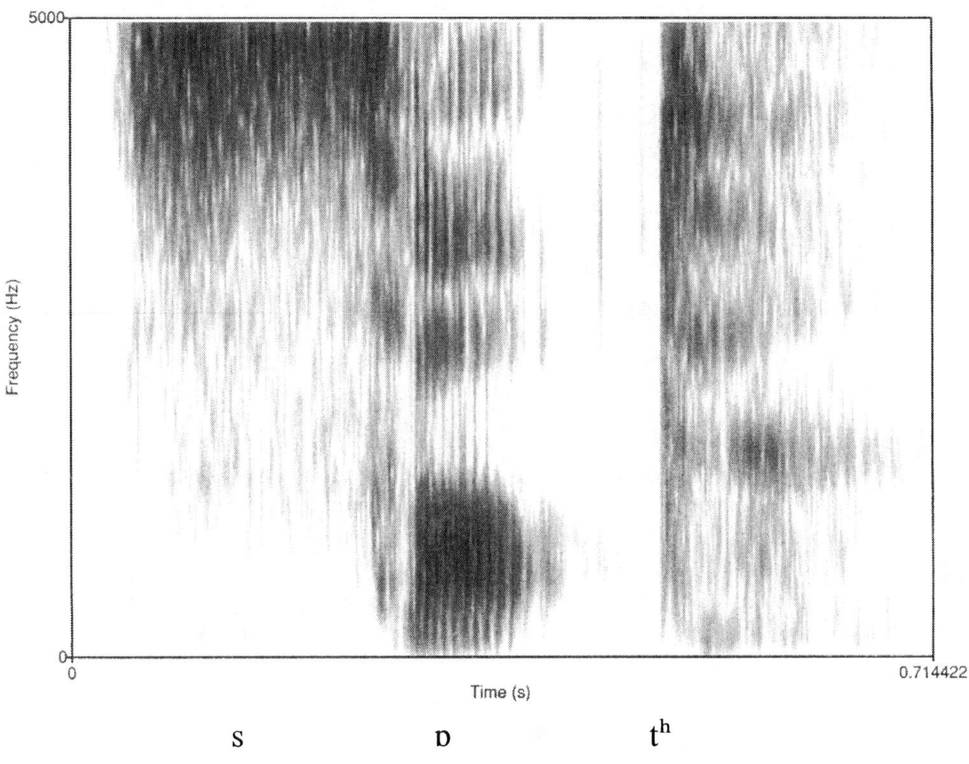

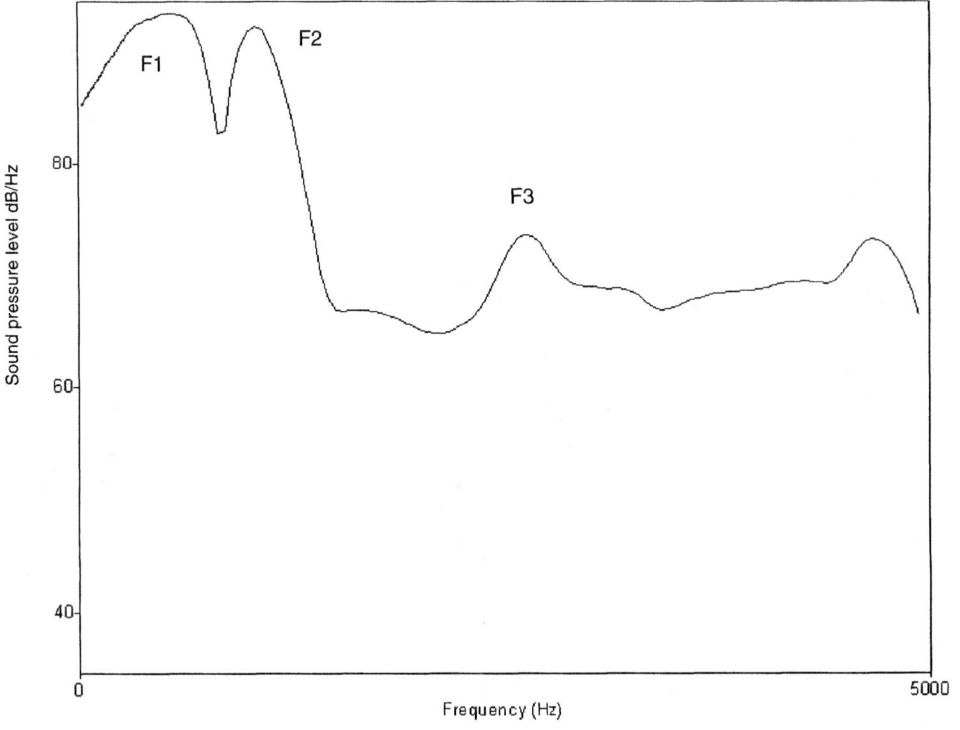

FIG 11.14. Wideband spectrogram and spectrum of the vowel in "sot."

TABLE 11.7
Typical Formant Values for /ɒ/

	F1	*F2*
Men	593	866
Women	602	994

English acoustics have, naturally, not included formant values for /ɒ/, so the data on values for F1–F2 of /ɒ/ in men and women in Table 11.7 are taken from Deterding (1997).

THE HIGH BACK VOWELS

The high back vowel pair consist of one tense and one lax vowel, and these are directly symmetrical to the two high front vowels.

The High Back Lax Vowel

/ʊ/

This vowel is usually described as being a high back lax rounded vowel. /ʊ/ cannot occur word-initially, but can before and after consonants, although not word-finally in open syllables. The symbol for this sound is derived from the Greek alphabet and can be called "oo" /ʊ/, or "upsilon."

Spelling
The most common ways of spelling /ʊ/ are:

<u> put butcher
<oo> book foot
<ou> could should

We also find:

<o> wolf woman

Note: Many of the spellings noted above can represent other vowels, and so may be listed in other entries.

The highest point of the tongue arch is positioned substantially in front of and below the highest frontest position possible for a vowel to produce the most frequently occuring allophone of this phoneme. The side rims of the tongue make no contact with the inner surfaces of the upper side teeth. The tongue is lax during the production of this vowel, which belongs to the group of short vowels. The lip shape for the vowel is closely and loosely rounded. In terms of the cardinal vowel system, English /ʊ/ would be plotted onto the vowel chart as seen in Figure 11.15, and with the symbolization [ŭ]. Some speakers produce a more centralized vowel.

The following are the main allophones of /ʊ/:

- [ʊ] full length vowel, found before voiced consonants (e.g., "hood").
- [ʊ̆] reduced length vowel, found before voiceless consonants (e.g., "put").

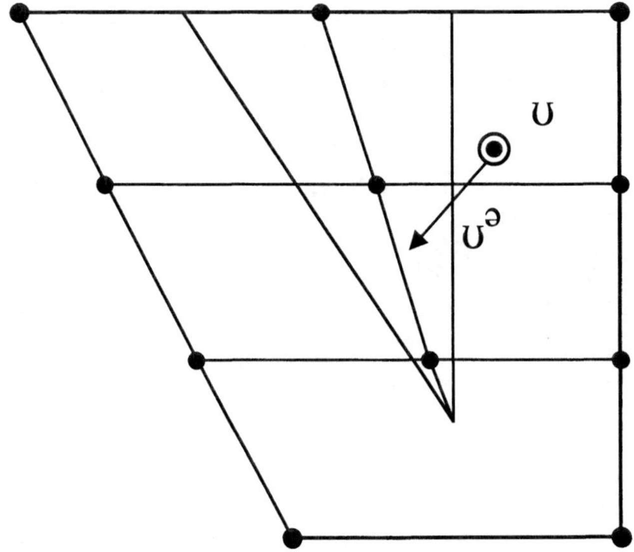

FIG 11.15. Cardinal vowel values of the main allophones of /ʊ/.

- [ʊᵊ] slight centralizing glide, found before dark-l (e.g., "bull"), imperceptible in many speakers.
- [ʊ̃] nasalized allophone found before nasal consonants (e.g., "woman").

Note, we use the vowel symbol /ʊ/ followed by /ɹ/ in rhotic contexts such as "tour" /tʊɹ/.

Figure 11.16 shows a spectrogram of the vowel /ʊ/ in the word "soot," together with a spectrum of the vowel taken halfway through the duration of the vowel. Table 11.8 gives typical values for the F0 and F1–F3 of /ʊ/ in men, women, and children.

The High Back Tense Vowel

/u/

This vowel is usually described as being a high back tense rounded vowel. /u/ can occur word-initially, before and after consonants, and word-finally in open syllables. Because the IPA symbol does not represent the same sounds as the traditional name of the letter of the alphabet <u>, we suggest calling the symbol "uu" /u/.

TABLE 11.8
Typical Formant Values for /ʊ/

	F0	*F1*	*F2*	*F3*
Men	133	469	1122	2434
Women	230	519	1225	2827
Children	243	568	1490	3072

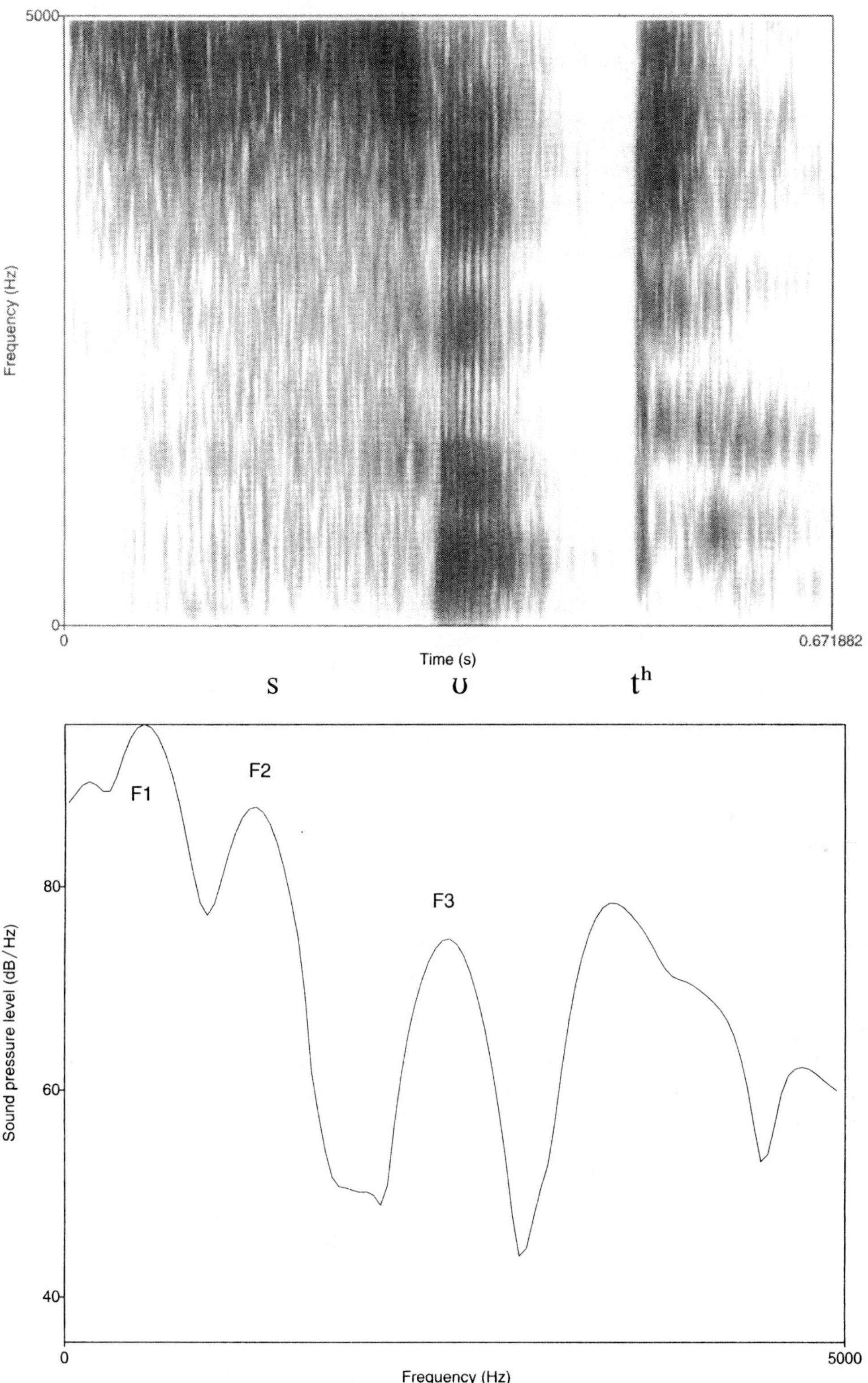

FIG 11.16. Wideband spectrogram and spectrum of the vowel in "soot."

Spelling

There are many different ways of spelling /u/, the most common are:

<u> (often with silent <e> after the consonant) crude crucial
<oo> soon food
<o> (often with silent <e> after the consonant) do prove
<ou> group

Other, less common, spellings also occur:

<oe> shoe
<ew> new
<ue> blue
<ui> juice
<ough> through
<wo> two

Note: Many of the spellings noted above can represent other vowels, and so may be listed in other entries.

The primary allophone of this phoneme is produced in the following way: The highest point of the tongue arch is raised to a position slightly in front of and below the highest backest position possible for a vowel. The side rims of the tongue make no contact with the inner surfaces of the upper side teeth. The tongue is tense during the production of this vowel, which belongs to the group of long vowels. The lip shape for the vowel is close rounded. In terms of the cardinal vowel system, English /u/ would be plotted onto the vowel chart as seen in Fig. 11.17, and with the symbolization [u̥+].

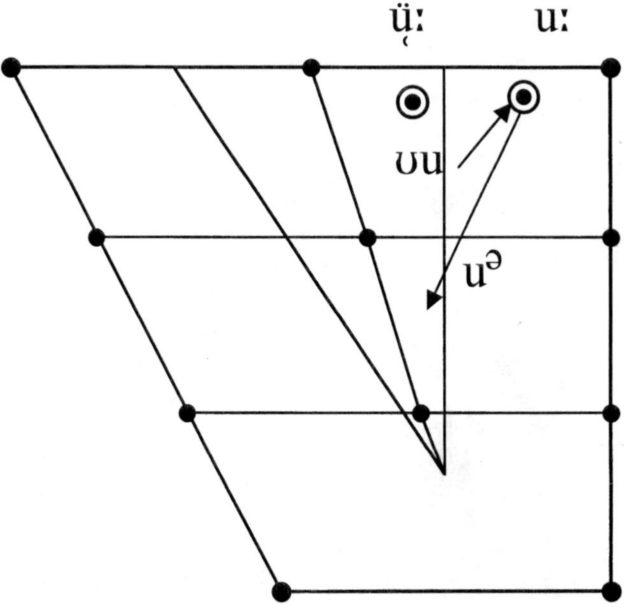

FIG 11.17. Cardinal vowel values of the main allophones of /u/.

TABLE 11.9
Typical Formant Values for /u/

	F0	*F1*	*F2*	*F3*
Men	143	300	997	2343
Women	235	459	1105	2735
Children	249	494	1345	2988

The following are the main allophones of /u/:

- [uː] full length vowel, found in open syllables and before voiced consonants (e.g., "sue," "sued").
- [uˑ] reduced length vowel, found before voiceless consonants (e.g., "suit").
- [ʊu] or [uʊ] vowel with diphthongal quality, variant realization in open syllables.
- [uᵊ] slight centralizing glide, found before dark-l (e.g., "rule"), imperceptible in many speakers.
- [ũ] nasalized allophone found before nasal consonants (e.g., "soon"). Less nasalization occurs after a nasal consonant ("moose").
- [ṵ] centralized realization with less rounding. A free variant more commonly heard from younger speakers today.

Figure 11.18 shows a spectrogram of the vowel /u/ in the word "sue," together with a spectrum of the vowel taken halfway through the duration of the vowel. Table 11.9 provides typical values for the F0 and F1–F3 of /u/ in men, women and children.

TRANSCRIPTION

In the exercises to this and following chapters, and in the exercises on the audio CD for these chapters, you will be called upon to transcribe English into phonetic symbols. In part I of the book, transcription exercises were mainly concerned with examples that were not English (or any language in most cases); those examples were to test your abilities to perceive sound differences. However, in this part we are specifically interested in English, and so that is what you will be transcribing for the most part.

When we transcribe a specific language, we can take two different approaches. We can concentrate on transcribing at a phonemic level or a phonetic level. Phonemic transcription requires us to note only the phoneme units used by the speaker; we do not write down the actual (allophonic) realizations of those phonemes. Taking an example from this chapter, in transcribing the words "seat" and "seed" we would write /sit/ and /sid/, not [siˑt] and [siːd]. In other words, the vowel length differences would be ignored because, if we know the rules of English phonology and if the speaker is abiding by those rules, the vowel length differences are predictable and do not need to be marked. This sort of transcription, then, is well suited to the speech of speakers who are using a phonology that is already recorded in detail, so that we can extract the actual realizations of the phoneme symbols by accessing the rules of the language or dialect in question.

Of course, if we are investigating a previously unanalyzed language, or perhaps a dialect of English that has not been closely studied, then we need to use as detailed a transcription as possible (often termed a *narrow* transcription) so that we can get the information we need to work out the phonemes and allophones of the variety being studied. Such narrow phonetic

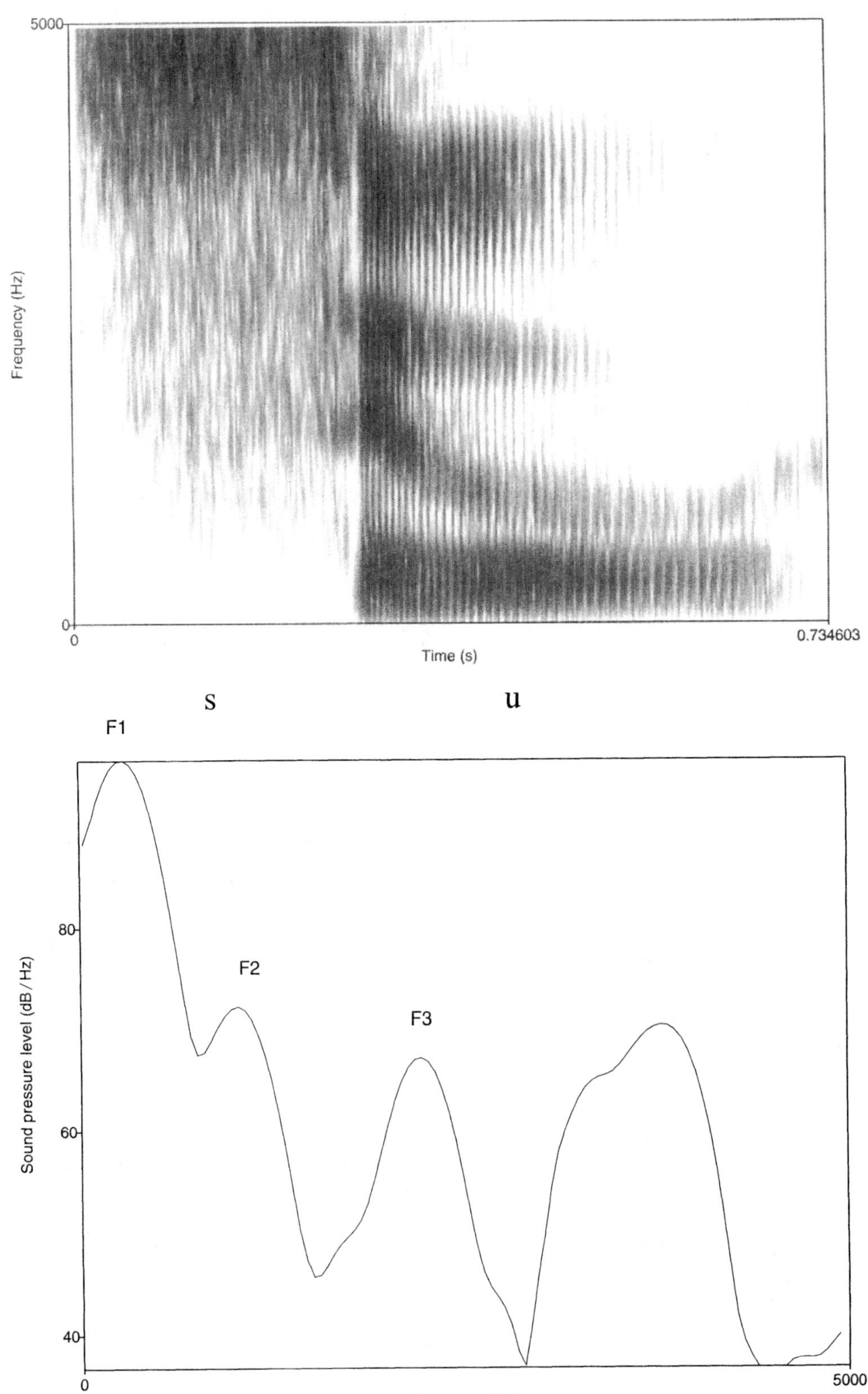

FIG 11.18. Wideband spectrogram and spectrum of the vowel in "sue."

transcriptions provide the building blocks of a phonological analysis that in turn gives us the phonemes of the variety.

Where does transcription in the speech clinic fit in? Clearly, if our clients used the normal phoneme system of their target language, then they would not require the resources of a speech clinic. We must assume, therefore, that they have problems at some level or other of their pronunciation. We cannot guess in advance what these are. This means that we must undertake as narrow and detailed a phonetic transcription as we can to discover where their problems lie. For example, if a child has a problem with vowel nasalization (perhaps using excessive nasalization even with no nasal consonant in the immediate context), transcribing this at a phonemic level without the nasal diacritic does not tell us a great deal: in fact, it would make the speech look normal.

The ability to transcribe narrowly is aided if you have started transcribing (as we have in this book) through a wide range of sounds, including those not found in your native language. To develop the ability to transcribe English narrowly we first start with mainly phonemic transcription. That means that most of the exercises in part II require you to transcribe into phonemic symbols using slant brackets. However, we do introduce some phonetic level transcription as we progress, where you will need to transcribe allophonic usage, within square brackets. The instructions to each task will make it clear what is required. In part III, the exercises will be mostly at the phonetic level and will include disordered and atypical speech sounds. An absolute rule in transcribing is that you should *never* transcribe first into ordinary orthography; doing so means that you lose time, and you may well guess wrongly what a client is actually trying to say, and so end up being distracted and confused in terms of the pronunciation you've heard.

BACKGROUND READING

Possibly the best in-depth treatment of English phonetics and phonology is Cruttenden (2001). Although this book deals primarily with British English, it does also cover American norms. Students may wish to consult a pronouncing dictionary. We recommend Wells (2000) and Landau (2000), though readers should be warned that neither follows exactly the choice of symbols we make, and they should, therefore, check the keys of these dictionaries carefully before using them.

EXERCISES

Transcription

(Answers to the transcription exercises are given at the end of the book.)

1. Transcribe the following into phonemic symbols using either GA or RP norms. These words use the vowels from this chapter, and some simple consonants. Note: We transcribe <r> as /ɹ/; RP does not use postvocalic-r.
   (a) need (b) writ
   (c) door (d) cool
   (e) foot (f) kept
   (g) bat (h) stop
   (i) tune (j) meat
   (k) head (l) paw
   (m) lamb (n) build
   (o) put (p) hot

2. Transcribe the following using either GA or RP norms, employing allophonic symbols to mark vowel length differences, nasalization, and centralizing before /l/, where appropriate.
   (a) feed (b) feat
   (c) queen (d) boot
   (e) fool (f) bell
   (g) bat (h) bad
   (i) booed (j) tin
   (k) spoon (l) awl
   (m) send (n) build
   (o) feel (p) hill
3. Convert the following GA transcriptions back into ordinary writing. (They all have more than one possible spelling—try to list all these.)
   (a) /nɑt/ (b) /sin/
   (c) /lɛd/ (d) /flu/
   (e) /ænt/ (f) /wʊd/
   (g) /nɪt/ (h) /sɔɹ/

Review Questions

1. What is vowel shortening, and where does it occur?
2. What is the difference between tense and lax vowels? Which vowels described in this chapter are tense and which are lax?
3. What context produces vowel centralization, and why does this happen?
4. List at least three spellings of vowels (either single letters or combinations of two letters) that can represent two or more different vowel phonemes.

Study Topics and Experiments

1. Either:
   (GA) Record yourself and your friends speaking words with "-aw," "-augh," and "-all" (e.g., "law," "caught," and "hall"). Find at least 10 different words and at least 6 speakers. Then check to see whether your speakers use /ɔ/ or /ɑ/ in these words. Are they consistent, or do some speakers switch from one vowel to the other?
   Or:
   (RP) Record yourself and your friends speaking words with "-ath," "-augh," and "-ance" (e.g., "path," "laugh," and "dance"). Find at least 10 different words and at least 6 speakers. Then check to see whether your speakers use /ɑ/ or /æ/ in these words. Are they consistent, or do some speakers switch from one vowel to the other?
2. Record yourself speaking all the vowels described in this chapter, and analyze the first three formants of each vowel using speech analysis software. How do your values compare to those listed in the chapter?

CD

Listen to the examples of different English vowels, and try to identify the test examples following the instructions on the CD. Answers to all the exercises on the CD are given at the end of the book.

12

English Central Vowels and Diphthongs

INTRODUCTION

In this chapter we continue our survey of the vocalic system of English started in chapter 11. Here, we turn our attention first to the central vowels, and then deal with the diphthongs. The central vowels fall into two groups, the nonrhotic (/ʌ/, /ə/) and the rhotic (/ɝ/, /ɚ/), each group having two phonemes. Interestingly, in each pair, one vowel occurs only in stressed syllables, whereas the other appears only in unstressed ones. Let us first consider the rhotic feature. As we noted in chapter 5, rhotic, or r-colored, vowels involve a raising (and possibly slight retroflexion) of the tongue tip during the production of the vowel, or a bunching of the tongue body (bunching is described in detail in chapter 15). We treat these vowels, then, not as a sequence of vowel+/ɹ/, but as a vowel with the /ɹ/ already built in, as it were. Why do we do this for the two central rhotic vowels, but not for any other vowels of English when followed by /ɹ/? Part of the reason is that the required tongue position for an /ɹ/ is very close to that for a central vowel, so that by raising the tongue tip when in the central vowel position, an /ɹ/-like quality is easy to add. When the tongue is in position for the front or back vowels, an /ɹ/-like quality is not so easy to add by simply curling up the tongue tip. So, with these vowels, the tongue adopts the normal vowel position and later moves into the right position and shape for /ɹ/. Therefore, in these cases we consider that we have a sequence of vowel plus /ɹ/.

Perhaps more of a problem is why we list separate vowels for stressed and unstressed syllables. It could be argued that these pairs of vowels could be treated as allophones of single vowel: one allophone for stressed syllables and one for unstressed ones. The reasons differ for the two groups. With the nonrhotics, /ʌ/ has a different tongue position than /ə/ (at least, it did originally, although for many speakers the tongue positions have become closer). Also, /ə/ has a very wide usage as a variant phoneme for many other vowels in nonemphatic pronunciation (compare emphatic "and" /ænd/ with nonemphatic /ən/), a point we return to in more detail in chapter 16. Because /ʌ/ has no similar role, it has been thought easiest to class the two vowels as separate phonemes.

In the case of the rhotics the situation is a little different. Both /ɝ/ and /ɚ/ have identical tongue positions and differ mainly in duration, so it would seem to be easier to class them together. However, there are a small number of minimal pairs that (at least for some speakers) contrast them. For example, if we compare the pronunciation of "foreword" /fɔɹwɝd/ with that of "forward" /fɔɹwɚd/, we can see the necessity of keeping these two vowels as separate phonemes.

Diphthongs, as we noted in chapter 5, are vocalic glides of the tongue, where we note the starting and finishing points and assume a smooth movement between the two. Diphthongs are completed within a single syllable, and so differ from the juxtaposition of two vowels across a syllable boundary; diphthongs are counted as single vowel phonemes of the language. In this chapter we divide the diphthongs into those with a mid starting position, those with a low starting position, and the one diphthong that crosses from back to front across the vowel area. We also include the centering diphthongs that are found in nonrhotic accents such as RP.

As in chapter 11, acoustic data on vowel formants is given. Some of this is based on work by Peterson and Barney (1952) and Hillenbrand et al. (1995); and for those vowels not dealt with by these authors we provide data from Cruttenden (2001). In each case, the dark bands on the spectrogram and the peaks on the spectrum clearly show the formant structure of the vowel.

For all the vowel variants described in this chapter, the vocal folds vibrate throughout the production of the vowel, producing voiced phonation; the soft palate is raised so that it blocks off the nasal cavity, resulting in purely oral airflow; and the tongue adopts a convex shape, except for the rhotic vowels, which may have a partly concave shape.

Except in the case of /ʊə/, all the diphthongs we describe can occur word-initially, before and after consonants, and word-finally in open syllables; and they all have a tense tongue during their production, and so belong to the group of long vowels.

THE NONRHOTIC CENTRAL VOWELS

These vowels are both unrounded. Some authorities consider that they are both lax, whereas others note that /ʌ/ is tenser than /ə/.

The Low Nonrhotic Central Vowel

/ʌ/

This vowel is usually described as being a half-low unrounded central vowel. /ʌ/ can occur word-initially, before and after consonants, but not word-finally in open syllables. The IPA symbol is derived from inverting the letter <v>, and we suggest calling the symbol "uh" /ʌ/, or "caret," or "upside-down v."

Spelling

There are many different ways of spelling /ʌ/; the most common are:

<u>	fun	hull	unhappy
<o>	love	other	
<ou>	couple	young	
<oo>	blood	flood	
<oe>	does		

Note: Many of the spellings noted above can represent other vowels, and so may be listed in other entries.

The commonest allophone of this phoneme is produced by raising the highest point of the tongue arch to a position centrally between front and back, and a quarter of the way from the lowest to the highest position. The side rims of the tongue make no contact with the inner

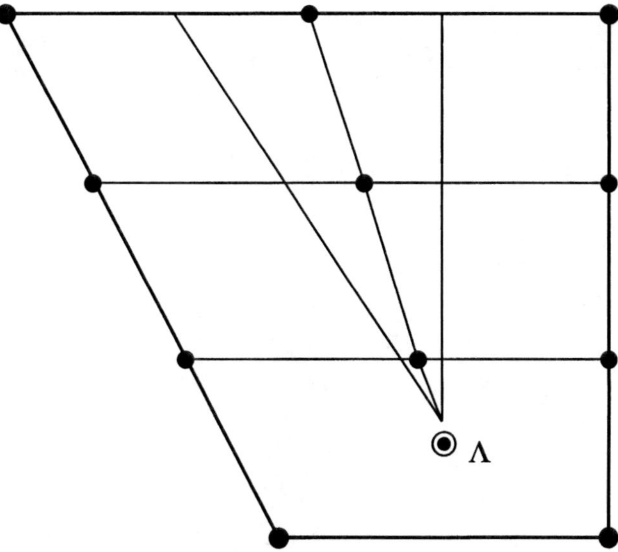

FIG 12.1. Cardinal vowel value of the main allophone of /ʌ/.

surfaces of the upper side teeth. The tongue is somewhat tenser than for schwa during the production of this vowel, which belongs to the group of short vowels. The lip shape for the vowel is neutrally open. In terms of the cardinal vowel system, English /ʌ/ would be plotted onto the vowel chart as seen in Fig. 12.1, and with the symbolization [ä̹]. In IPA terms, the lax vowel symbol [ɐ] would be a more relevant symbol for the current quality of the vowel, but all traditions of English transcription currently use the [ʌ], which reflects more posterior pronunciations found earlier in the last century. For those speakers who use a higher version of /ʌ/, a cardinal vowel notation would be [ʌ̈].

The following are the main allophones of /ʌ/:

- [ʌ] full length vowel, found before voiced consonants (e.g., "bud").
- [ʌ̆] reduced length vowel, found before voiceless consonants (e.g., "but").
- [ʌ̃] nasalized allophone found before nasal consonants (e.g., "sun"). Less nasalization occurs after a nasal consonant ("mug").

Note: No centralizing glides before dark-l are found with central vowels, because they are already in a good position to move to the dark-l position.

Figure 12.2 shows a spectrogram of the vowel /ʌ/ in the word "sud," together with a spectrum of the vowel taken halfway through the duration of the vowel. Table 12.1 gives typical values for the F0 and F1–F3 of /ʌ/ in men, women, and children.

TABLE 12.1
Typical Formant Values for /ʌ/

	F0	*F1*	*F2*	*F3*
Men	133	623	1200	2550
Women	218	753	1426	2933
Children	236	749	1546	3145

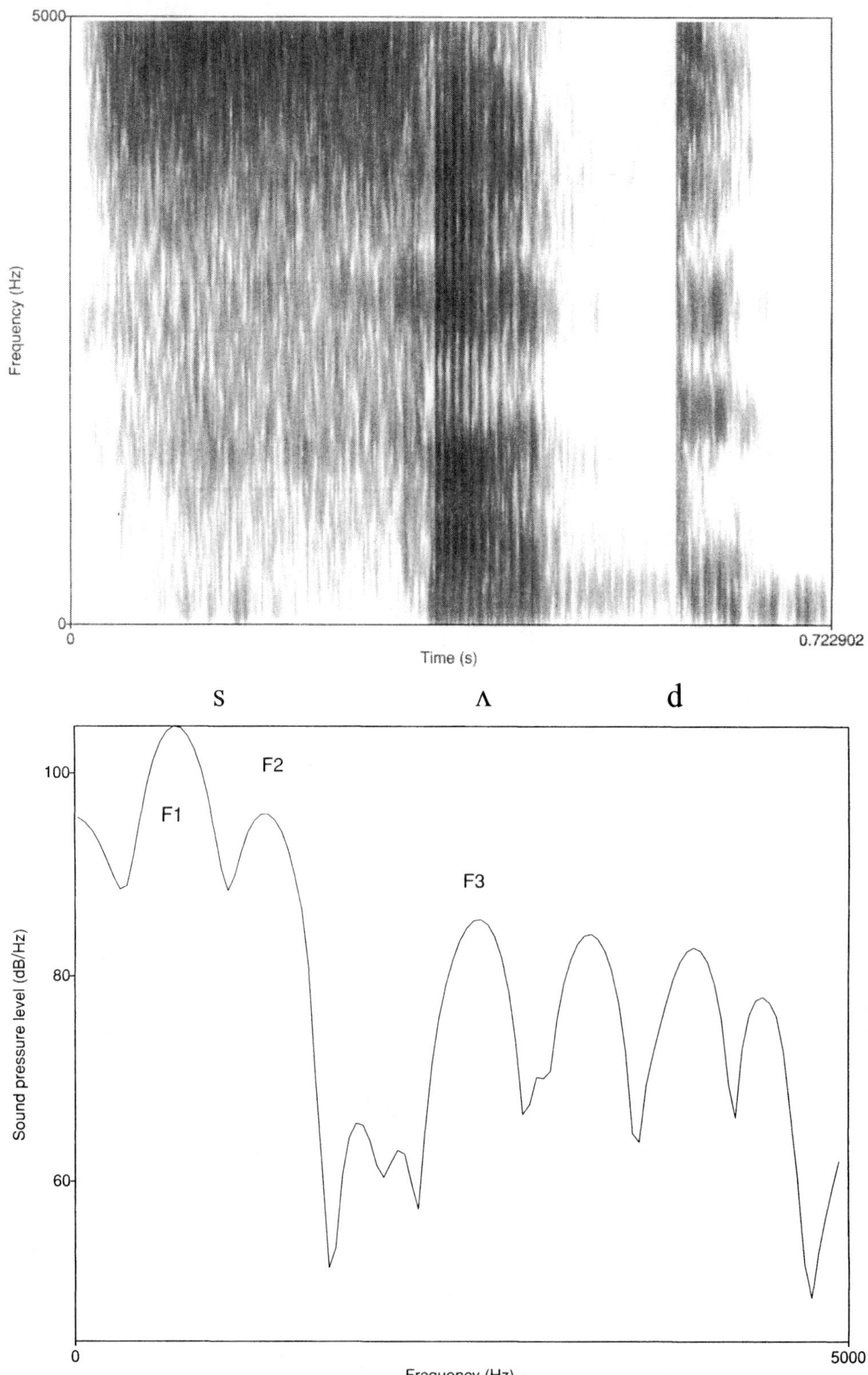

FIG 12.2. Wideband spectrogram and spectrum of the vowel in "sud."

The Mid Nonrhotic Lax Central Vowel

/ə/

This vowel is usually described as being a mid unrounded central vowel. /ə/ can occur word-initially, before and after consonants, and word-finally in open syllables. The IPA symbol is derived from inverting the letter <e>, and its universal name is "schwa" (/ʃwɑ/), derived from the Hebrew name for a similar vowel.

> Spelling
>
> Because historically /ə/ came to be used in unstressed syllables that once had a range of other vowels, and it is used today in connected speech for many other vowels that are still pronounced in emphatic speech, a large number of possible spellings are found. The most common are:
>
> <o> oblige besom
> <a> around woman
> <i> possible
> <e> postmen
> <u> suppose
>
> Other spellings include:
>
> <ou> famous
> <eo> luncheon
> <ie> mischievous
> <ia> parliament
>
> Note: Many of the spellings noted above can represent other vowels, and so may be listed in other entries.

To produce the most frequent allophone of this phoneme the highest point of the tongue arch is positioned centrally between front and back, and midway from the lowest to the highest position (i.e., virtually in the center of the vowel area). The side rims of the tongue make no contact with the inner surfaces of the upper side teeth. The tongue is lax during the production of this vowel, which belongs to the group of short vowels. The lip shape for the vowel is neutrally open. In terms of the cardinal vowel system, English /ə/ would be plotted onto the vowel chart as seen in Fig. 12.3, and with the symbolization [ɜ̝] or [ə̞]. The restriction of /ə/ to unstressed syllables and its very short duration mean that we do not record any length differences connected to following consonant voicing in the allophones.

The following are the main allophones of /ə/:

- [ə] mid central tongue position found in most contexts (e.g., "obey").
- [ə̞] lowered tongue position, found in final open syllables (e.g., "sofa").
- [ə̝] raised tongue position, found before velars (e.g., "agree").
- [ə̃] nasalized allophone found before nasal consonants (e.g., "anew," "second"). Less nasalization occurs after a nasal consonant ("manacle").

Figure 12.4 shows a spectrogram of the vowel /ə/ in the word "destroy," together with a spectrum of the vowel taken halfway through the duration of the vowel. Studies on American English acoustics have generally ignored formant values for /ə/, so the data in

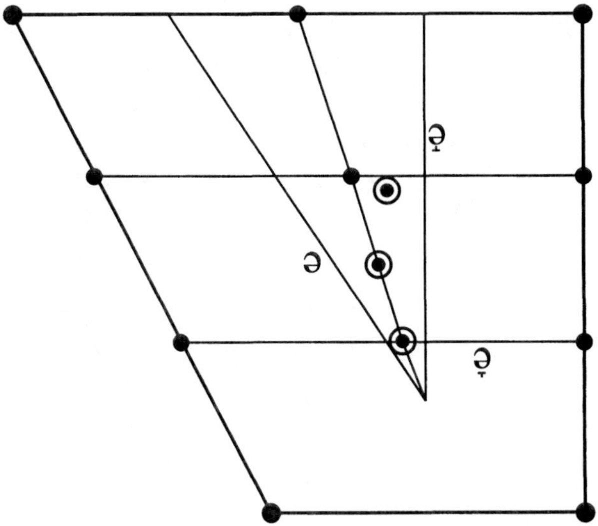

FIG 12.3. Cardinal vowel values of the main allophones of /ə/.

TABLE 12.2
Typical Formant Values for /ə/

	F1	*F2*
Men	478	1436
Women	606	1695

Table 12.2 are taken from Deterding (1997) for the stressed schwa, but will be close enough for the main allophone of schwa. Table 12.2 gives typical values for F1–F2 of /ə/ in men and women.

THE RHOTIC CENTRAL VOWELS, (GA)

These vowels are both unrounded, and both pronounced with tongue tip raising or tongue body bunching. As we noted above, the main difference between these two vowels is one of duration: /ɝ/ is long and tense, while /ɚ/ is short and lax. These rhotic vowels are not found in RP, though similar articulations are found in some British rhotic accents.

The Mid, Long Rhotic Central Vowel

/ɝ/

This vowel is usually described as being a mid, unrounded, long, rhotic central vowel. /ɝ/ can occur word-initially, before and after consonants, and finally in open syllables. The IPA symbol is derived from reversing the Greek letter <ε> and adding the rhoticity diacritic, and we suggest calling the symbol "er" /ɝ/, "stressed schwar," or "hooked reverse epsilon," or "hooked reverse Greek e."

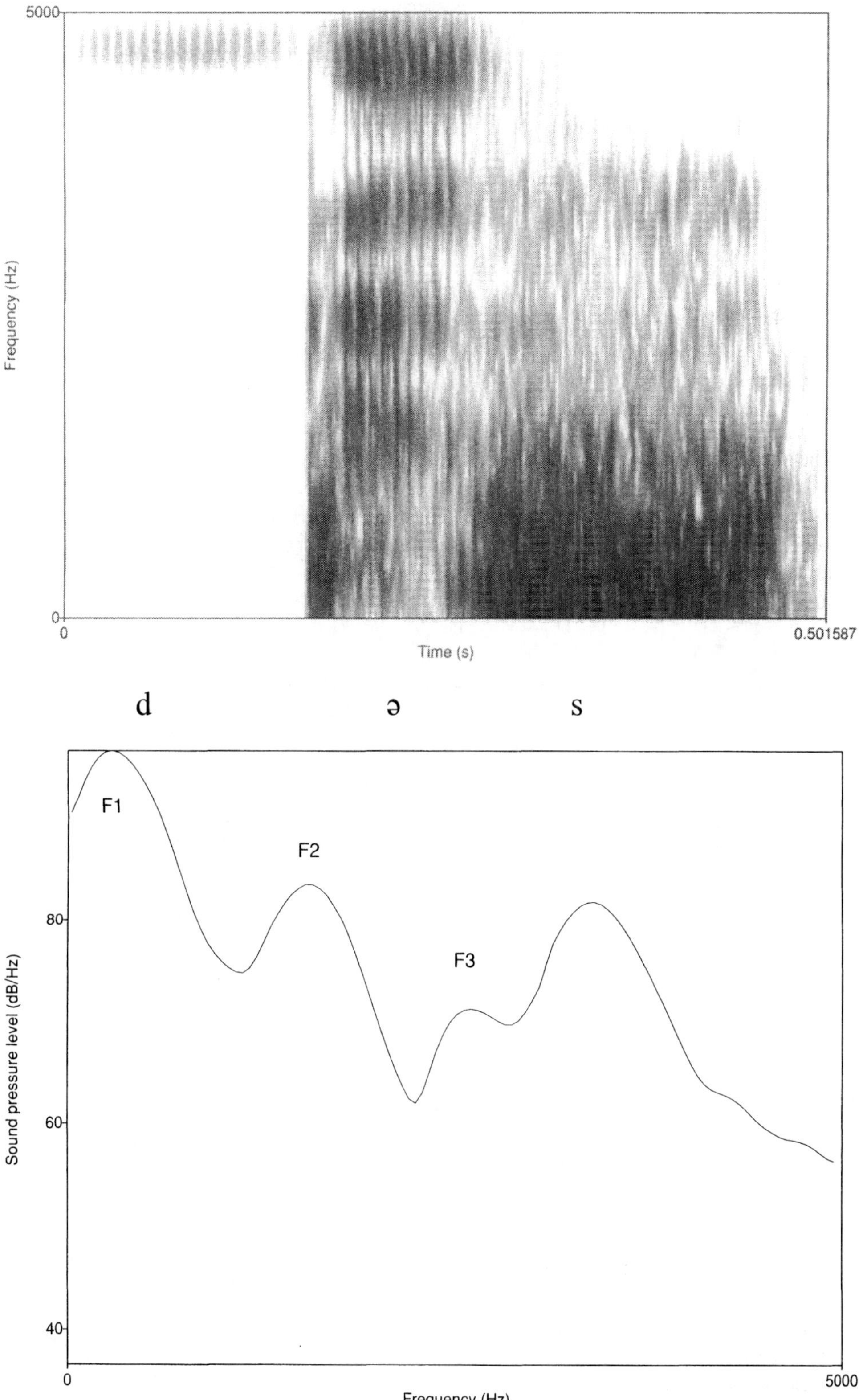

FIG 12.4. Wideband spectrogram and spectrum of the vowel in "des(troy)."

Spelling

There are many different ways of spelling /ɝ/, but all require a following <r>. The most common are:

<er(r)> her err perfect
<ur(r)> fur nurse purr
<ir>/<yr> fir bird myrtle

Other spellings include:

<(w)or> word worse
<ear> earth heard
<our> scourge journey

Note: Many of the spellings noted above can represent other vowels, and so may be listed in other entries.

The main allophone of this phoneme is made by positioning the highest point of the tongue arch centrally between front and back, and halfway between the lowest to the highest position (i.e., virtually in the center of the vowel area). For some speakers the tongue tip is raised toward the alveolar ridge throughout the production of the vowel, whereas others use an articulation involving bunching the back of the tongue dorsum up into the back of the mouth and placing the tongue tip inside the lower front teeth. The side rims of the tongue make no contact with the inner surfaces of the upper side teeth. The tongue is tense during the production of this vowel, which belongs to the group of long vowels. The lip shape for the vowel is neutrally open, although some speakers may always use a certain amount of loose rounding. In terms of the cardinal vowel system, English /ɝ/ would be plotted onto the vowel chart as seen in Fig. 12.5, with the symbolization [ɝ̝] or [ɝ̞].

The following are the primary allophones of /ɝ/:

- [ɝː] full length vowel, found before voiced consonants (e.g., "heard").
- [ɝˑ] reduced length vowel, found before voiceless consonants (e.g., "hurt").

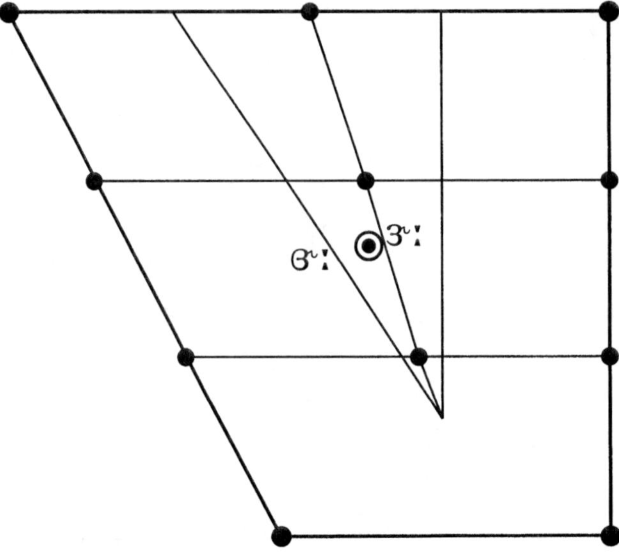

FIG 12.5. Cardinal vowel values of the main allophones of /ɝ/.

TABLE 12.3
Typical Formant Values for /ɝ/

	F0	*F1*	*F2*	*F3*
Men	130	474	1379	1710
Women	217	523	1588	1929
Children	237	586	1719	2143

- [ɝ̃] nasalized allophone found before nasal consonants (e.g., "learn"). Less nasalization occurs after a nasal consonant ("nurse").
- [ɵ˞] lip-rounded free variant.

It should be noted that nonrhotic accents of English lack this vowel, and replace it with /ɜ/, which is similar in most respects apart from the tongue tip position. We return to regional differences in chapter 18.

Figure 12.6a shows a spectrogram of the vowel /ɝ/ in the word "surge," together with a spectrum of the vowel taken halfway through the duration of the vowel. Table 12.3 gives typical values for the F0 and F1–F3 of /ɝ/ in men, women, and children. We can note the effect of retroflexion on the F3 values; as noted in chapter 10, we expect these to be depressed, and the table confirms this. Figure 12.6b shows the spectrogram and spectrum for the nonrhotic /ɜ/ in the same word spoken with a British RP accent.

The Mid, Short Rhotic Central Vowel

/ɚ/

This vowel is usually described as being a mid, unrounded, short, rhotic central vowel. /ɚ/, with a few exceptions, can only occur syllable-finally in open syllables, or followed by /z/ and /d/ as plural, possessive, or past tense morphemes. Some books will list /ɚ/ in words such as "urbane," but as the first syllable here is at least partially stressed, it is better to treat this vowel as being /ɝ/ (see further below). The IPA symbol is derived from adding the rhoticity diacritic to schwa, and so a common name for the symbol is "(unstressed) schwar."

Spelling

There are many different ways of spelling /ɚ/, but all require a following <r>. The most common are:

<er> waiter
<or> color
<ar> burglar

Other spellings include:

<ir> elixir
<our> glamour (non-US spelling)
<re> theatre (non-US spelling)
<ure> picture
<yr> martyr

Note: Many of the spellings noted above can represent other vowels, and so may be listed in other entries.

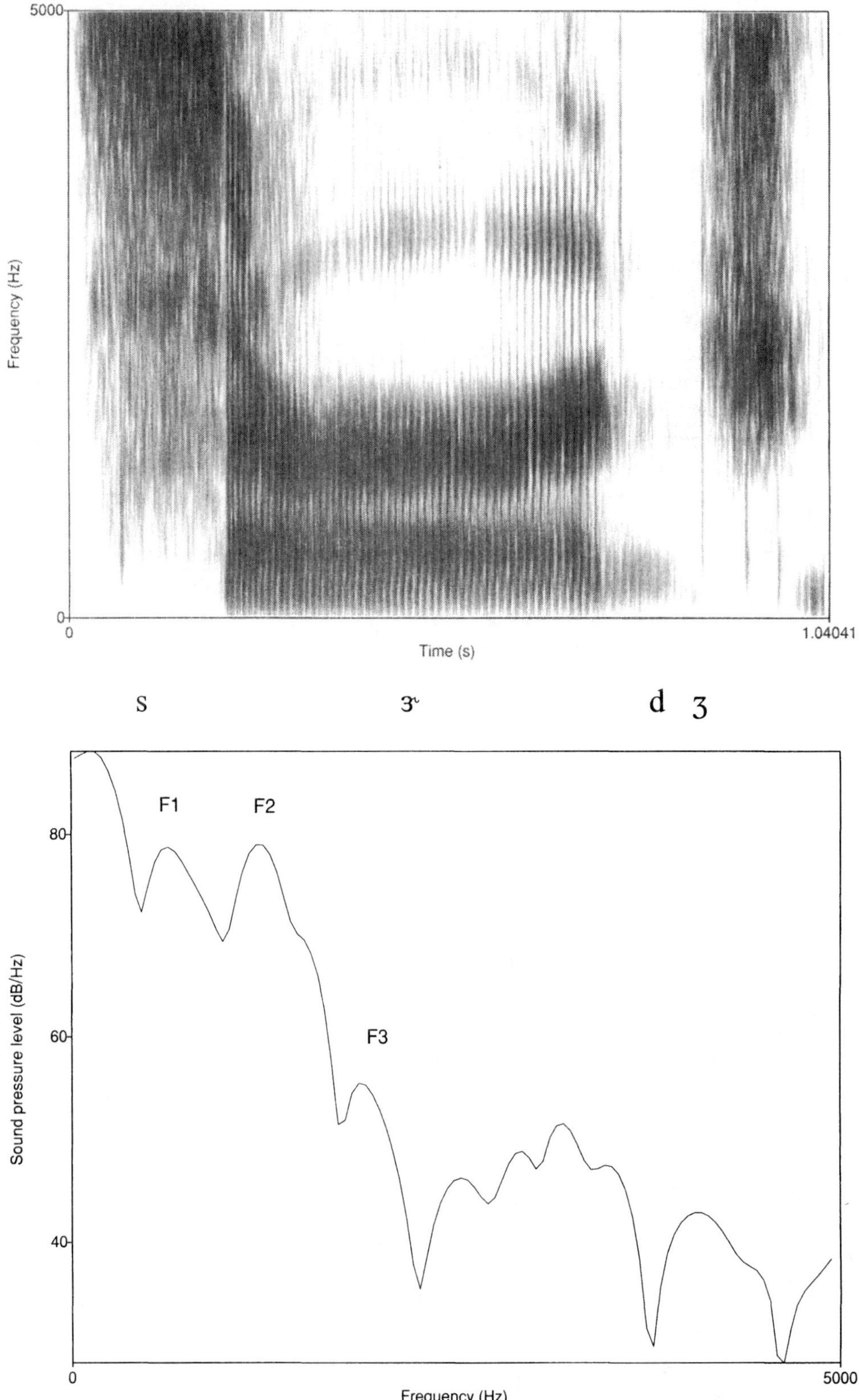

FIG 12.6a. Wideband spectrogram and spectrum of the vowel in "surge" (rhotic).

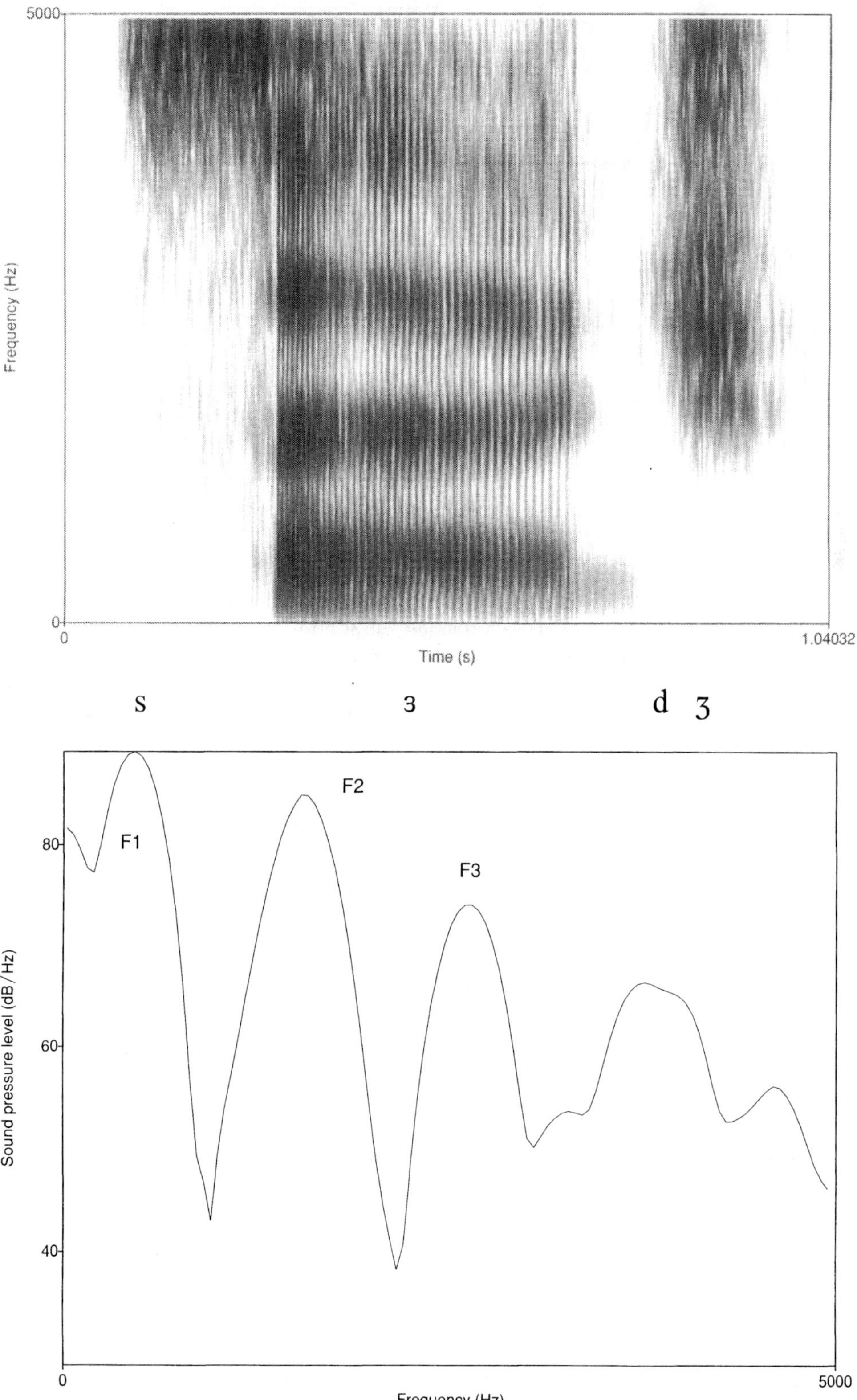

FIG 12.6b. Wideband spectrogram and spectrum of the vowel in "surge" (nonrhotic).

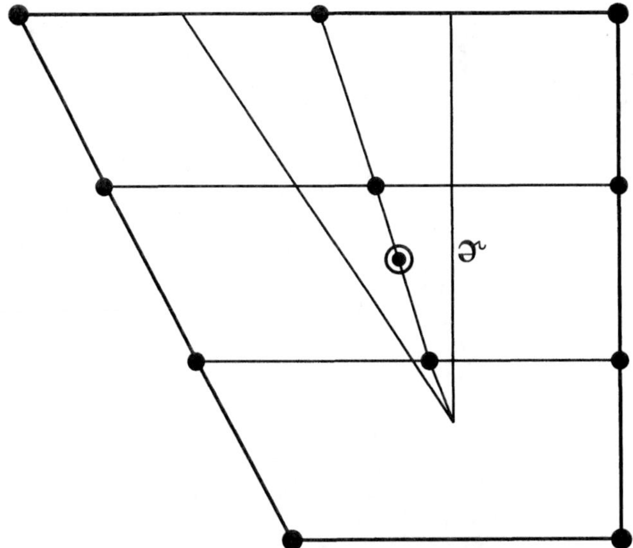

FIG 12.7. Cardinal vowel value of the main allophone of /ɚ/.

The highest point of the tongue arch is raised to a position centrally between front and back, and halfway between the lowest to the highest position (i.e., virtually in the center of the vowel area) to make the commonest allophone of this phoneme. The tongue tip is raised toward the alveolar ridge throughout the production of the vowel for some speakers, whereas others bunch the back of the tongue dorsum up into the back of the mouth and place the tongue tip inside the lower front teeth. The side rims of the tongue make no contact with the inner surfaces of the upper side teeth. The tongue is lax during the production of this vowel, which belongs to the group of short vowels. The lip shape for the vowel is neutrally open, although some speakers do use a certain amount of lip rounding. In terms of the cardinal vowel system, English /ɚ/ would be plotted onto the vowel chart, as seen in Fig. 12.7, and with the symbolization [ɝ̝] or [ɚ̝].The restriction of /ɚ/ to unstressed syllables and its very short duration mean that we do not record any length differences connected to following consonant voicing in the allophones.

The following are the main allophones of /ɚ/:

- [ɚ] the mid central tongue position, found in most contexts (e.g., "paper," "papers").
- [ɚ̃] nasalized allophone found before nasal consonants (e.g., "afternoon"). Less nasalization occurs after a nasal consonant ("runner").

It should be noted that nonrhotic accents of English lack this vowel, and replace it with /ə/, which is similar in most respects, apart from the tongue tip position. We return to regional differences in chapter 18.

Acoustic studies of the vowels of English have traditionally not compared stressed and unstressed schwar but, because the main difference between these vowels is one of duration, we can assume that formant values for /ɚ/ will be similar to those for /ɝ/. Figure 12.8 shows a spectrogram of the vowel /ɚ/ in the word "waiter," together with a spectrum of the vowel taken halfway through the duration of the vowel. The dark bands on the spectrogram, and the peaks on the spectrum clearly show the formant structure of the vowel and the depressed F3 characteristic of rhotic vowels.

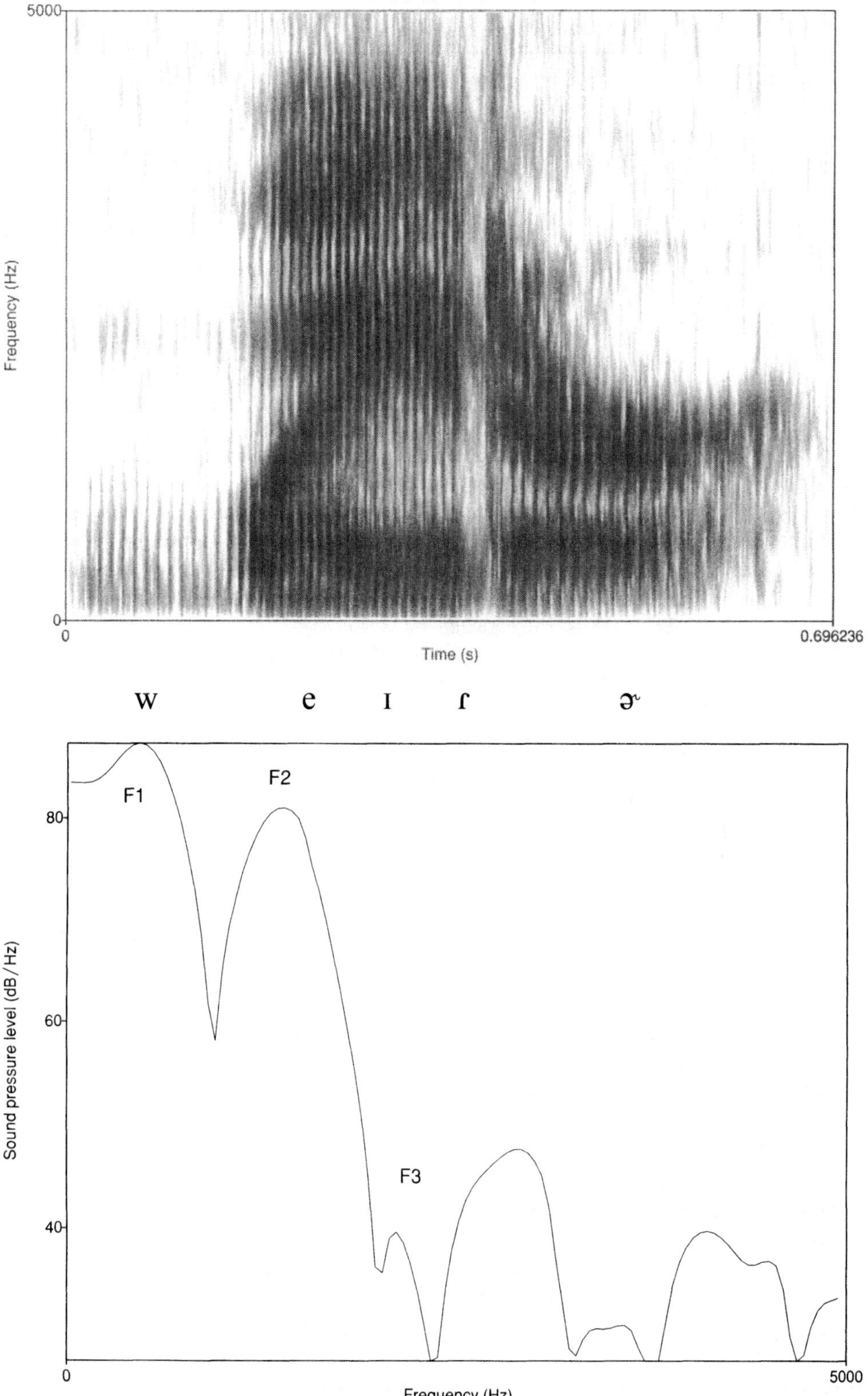

FIG 12.8. Wideband spectrogram and spectrum of the vowel in "waiter."

TABLE 12.4
Usage of Stressed and Unstressed Schwar

	Fully stressed	*Secondary stress*	*Unstressed*
ˈerr	ɝ		
ˈword	ɝ		
reˈfer	ɝ		
ˈfurnace	ɝ		
ˌurˈbane		ɝ	
ˈforeˌword		ɝ	
ˌflirˈtatious		ɝ	
ˌergoˈnomic		ɝ	
ˈforward			ɚ
perˈtain			ɚ
ˈmustard			ɚ
ˈtreasure			ɚ

As we noted above, there is some disagreement over when to use /ɚ/ and when to use /ɝ/. Wells (2000) prefers to keep /ɚ/ for fully unstressed syllables and to use /ɝ/ in both fully stressed syllables and syllables with secondary stress (see chaps. 9 and 16 for a discussion of these differences). We follow that usage here, because if we used /ɚ/ for both unstressed and secondary stressed syllables, then we could not mark the difference between "foreword" and "forward" that we noted earlier. Table 12.4 may help to show the usage we recommend; ˈ and ˌ denote full and secondary stress, respectively.

Another problem arises when we have schwa followed by <r> in the spelling, and then followed by another syllable starting with a vowel. Examples of such words are "parade," "peruse," and "surround." The rules for syllable boundaries in English are not always obvious, but one strong tendency is to assume that most syllables should start with a consonant if possible. Taking "peruse" as our example (and using the period to show syllable boundaries), this would suggest that we should transcribe this combination as /pə.ɹuz/ (as is indeed done for American English by Wells, 2000). On the other hand, as we have just seen in this subsection, we treat schwa plus /ɹ/ as schwar, and this suggests a transcription of /pɚ.uz/ (as recommended, for example, by Small, 1999). We feel that this suggestion does not reflect actual pronunciations, although we do recognize that some speakers may use both a schwar *and* a syllable-initial /ɹ/. For these words, then, we recommend /pə.ɹuz/ for speakers whose first syllable vowel is nonrhotic, and /pɚ.ɹuz/ for those whose first syllable vowel is rhotic.

THE MID-CLOSING DIPHTHONGS

This pair of diphthongs is symmetrical: /eɪ/ has a tongue glide from mid front, upward and backward, whereas /oʊ/ has a tongue glide from mid back, upward and forward. As we have noted previously, certain texts treat these two vowels as monophthongs (/e/ and /o/, respectively), with diphthongal allophones. However, as more contexts require the diphthong than the monophthongal realizations, it would appear to us to make more sense to stick with the long tradition of treating these sounds as diphthongs.

The Front Mid-Closing Diphthong

/eɪ/

This diphthong is a glide from a mid front tongue position toward a higher, backer position similar to that of /ɪ/. The IPA symbol is derived from combining a symbol for the initial position of the tongue with one for the final position. To show the diphthongal nature, some authorities add a tie-bar to all diphthongs (e.g., /e͡ɪ/), but we do not adopt that convention in this book, because the absence of the tie-bar is not likely to cause confusion. We can call the symbols "ay-diphthong."

> **Spelling**
>
> There are several different ways of spelling /eɪ/. The most common are:
>
> <a> (with following silent <e>) face plate waste
> <ai> train aim waist
> <ay> play hay crayon
> <ei> eight rein
> <ey> they whey
> <ea> break great
>
> Other spellings include:
>
> <au> gauge
> <e> (with following silent <e>) fete suede
> <e> cafe
> <et> ballet
> <ee> puree
> <er> dossier
>
> Note: Many of the spellings noted above can represent other vowels, and so may be listed in other entries.

The most frequent allophone of this phoneme has the highest point of the tongue arch raised to a fully front position halfway between the lowest and the highest positions. The tongue glides from here upward and backward toward the position of /ɪ/, this glide being accompanied by a slight closing of the jaw. The side rims of the tongue make light contact with the inner surfaces of the upper side teeth. As with all the English diphthongs, the tongue is tense during the production of this vowel, which belongs to the group of long vowels. The lip shape for the vowel is spread. In terms of the cardinal vowel system, English /eɪ/ would be plotted onto the vowel chart, as seen in Fig. 12.9.

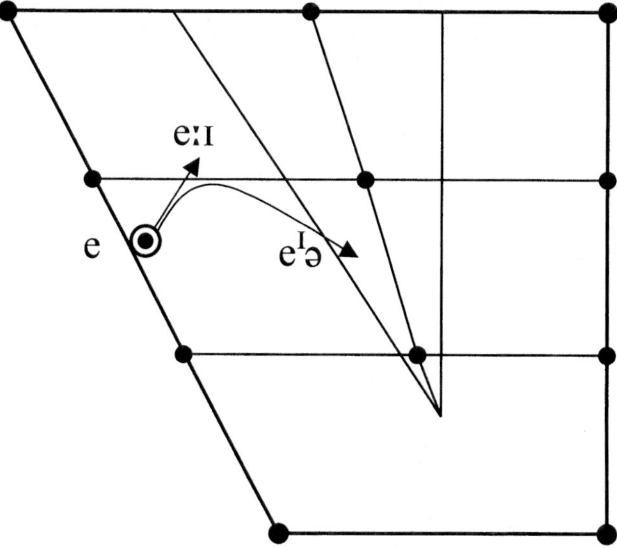

FIG 12.9. Cardinal vowel values of the main allophones of /eɪ/.

The following are the main allophones of /eɪ/:

- [eːɪ] full length vowel, found in final open syllables and before voiced consonants (e.g., "play," "played").
- [eˑɪ] reduced length vowel, found before voiceless consonants (e.g., "plate").
- (GA, not RP) [e] short monophthong, found in unstressed syllables (e.g., "mandate").
- [eˡə] or [eə] centralizing variant, found before dark-l (e.g., "snail").
- [ẽɪ̃] nasalized allophone found before nasal consonants (e.g., "gain"). Less nasalization occurs after a nasal consonant ("make").

Note that we mark length on the first element of the diphthong because, in longer realizations, it tends to be the first element that is drawn out.

Figure 12.10 shows a spectrogram of the vowel /eɪ/ in the word "say," together with two spectra of the vowel taken toward the beginning and the end of the vowel. (For the remaining diphthongs we show only the spectrogram, and not the spectra.) Note how the formants change from the early to the late part of the vowel. Table 12.5 gives typical values for F1–F2 /eɪ/ in men and women taken from Cruttenden (2001). The values are given for both the initial and final components of the diphthong.

The Back Mid-Closing Diphthong (GA)

/oʊ/

This diphthong is a glide from a mid back tongue position toward a higher, fronter position similar to that of /ʊ/. As with all the diphthongs, the IPA symbol is derived from combining a symbol for the initial position of the tongue with one for the final position. We can call the symbols "oh-diphthong."

Spelling

There are several different ways of spelling /oʊ/. The most common are:

<o> so old both home
<oe> toe foe
<ow> know meadow
<oa> soap roam
<ou> though boulder

Other spellings include:

<au> gauche
<oo> brooch
<eau> beau
<ew> sew

Note: Many of the spellings noted above can represent other vowels, and so may be listed in other entries.

To produce the most usual allophone of this phoneme the highest point of the tongue arch is raised to a fully back position halfway between the lowest and the highest positions. The tongue glides from here upward and forward toward the position of /ʊ/, this glide being accompanied by a slight closing of the jaw. The side rims of the tongue make no contact with the inner surfaces of the upper side teeth. The lip shape for the vowel is open rounded. In terms

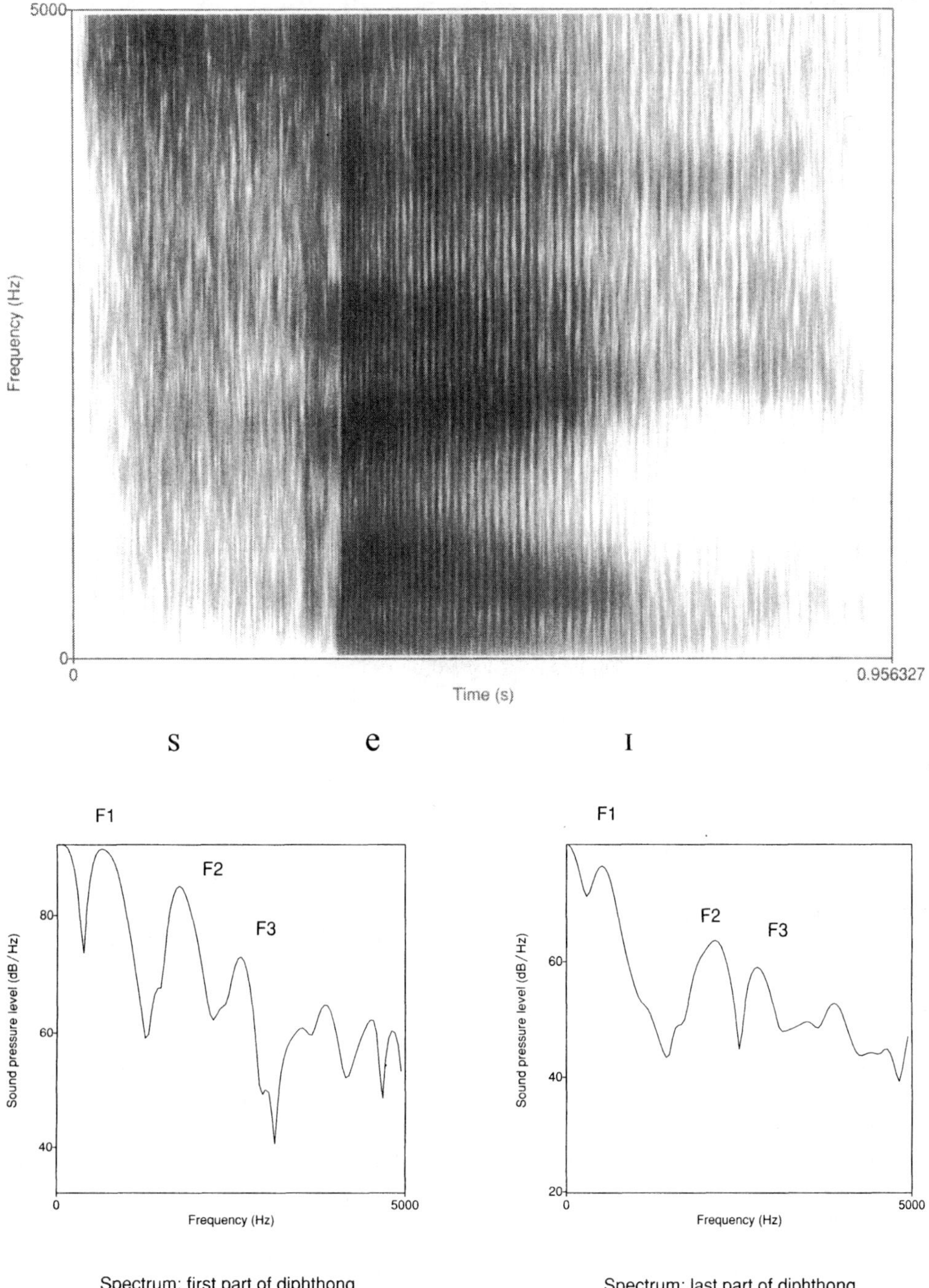

FIG 12.10. Wideband spectrogram and spectra of the vowel in "say."

TABLE 12.5
Typical Formant Values for /eɪ/

	F1 initial	*F2 initial*	*F1 final*	*F2 final*
Men	587	1945	413	2130
Women	581	2241	416	2204

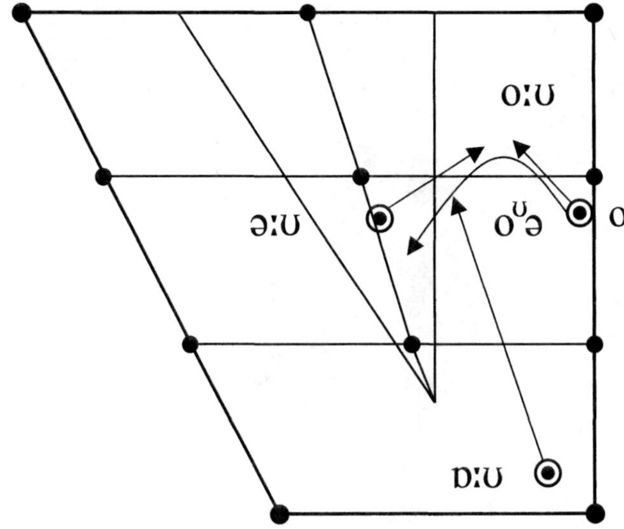

FIG 12.11. Cardinal vowel values of the main allophones of /oʊ/.

of the cardinal vowel system, English /oʊ/ would be plotted onto the vowel chart as seen in Fig. 12.11.

The following are the main allophones of /oʊ/:

- [o:ʊ] full length vowel, found in final open syllables and before voiced consonants (e.g., "roe," "road").
- [o'ʊ] reduced length vowel, found before voiceless consonants (e.g., "wrote").
- [o] short monophthong, found in unstressed syllables (e.g., "rotation").
- [oᵘə] or [oə] centralizing variant, found before dark-l (e.g., "goal").
- [õʊ̃] nasalized allophone found before nasal consonants (e.g., "roam"). Less nasalization occurs after a nasal consonant ("motor").

Note that, as with all diphthongs in English, we mark length on the first element of the diphthong because, in longer realizations, it tends to be the first element that is drawn out.

Figure 12.12 shows a spectrogram of the vowel /oʊ/ (GA pronunciation) and the vowel /əʊ/ (RP pronunciation) in the word "sew." Again, note how the formants change from the early to the late part of the vowel. Table 12.6 gives typical values for F1 and F2 of this vowel in men and women taken from Cruttenden (2001). The values are given for both the initial and final components of the diphthong.

TABLE 12.6
Typical Formant Values for /əʊ/

	F1 initial	*F2 initial*	*F1 final*	*F2 final*
Men	537	1266	379	1024
Women	545	1573	380	1267

Note: These values are derived from British English, where the starting point of the diphthong is more centralized. We would expect somewhat lower F2 values in the initial component in American English.

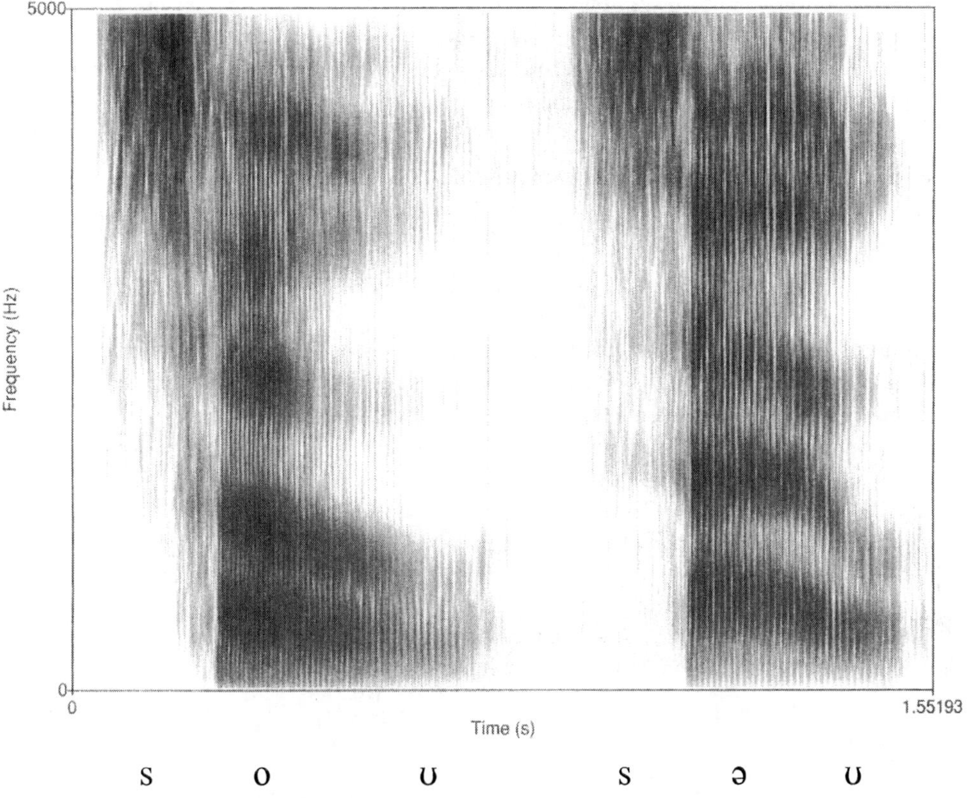

FIG 12.12. Wideband spectrogram of the GA and RP vowels in "sew."

The Central Mid-Closing Diphthong (RP)

/əʊ/

This diphthong is a glide from a mid central tongue position toward a higher, backer position similar to that of /ʊ/. We can call the symbols "schwa-upsilon-diphthong."

> Spelling
>
> The spellings for /əʊ/ are the same as those for /oʊ/.

The highest point of the tongue arch is raised to a central position halfway between the lowest and the highest positions to produce the main allophone of this phoneme. The tongue glides from this position upward and backward toward the position of /ʊ/, this glide being accompanied by a slight closing of the jaw. The side rims of the tongue make no contact with the inner surfaces of the upper side teeth. The lip shape for the vowel is neutral at the start, changing to open rounded. In terms of the cardinal vowel system, English /əʊ/ would be plotted onto the vowel chart as seen in Fig. 12.11.

The following are the most frequent allophones of /əʊ/:

- [əːʊ] full length vowel, found in final open syllables and before voiced consonants (e.g., "roe," "road").

- [ə'ʊ] reduced length vowel, found before voiceless consonants (e.g., "wrote").
- [ɒːʊ], [ɒᶷə] or [ɒə] centralizing variant, found before dark-l (e.g., "goal").
- [ə̃ʊ̃] nasalized allophone found before nasal consonants (e.g., "roam"). Less nasalization occurs after a nasal consonant ("motor").

Formant values of this vowel are given in Table 12.6, and a spectrogram in Fig. 12.12.

THE LOW-CLOSING DIPHTHONGS

This pair of diphthongs is symmetrical: /aɪ/ has a tongue glide from low front upward, while /aʊ/ has a tongue glide from low central, upward and backward. Because /aʊ/ starts further back than /aɪ/, some texts prefer to transcribe it /ɑʊ/, but /aʊ/ appears to be the current standard transcription.

The Front Low-Closing Diphthong

/aɪ/

This diphthong is a glide from a low front tongue position towards a higher position similar to that of /ɪ/. We can call the symbols "eye-diphthong."

Spelling

There are several different ways of spelling /aɪ/. The most common are:

<i> (with following silent <e>) white mime
<ie> die cried
<y> my shy
<y> (with following silent <e>) type
<ye> dye
<igh> high night
<eigh> height

Other spellings include:

<ia> diamond
<ui> guide
<ei> either (can also be /i/)
<ai> aisle
<uy> buy

Note: Many of the spellings noted above can represent other vowels, and so may be listed in other entries.

For the most common allophone of this phoneme the highest point of the tongue arch is placed at a fully low position somewhat retracted from the frontest possible one. The tongue glides from there almost directly upward toward the position of /ɪ/, this glide being accompanied by a considerable closing of the jaw. Especially in rapid speech, the tongue glide may not always reach the /ɪ/ position. The side rims of the tongue make light contact with the inner surfaces of the upper side teeth toward the end of the glide. The lip shape for the vowel starts neutrally

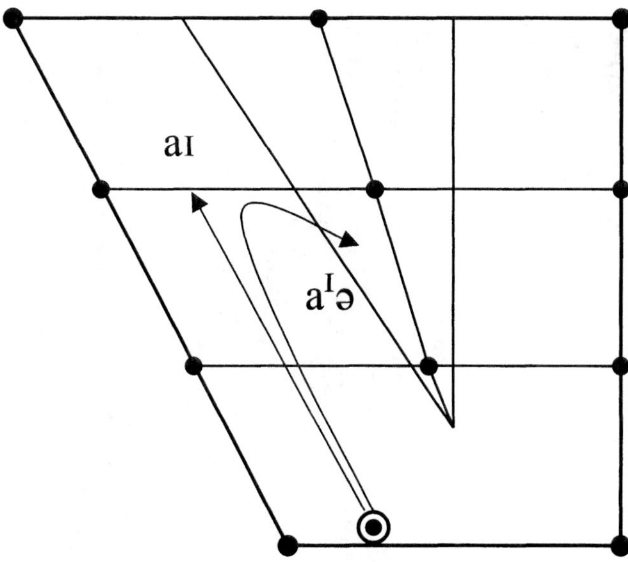

FIG 12.13. Cardinal vowel values of the main allophones of /aɪ/.

open and ends loosely spread. In terms of the cardinal vowel system, English /aɪ/ would be plotted onto the vowel chart as seen in Fig. 12.13.

The following are the main allophones of /aɪ/:

- [aːɪ] full length vowel, found in final open syllables and before voiced consonants (e.g., "fry," "fried").
- [aˑɪ] reduced length vowel, found before voiceless consonants (e.g., "fright").
- [aᴵə] or [aə] centralizing variant, found before dark-l (e.g., "smile").
- [ãĩ] nasalized allophone found before nasal consonants (e.g., "sign"). Less nasalization occurs after a nasal consonant ("mike").

Figure 12.14 shows a spectrogram of the vowel /aɪ/ in the word "sigh." Table 12.7 gives typical values for F1 and F2 of /aɪ/ in men and women taken from Cruttenden (2001). The values are given for both the initial and final components of the diphthong.

The Back Low-Closing Diphthong

/aʊ/

This diphthong is a glide from a low nearly central tongue position toward a higher, backer position similar to that of /ʊ/. We can call the symbols "ow-diphthong."

TABLE 12.7
Typical Formant Values for /aɪ/

	F1 initial	*F2 initial*	*F1 final*	*F2 final*
Men	734	1117	439	2058
Women	822	1275	359	2591

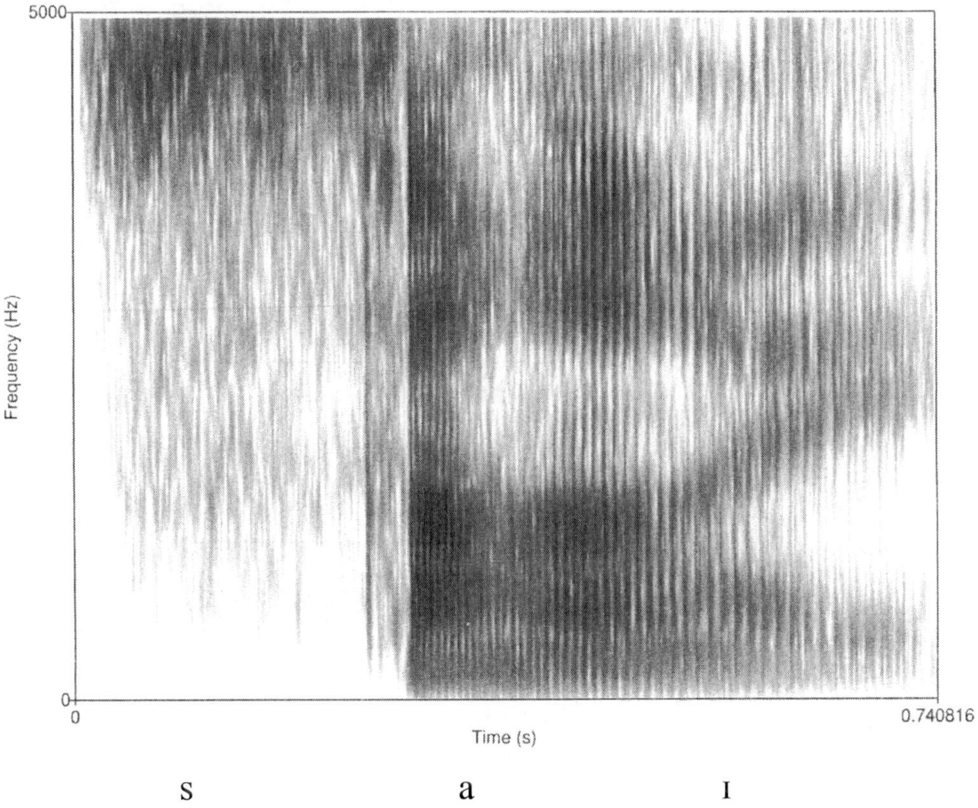

FIG 12.14. Wideband spectrogram of the vowel in "sigh."

Spelling

There are several different ways of spelling /aʊ/. The two most common are:

<ou> out mouse counsel
<ow> now powder cloud

Other spellings include:

<ough> bough

Note: All of the spellings noted above can represent other vowels, and so may be listed in other entries.

The primary allophone of this phoneme is produced by placing the highest point of the tongue arch at a fully low position retracted from the frontest possible one to a near central one. The tongue glides from this position upward and backward toward the position of /ʊ/, this glide being accompanied by a considerable closing of the jaw.

Especially in rapid speech, the tongue glide may not always reach the /ʊ/ position. The side rims of the tongue make no contact with the inner surfaces of the upper side teeth during the glide. The lip shape for the vowel starts neutrally open and ends loosely rounded. In terms of the cardinal vowel system, English /aʊ/ would be plotted onto the vowel chart as seen in Fig. 12.15.

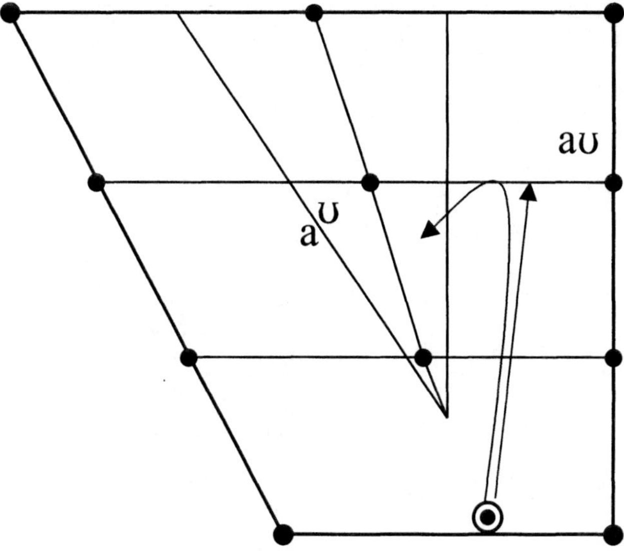

FIG 12.15. Cardinal vowel values of the main allophones of /aʊ/.

TABLE 12.8
Typical Formant Values for /aʊ/

	F1 initial	*F2 initial*	*F1 final*	*F2 final*
Men	734	1117	439	2058
Women	822	1275	359	2591

The following are the main allophones of /aʊ/:

- [aːʊ] full length vowel, found in final open syllables and before voiced consonants (e.g., "bow," "bowed").
- [aˑʊ] reduced length vowel, found before voiceless consonants (e.g., "bout").
- [aᵘə] or [aə] centralizing variant, found before dark-l (e.g., "growl").
- [ãʊ̃] nasalized allophone found before nasal consonants (e.g., "frown"). Less nasalization occurs after a nasal consonant ("mouse").

Figure 12.16 shows a spectrogram of the vowel /aʊ/ in the word "sow." Note how the formants change from the early to the late part of the vowel. Table 12.8 gives typical values for F1 and F2 of /aʊ/ in men and women taken from Cruttenden (2001). The values are given for both the initial and final components of the diphthong.

THE FRONTING-CLOSING DIPHTHONG

There is only a single diphthong that crosses the vowel area in English: /ɔɪ/. This is one of the least frequent vowel sounds of the language, and most examples derive from borrowings from Norman French in the period following the Norman conquest of England in the 11th century.

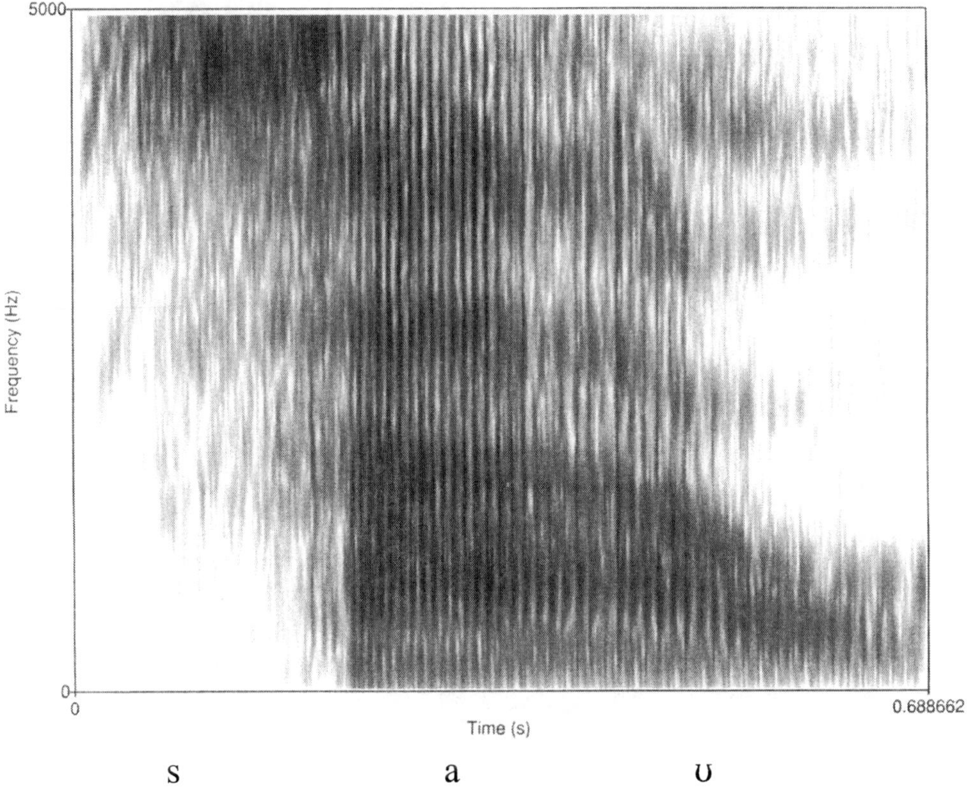

FIG 12.16. Wideband spectrogram of the vowel in "sow."

The Fronting Low-Closing Diphthong

/ɔɪ/

This diphthong is a glide from a mid-low back tongue position toward a higher, fronter position similar to that of /ɪ/. We can call the symbols "oy-diphthong."

> Spelling
>
> There are only two main ways of spelling /ɔɪ/:
>
> <oi> coin voice
> <oy> toy oyster

To produce the main allophone of this phoneme the highest point of the tongue arch is set at a mid-low, back position. The tongue glides from there upward and forward toward the position of /ɪ/, this glide being accompanied by a considerable closing of the jaw. Especially in rapid speech, the tongue glide may not always reach the /ɪ/ position. The side rims of the tongue make light contact with the inner surfaces of the upper side teeth toward the end of the glide. The lip shape for the vowel starts open rounded and ends loosely spread. In terms of the cardinal vowel system, English /ɔɪ/ would be plotted onto the vowel chart as seen in Fig. 12.17.

The following are the commonest allophones of /ɔɪ/:

- [ɔːɪ] full length vowel, found in final open syllables and before voiced consonants (e.g., "joy," "joys").
- [ɔˑɪ] reduced length vowel, found before voiceless consonants (e.g., "Joyce").

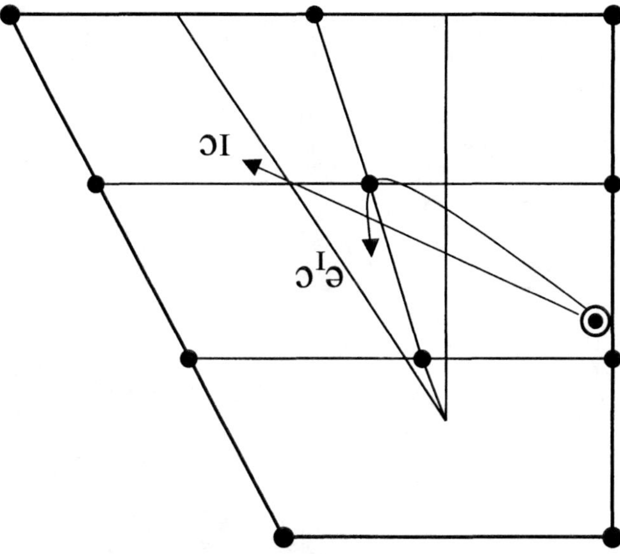

FIG 12.17. Cardinal vowel values of the main allophones of /ɔɪ/.

TABLE 12.9
Typical Formant Values for /ɔɪ/

	F1 initial	*F2 initial*	*F1 final*	*F2 final*
Men	477	824	443	1924
Women	428	879	334	2520

- [ɔᴵə] or [ɔə] centralizing variant, found before dark-l (e.g., "boil").
- [ɔ̃ɪ̃] nasalized allophone found before nasal consonants (e.g., "coin"). Less nasalization occurs after a nasal consonant ("noise").

Figure 12.18 shows a spectrogram of the vowel /ɔɪ/ in the word "soy." Table 12.9 gives typical values for F1 and F2 of /ɔɪ/ in men and women taken from Cruttenden (2001). The values are given for both the initial and final components of the diphthong.

THE CENTERING DIPHTHONGS (RP)

These are found in nonrhotic accents of English and, consequently, are found in RP. They derive from /ɪ, ɛ, ɔ, ʊ/ plus /ɹ/, where the /ɹ/ was replaced by schwa. In current RP the centering diphthong /ɔə/ has been replaced by /ɔ/, except in speakers who use a rather old-fashioned variant of RP. The replacement of /ʊə/ by /ɔ/ and /ɛə/ by /ɛ/ also seem to be occurring in younger people's speech, but these diphthongs are still considered part of the vowel system.

The High Front Centering Diphthong

/ɪə/

This diphthong is a glide from a high front tongue position similar to that of /ɪ/ toward a mid central position. We can call the symbols "ear-diphthong."

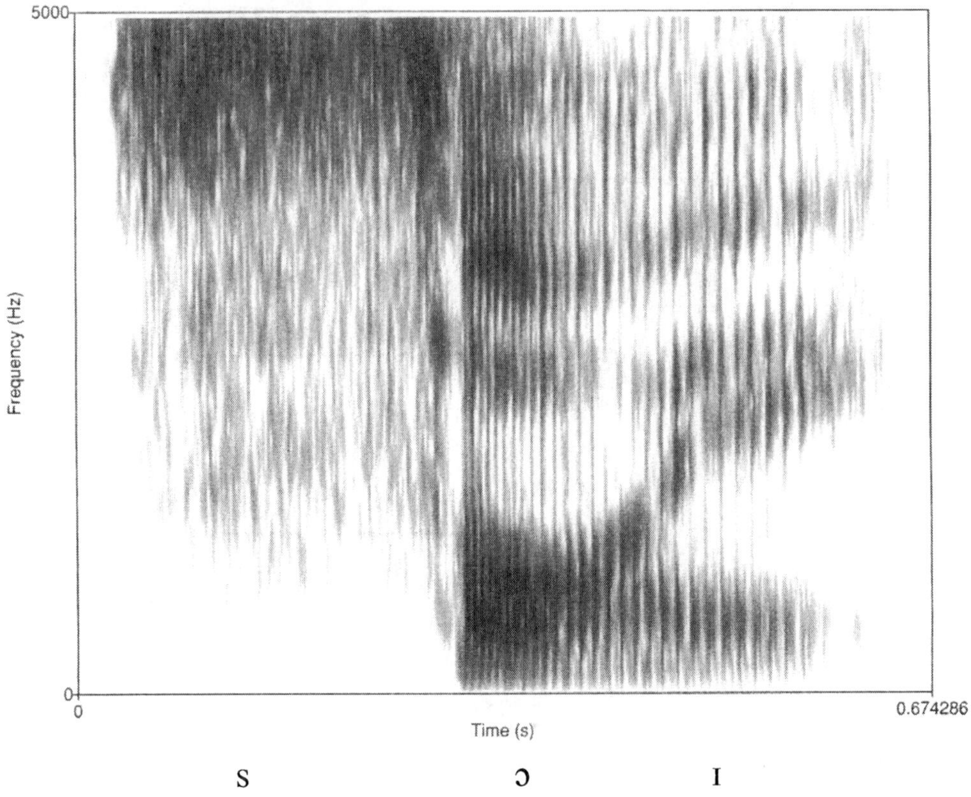

FIG 12.18. Wideband spectrogram of the vowel in "soy."

Spelling

These are the main ways of spelling /ɪə/:

<er>/<ere>	zero	here	sincere
<ear>/<eer>	fear	nuclear	deer
*<ia>	media	familiar	
*<ea>	idea	area	
*<eu>/<eo>	museum	theological	
*<ie>	salient	spaniel	
*<io>/<iou>	period	previous	
*<iu>	union	stadium	

*In GA and also many non-RP British accents, these spellings represent bisyllabic /i.ə/.

The most frequently occuring allophone of this phoneme is produced as follows: The highest point of the tongue arch is set at the position of /ɪ/; the tongue glides from there downward and backward toward a mid central position, this glide being accompanied by a slight opening of the jaw. Especially in rapid speech, the tongue glide may not always reach the absolute mid central position. The side rims of the tongue make light contact with the inner surfaces of the upper side teeth at the start of the glide. The lip shape for the vowel starts loosely spread and ends in a neutral shape. In terms of the cardinal vowel system, English /ɪə/ would be plotted onto the vowel chart as seen in Fig. 12.19.

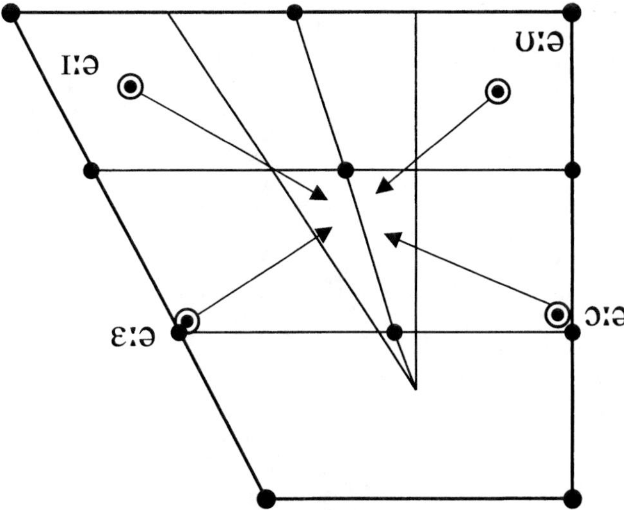

FIG 12.19. Cardinal vowel values of allophones /ɪə/, /ɛə/, and /ʊə/.

The following are the main allophones of /ɪə/:

- [ɪːə] full length vowel, found in final open syllables and before voiced consonants (e.g., "fear," "fears").
- [ɪˑə] reduced length vowel, found before voiceless consonants (e.g., "fierce").
- [ɪː]/[ɪˑ] long monophthong variant being adopted by some younger speakers.
- [ɪ̆ə] rising diphthong found in unstressed syllables (e.g., "period" [ˈpɪːəɹɪ̆əd]). Some speakers will use a glide plus schwa in these contexts: [ˈpɪːəɹjəd].
- [ɪ̃ə̃] nasalized allophone found before nasal consonants (e.g., "medium"). Less nasalization occurs after a nasal consonant ("near").

Figure 12.20 shows a spectrogram of the diphthong /ɪə/ in the word "tier," together with the diphthongs in "tare" and "tour." Table 12.10 gives typical values for F1 and F2 of /ɪə/ in men and women taken from Cruttenden (2001). The values are given for both the initial and final components of the diphthong.

The Mid Front Centering Diphthong

/ɛə/

This diphthong is a glide from a mid front tongue position similar to that of /ɛ/ toward a mid central position. We can call the symbols "air-diphthong." Some texts on RP transcribe this diphthong as /eə/.

TABLE 12.10
Typical Formant Values for /ɪə/

	F1 initial	*F2 initial*	*F1 final*	*F2 final*
Men	382	2096	578	1643
Women	399	2514	417	1846

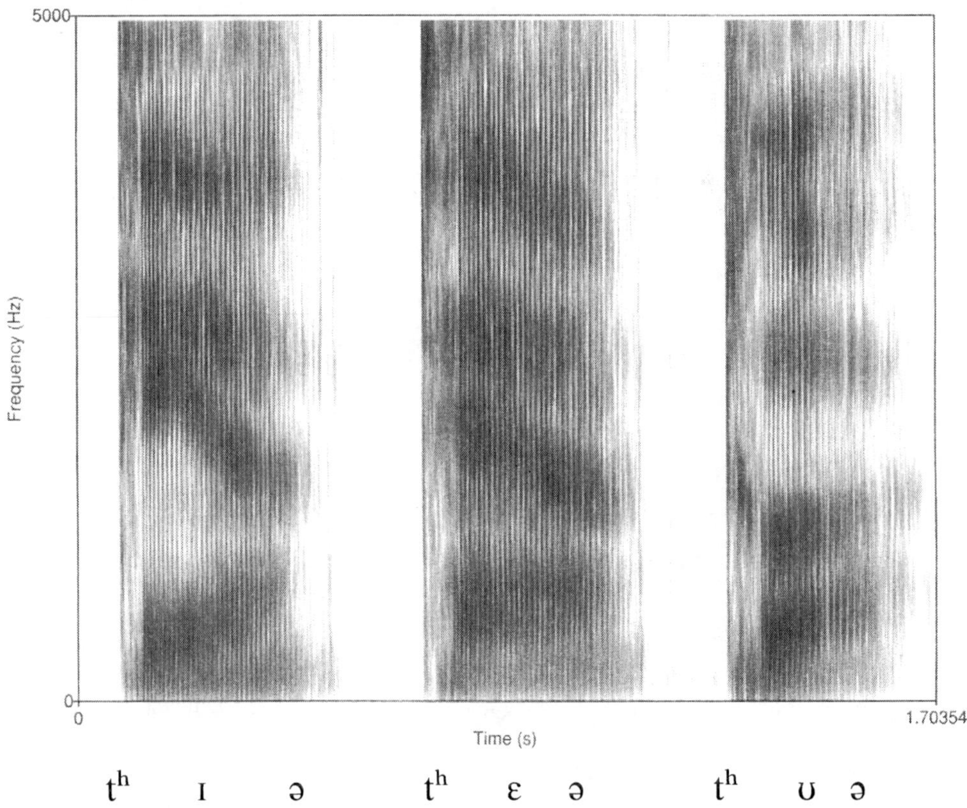

FIG 12.20. Wideband spectrogram of the vowels in "tier," "tare," and "tour."

Spelling

These are the main ways of spelling /ɛə/:

<ar>/<are> scarce care aware
<air> air stair impair
<ear> bear swear
<aer> aerial aerobics
<eir> heir their
<ere> there
<ayor>/<ayer> mayor prayer

The highest point of the tongue arch is set at the position of /ɛ/ for the primary allophone of this phoneme. The tongue glides from this position upward and backward toward a mid central position, this glide being accompanied by very slight closing of the jaw. Especially in rapid speech, the tongue glide may not always reach the absolute mid central position. The side rims of the tongue make light contact with the inner surfaces of the upper side teeth at the start of the glide. The lip shape for the vowel remains neutral throughout. In terms of the cardinal vowel system, English /ɛə/ would be plotted onto the vowel chart as seen in Fig. 12.19.

TABLE 12.11
Typical Formant Values for /ɛə/

	F1 initial	*F2 initial*	*F1 final*	*F2 final*
Men	538	1864	655	1594
Women	691	2210	751	1883

The following are the main allophones of /ɛə/:

- [ɛːə] full length vowel, found in final open syllables and before voiced consonants (e.g., "scare," "scares").
- [ɛˑə] reduced length vowel, found before voiceless consonants (e.g., "scarce").
- [ɛː]/[ɛˑ] long monophthong, increasingly common in all contexts, especially final open syllables.
- [ɛ̃ə̃] nasalized allophone found before nasal consonants (e.g., "Mearns": place-name; nasal stops rarely follow this sound). Less nasalization occurs after a nasal consonant ("mare").

Figure 12.20 shows a spectrogram of the diphthong /ɛə/ in the word "tare," together with the diphthongs in "tier" and "tour." Table 12.11 gives typical values for F1 and F2 of /ɛə/ in men and women taken from Cruttenden (2001). The values are given for both the initial and final components of the diphthong.

The High Back Centering Diphthong

/ʊə/

This diphthong is a glide from a high back tongue position similar to that of /ʊ/ toward a mid central position. It can occur before and after consonants, and word-finally in open syllables, but not initially. We can call the symbols "oo-er-diphthong."

Spelling

These are the main ways of spelling /ʊə/:

<oor>	poor	moor	
<our>	tour	gourd	bourgeois
<ure>	cure	endure	secure
<ur>	during	furious	
*<ue>	cruel	puerile	
*<ua>	usual	actual	

*In GA and also many non-RP British accents, these spellings represent bisyllabic /u.ə/

The highest point of this tongue arch is set at the position of /ʊ/ in producing the commonest allophone of this phoneme. The tongue glides from there downward and forward toward a mid central position, this glide being accompanied by very slight opening of the jaw. Especially in rapid speech, the tongue glide may not always reach the absolute mid central position. The

TABLE 12.12
Typical Formant Values for /ʊə/

	F1 initial	*F2 initial*	*F1 final*	*F2 final*
Men	426	1028	587	1250
Women	420	1157	485	1258

lips for the vowel start loosely rounded and finish in a neutral shape. In terms of the cardinal vowel system, English /ʊə/ would be plotted onto the vowel chart as seen in Fig. 12.19.

The following are the main allophones of /ʊə/:

- [ʊːə] full length vowel, found in final open syllables and before voiced consonants (e.g., "tour," "tours").
- [ʊˑə] reduced length vowel, found before voiceless consonants (e.g., "Ewart": personal name; /ʊə/ rarely occurs before voiceless consonants).
- [ʊ̆ə] rising diphthong found in unstressed syllables (e.g., "influence" [ˈɪnflʊ̆ə ns]). Some speakers will use a glide plus schwa in these contexts: [ˈɪnflwə ns].
- [ʊː]/[ʊˑ] long monophthong, used by some RP speakers in all contexts.
- [ʊ̃ə̃] nasalized allophone found before nasal consonants (e.g., "fluent"). Less nasalization occurs after a nasal consonant ("moor").

The use of the vowel /ɔ/ instead of /ʊə/ is increasingly common in most contexts, except following /j/ and in those contexts where there is no <r> in the spelling.

Figure 12.20 shows a spectrogram of the diphthong /ʊə/ in the word "tour," together with the diphthongs in "tier" and "tare." Table 12.12 gives typical values for F1 and F2 of /ʊə/ in men and women taken from Cruttenden (2001). The values are given for both the initial and final components of the diphthong.

The Mid Back Centering Diphthong

/ɔə/

This diphthong is the back equivalent of /ɛə/, but is no longer deemed to be part of the system of RP, being replaced everywhere by /ɔ/. Those nonrhotic accents that retain this diphthong use it in such words as "door," "pore," "pour," and "shore." The merger of this diphthong with /ɔ/, and the tendency to a similar merger we noted above for /ʊə/, may result in the words "Shaw," "sure," and "shore" all being pronounced as /ʃɔ/. Older RP speakers would distinguish them as /ʃɔ/, /ʃʊə/, /ʃɔə/.

BACKGROUND READING

As for the previous chapter, we recommend further study of Cruttenden (2001). Both Small (1999) and Edwards (2003) cover vowels and consonants, but do not deal with the full range of allophonic variation, and Edwards sometimes combines allophones with regional variants and with phonemic substitutions.

EXERCISES

Transcription

(Answers to the transcription exercises are given at the end of the book.)

1. Transcribe the following into phonemic symbols using either GA or RP norms. These words use the vowels from this chapter, and some simple consonants. Note: We transcribe <r> as /ɹ/; remember that RP does not use postvocalic-r.
   (a) purred (b) cut
   (c) why (d) join
   (e) loud (f) stay
   (g) slow (h) player
   (i) attend (j) curse
   (k) mower (l) tailor
   (m) mother (n) kite
   (o) louse (p) annoy

2. Transcribe the following using either GA or RP norms, employing allophonic symbols to mark vowel length differences, nasalization, and centralizing before /l/, where appropriate.
   (a) bide (b) spurt
   (c) turn (d) foal
   (e) owl (f) town
   (g) bite (h) loud
   (i) state (j) isle
   (k) lout (l) stun
   (m) spurred (n) staid
   (o) spoil (p) pail

3. Convert the following GA transcriptions back into ordinary writing. (All of them have more than one possible spelling—try to list all these.)
   (a) /ɹaɪt/ (b) /baʊ/
   (c) /hɝd/ (d) /steɪd/
   (e) /moʊn/ (f) /əsɛnt/
   (g) /mænɚ/ (h) /kɔɪ/
   (i) /ɹʌf/

Review Questions

1. What are rhotic vowels and how are they made?
2. What is the definition of a diphthong?
3. (GA) When do we use /ɚ/ and when /ɝ/? Give examples.
4. (RP) When do we use /ə/ and when /ɜ/? Give examples.
5. When do we use /ʌ/ and when /ə/? Give examples.

Study Topics and Experiments

1. Record yourself and your friends speaking words with initial schwa (but not before velars) and final schwa (e.g., "annoy," "obtain," versus "China," "sofa"). Find at least 10 different words (5 each) and at least 6 speakers. Then check to see whether your speakers use a lower schwa in final position than in initial position. You can use speech analysis software to help

if you're not sure. Are they consistent, or do some speakers switch from one vowel to the other?

2. Record yourself speaking all the vowels described in this chapter, and analyze the first three formants of each vowel using speech analysis software. How do your values compare to those listed in the chapter?

CD

Listen to the examples of various English vowels, and attempt the test examples following the instructions on the CD.

13

English Plosives and Affricates

INTRODUCTION

In this chapter we will be looking closely at the six plosive phonemes of English and the two affricate phonemes. We will also examine the use and status of the glottal stop, although this sound is not a phoneme of English. Although each section will examine the individual sounds in detail, some phonetic factors are held in common by this group of sounds, or by subsets of the group. We can look at these in this first section, and then proceed to the individual phonemes.

We will consider first the six plosives: /p, b, t, d, k, g/. These sounds all consist of the three stages of stop production we described in chapter 8; that is to say, a shutting phase, where the articulators come together to produce an air-tight seal somewhere in the oral cavity; a closure phase lasting some 40–150 ms, where the air from the lungs is stopped in the mouth, resulting in a build-up of air pressure behind the closure; and the release phase, when the articulators part and the compressed air rushes out with a popping noise. We commented in chapter 8 that some of these phases can be modified, and we will describe when this occurs in the sections below dealing with the individual sounds.

If these articulatory facts unite these six sounds, what can we use to distinguish between them? The following are the features we can utilize in this respect: place of articulation, force of articulation, voicing, aspiration, and length of preceding sound.

The six plosives are produced at three different places of articulation. /p, b/ are normally articulated at the bilabial place, with a closure between the upper and lower lips; /t, d/ are usually produced at the alveolar place, with a closure between the tongue tip and/or blade and the alveolar ridge; and /k, g/ have as their most common place of articulation a closure between the back of the tongue and the velum. As we will see later, all these phonemes have context dependent allophones with slightly differing places of articulation than those listed here.

Place of articulation differences, then, divide the six plosives into three pairs: bilabial, alveolar, and velar. We can now turn our attention to how we distinguish between the members of each pair. Most consonants can be assigned to two broad categories derived from how much force (both muscular energy and aerodynamic force) is expended in producing them. The categories are strong sounds (called *fortis*) and weak sounds (or *lenis*). The English plosives /p, t, k/ are all fortis, whereas /b, d, g/ are lenis. Fortis sounds are generally of longer duration than lenis, and louder. However, these differences are not so great that a distinction based purely on force of articulation would be sufficient for listeners to perceive consistently a contrast between the pairs of plosives. Other factors also have a part to play.

> The IPA has no diacritics to mark the fortis–lenis distinction. This is partly because it is difficult to make clear measurements that mark a sound as either one or the other. In disordered speech, however, we may well need to distinguish very strong from very weak articulations, and we return to the topic of how to mark these later in the book.

The English plosives are often described as being divided into a voiceless group (/p, t, k/) and a voiced group (/b, d, g/). These groups correspond with the force of articulation distinction: voiceless sounds are fortis, voiced are lenis. However, in English the sounds described as voiced often do not have vocal fold vibration throughout the duration of the sound. This is especially noted word-initially (where voicing may start partway through the sound) and word-finally (where voicing may end early). It seems that it is only in intervocalic position (i.e., between two vowel sounds) that /b, d, g/ are fully voiced throughout their duration. Word-initial and word-final lenis plosives may show full voicing, however, in connected speech if preceded or followed by a fully voiced segment.

Aspiration was described in chapter 6. With voiceless, fortis plosives, if there is a long voice onset time (that is, the time it takes for the voicing of the following sound to commence after the release phase of the plosive) we hear the resultant flow of voiceless air as aspiration. In English, /p, t, k/ are generally aspirated; that is, there is generally an audible puff of voiceless air on the release of the stop. As such aspiration doesn't occur with the voiced, lenis plosives, this aspiration is another cue for listeners to help distinguish the fortis and lenis pairs. However, the strength of the aspiration does differ depending upon the context of the sound. In syllable-initial position in a stressed syllable, aspiration is quite strong (because the voice onset time is quite long). In unstressed syllables, aspiration is weaker, and in word-final position there may be little or no aspiration (as we will see later, other variants may be used in final position). Interestingly, when /p, t, k/ follow /s/ in clusters (such as "spot," "stop," and "scot"), there is no aspiration at all.

Length of the preceding sound is a good distinguishing cue for syllable-final plosives. For example, a vowel before a fortis plosive is noticeable shorter than the same vowel before a voiced plosive: say the words "seat" and "seed" aloud a few times and listen for the difference. It would appear that slight durational differences are found in all languages before fortis and lenis plosives, but only in a few (including English) have these differences been drawn out to become noticeable by listeners.

Summarizing the differences in English between the pairs of plosives, we see that the overall force of articulation difference is augmented in different ways at different positions within the syllable and word. Word-initially, the main difference is in the presence versus the absence of aspiration; medially the main difference will be the presence versus absence of vocal fold vibration; and finally the main distinction is carried by the length of the preceding segment.

Do the affricates differ from the plosives? The lenis affricate /dʒ/ is similar to the lenis plosives in that it is only fully voiced intervocalically. The fortis affricate /tʃ/ is similar to the fortis plosives in that it reduces the length of preceding segments. However, due to the fricative release of the affricates, any voice onset time differences are masked: The fricative portion of the release takes place at the time when aspiration occurs with the plosives. The duration of the frication in the fortis affricate is markedly longer and louder than that with the lenis, though. It would appear, then, that initially in the word or syllable /tʃ/ is distinguished from /dʒ/ by the acoustic characteristics of the frication; medially the sounds are distinguished by vocal fold vibration; and finally, by the effect on preceding segments.

For all the consonants described in this chapter the soft palate is in the raised position, thus directing the pulmonic egressive airflow into the oral cavity and blocking off the nasal cavity.

THE BILABIAL PLOSIVES

/p/

This sound is described as a voiceless, bilabial plosive, and the name of the symbol is the same as the letter name (/pi/). As we saw in chapter 10, /p/ can occur in word-initial and word-final position and can be found in both initial and final clusters. The sound can also occur word-medially, but it should be noted that this term is potentially misleading, because a word-medial consonant is actually either syllable-final for the previous syllable (e.g., "cap.size") or syllable-initial for the following syllable ("re.peal").

Spelling

/p/ The most common spelling is to use <p> or <pp> (this latter is common in the middle of words but does *not* mean that /p/ is lengthened):

<p>	put	cup	repair
<pp>	pepper		support

Some exceptional forms are also found in individual words:

<ph>	shepherd
<gh>	hiccough

In a range of words with <p>, no /p/ is pronounced:

pneumonia psychiatry ptarmigan receipt cupboard raspberry

The main allophone of /p/ is produced in the following way. The vocal folds are abducted (held apart) in the voiceless phonation posture throughout the sound. The upper and lower lips are brought together, mainly through a closing movement of the lower jaw, and an air-tight seal is formed between them (see Fig. 13.2). Air from the lungs is pressurized behind this closure, which lasts for around 100–140 ms. At the end of this period, the lips are parted (mainly through movement of the lower jaw), and the compressed air rushes out with a popping noise. After the release of the articulators, some time will pass (perhaps about 60 ms) before vocal fold vibration commences for the following segment, resulting in the aspiration we described earlier. Throughout the articulation, the tongue is likely to be moving into position for the following segment.

The commonest allophones of /p/ are as follows:

- [pʰ] voiceless aspirated bilabial plosive. This is found initially in stressed syllables. A less strongly aspirated allophone is found initially in unstressed syllables and is one choice for syllable final position. This can be shown either by [p^{h}] or [pʿ], but the use of stress marks in a transcription normally tells us the degree of aspiration being used. When /p/ is followed by an approximant, the aspiration takes the form of devoicing of part of the approximant (see also chap. 15).
- [p⁼] voiceless unaspirated bilabial plosive. This allophone is found syllable-initially after /s/ in clusters. This is both in two-member clusters such as "spin," and in three-member clusters such as "splash."

- [p̪] voiceless labiodental plosive. This allophone is found when /p/ is immediately followed by /f/, in words such as "cupful," or even across word boundaries such as "up from." Although not all speakers will use this context-dependent allophone, it clearly reduces articulatory complexity if a single labiodental articulation is formed for the plosive and then slightly adjusted to provide for the following fricative, instead of starting with a bilabial gesture and having to transform it into a labiodental one.
- [p^{wh}] labialized aspirated voiceless bilabial plosive. This allophone is found before rounded vowels, because the bilabial closure is characterized by a protruded lip shape. Compare "pool" with "peel." In fact the latter may be characterized as an allophone with marked spread lip shape. The IPA has no diacritic for this, however.
- [p˺] voiceless bilabial plosive with no audible release. This occurs when /p/ is the first member of a two-plosive combination (e.g., "apt"), or as another choice for word-final position ("cap").
- [p^{l}] voiceless bilabial plosive with lateral release. Examples include "apple" and "couple."
- [p^{n}] voiceless bilabial plosive with nasal release. Examples include "happen" and "topmost."
- [p͡ʔ] voiceless bilabial plosive with glottal reinforcement. In syllable-final position some speakers use a plosive reinforced by a simultaneous glottal stop. Indeed, the glottal stop may occasionally be used alone.

Figure 13.1 shows a wideband spectrogram of the word "upper" (in this chapter, all the spectrograms have a maximum frequency of 5000 Hz). The most salient feature is the closure phase of the stop, shown as an unmarked band roughly in the center of the spectrogram. Also noticeable is the period of aspiration, marked on the spectrogram as pale markings immediately

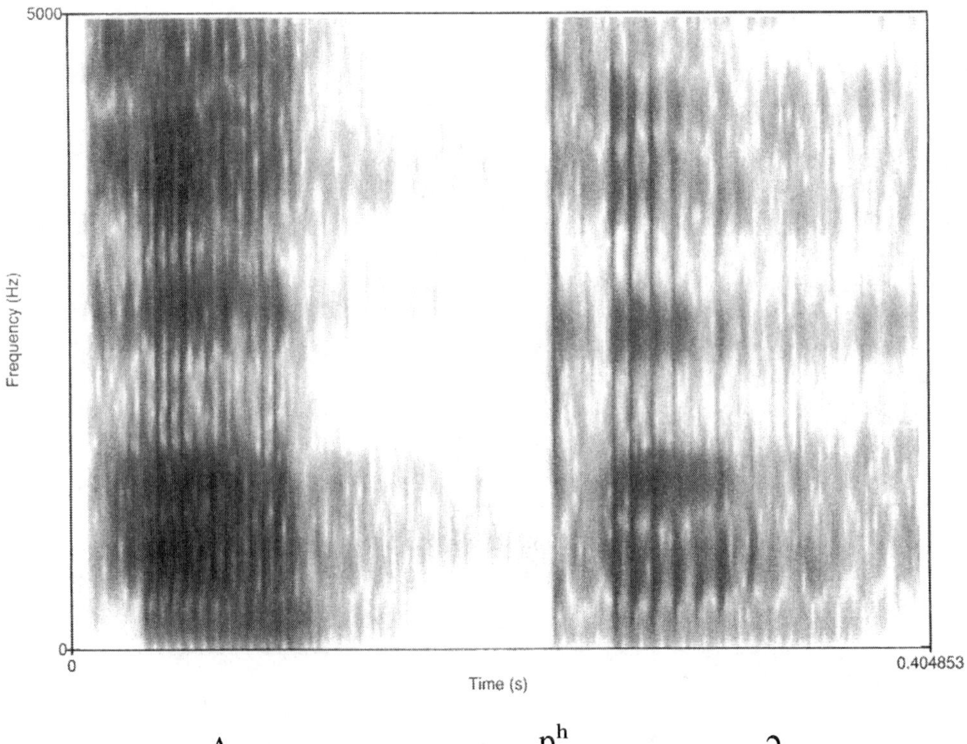

FIG 13.1. Wideband spectrogram of "upper" (RP pronunciation).

after the unmarked band. Distinctions between plosives at different places of articulation are carried by the formants of the preceding and following sounds. Bilabial plosives cause the second formant of a following vowel to move upward, and this can be seen in the figure. These movements are termed *formant transitions*.

/b/

This sound is described as a voiced, bilabial plosive, and the name of the symbol is the same as the letter name (/bi/). The sound /b/ can occur in word-initial and word-final position, and can be found in initial and final clusters. The sound can also occur word-medially, both as a word-medial syllable-final (e.g., "rib.cage") and as a word-medial syllable-initial ("de.bate").

Spelling

/b/ The most common spelling is to use <b> or <bb> (this latter is common in the middle and at the end of words but does *not* mean that /b/ is lengthened):

<b>	bid	sob	rebate
<bb>	robber	ebb	

Some exceptional forms are also found in individual words:

<pb> cupboard

In a range of words with final or near final <b>, no /b/ is pronounced:

bomb thumb debt doubt subtle

For the main allophone of /b/ the vocal folds are vibrating in the voiced phonation posture, throughout all (or most) of the sound. The upper and lower lips are brought together, mainly through a closing movement of the lower jaw, and an air-tight seal is formed between them (see Fig. 13.2). Air from the lungs is pressurized behind this closure, which lasts for around 60 ms. At the end of this period, the lips are parted (mainly through movement of the lower jaw), and the compressed air rushes out with a popping noise. Throughout the articulation, the tongue is likely to be moving into position for the following segment.

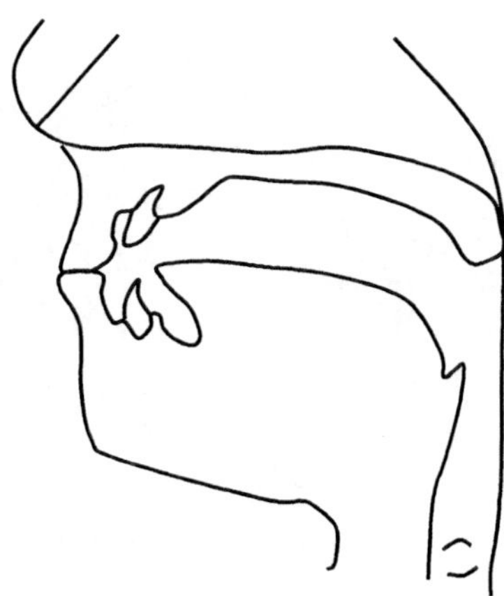

FIG 13.2. Articulator positions for /p, b/.

The most frequently occuring allophones of /b/ are as follows:

- [b] voiced unaspirated bilabial plosive. This is found intervocalically and has voicing lasting throughout the closure and release stages of the stop.
- [b̥] devoiced unaspirated bilabial plosive. This allophone is found word-initially and finally. In word-initial position the devoicing is found at the beginning of the sound; in word-final position it is found at the end of the sound. This can, if need be, be transcribed as [̥b] and [b̥], respectively.
- [b̪] voiced labiodental plosive. This allophone is found when /b/ is immediately followed by /v/ or /f/, in words such as "obvious," or even across word boundaries such as "rob from." Although not all speakers will use this context-dependent allophone, it clearly reduces articulatory complexity if a single labiodental articulation is formed for the plosive and then slightly adjusted to provide for the following fricative, instead of starting with a bilabial gesture and having to transform it into a labiodental one.
- [bʷ] labialized voiced bilabial plosive. This allophone is found before rounded vowels, as the bilabial closure is characterized by a protruded lip shape. Compare "boot" with "beat." In fact the latter may be characterized as an allophone with marked spread lip shape. As noted previously, the IPA has no diacritic for this, however.
- [b˺] voiced bilabial plosive with no audible release. This occurs when /b/ is the first member of a two-plosive combination (e.g., "obtain").
- [bˡ] voiced bilabial plosive with lateral release. Examples include "rubble" and "trouble."
- [bⁿ] voiceless bilabial plosive with nasal release. Examples include "ribbon" and "submarine."

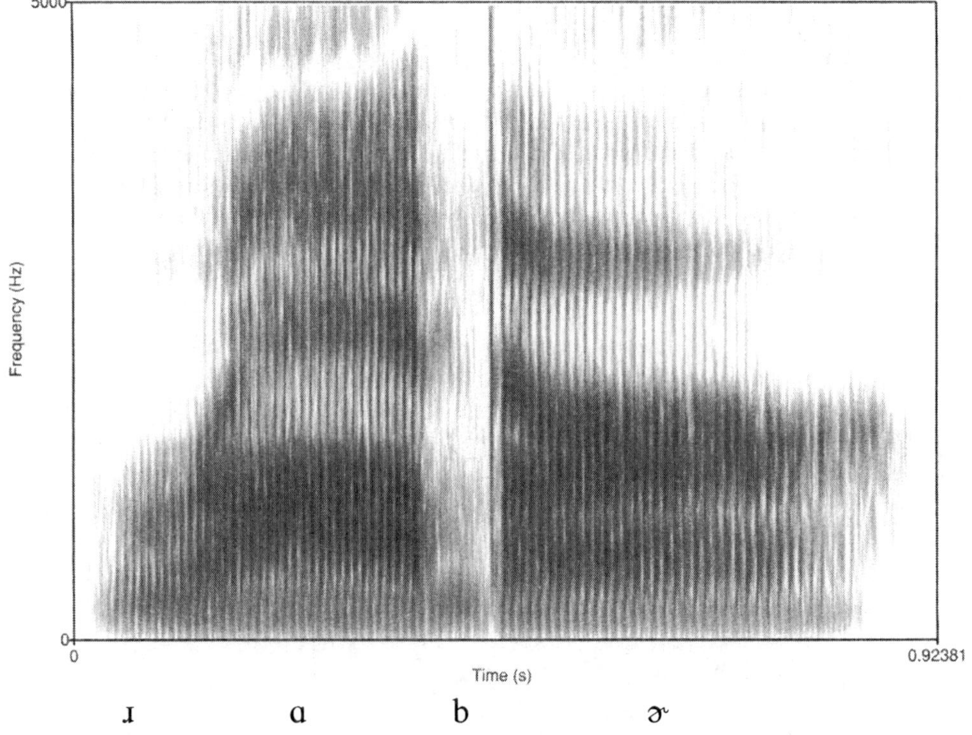

FIG 13.3. Wideband spectrogram of "robber" (GA pronunciation).

Figure 13.3 shows a wideband spectrogram of the word "robber." The most salient feature is the closure phase of the stop, shown as a mostly unmarked band roughly in the center of the spectrogram, but having the voicing bar at foot of the spectrogram. Notice that there are no aspiration markings on the spectrogram. The same formant transitions we noted for /p/ occur in the surrounding vowels for /b/.

THE ALVEOLAR PLOSIVES

/t/

This sound is described as a voiceless, alveolar plosive, and the name of the symbol is the same as the letter name (/ti/). The sound /t/ can occur in word-initial and word-final position and can be found in initial and final clusters. The sound can also occur word-medially, both as a word-medial syllable-final (e.g., "foot.ball") and as a word-medial syllable-initial ("re.tell").

Spelling

/t/ The most common spelling is to use <t> or <tt> (this latter is common in the middle of words but does *not* mean that /t/ is lengthened):

<t>	sit	seat	debate
<tt>	better	little	

The past tense marker <ed> is pronounced /t/ when following a voiceless consonant:

<ed>	hoped	laughed	booked

Some exceptional forms are also found:

<pt>	receipt	
<bt>	debt	
<th>	Thomas	Thames

In a range of words with <t>, no /t/ is pronounced:

castle mortgage soften Christmas postman

To produce the main allophone of /t/ the vocal folds are abducted in the voiceless phonation posture, throughout the sound. The tongue tip and/or blade (an individual preference) is raised until it touches the alveolar ridge, and an air-tight seal is formed between the tongue and the alveolar ridge, and between the side rims of the tongue and inner surface of the upper side teeth (see Fig. 13.5). Air from the lungs is pressurized behind this closure, which lasts for around 100–140 ms. At the end of this period, the tongue lowers, and the compressed air rushes out with a popping noise. After the release of the articulators, some time will pass (perhaps about 65 ms) before vocal fold vibration commences for the following segment, resulting in the aspiration we described earlier. Throughout the articulation, the lip shape is likely to be influenced by the following segment.

The range of allophones for /t/ is as follows:

- [t^h] voiceless aspirated alveolar plosive. This is found initially in stressed syllables. A less strongly aspirated allophone is found initially in unstressed syllables and is one choice

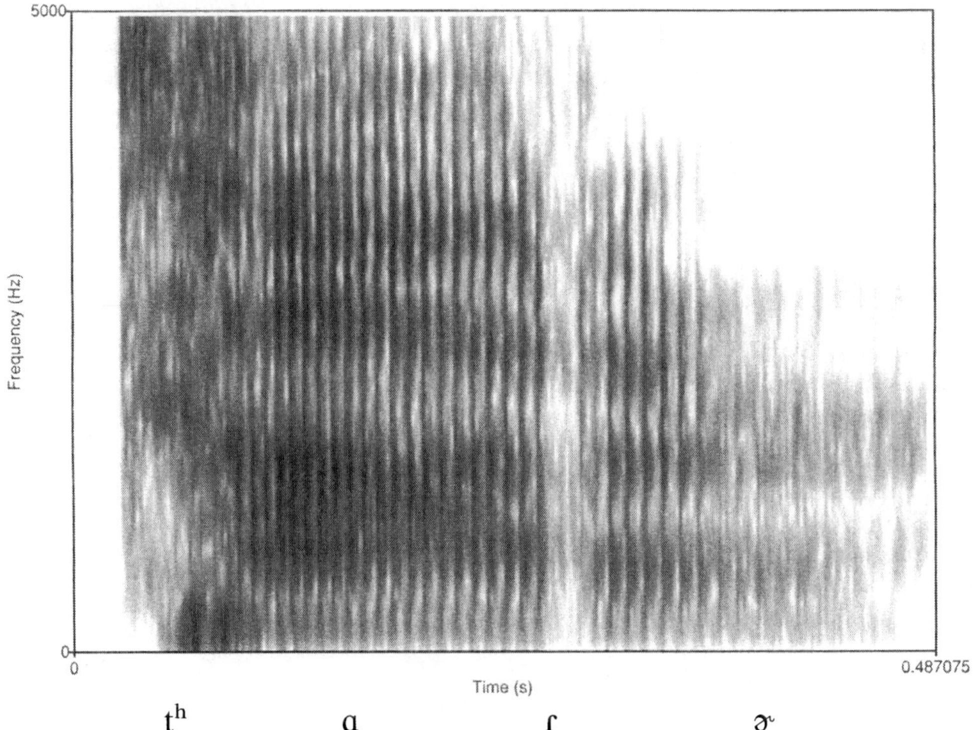

FIG 13.4. Wideband spectrogram of "totter" (GA pronunciation).

for syllable final position. This can be shown by either [tʰ] or [tʿ], but the use of stress marks in a transcription normally tells us the degree of aspiration being used. When /t/ is followed by an approximant, the aspiration takes the form of devoicing of part of the approximant (see also chap. 15).

- [t⁼] voiceless unaspirated alveolar plosive. This allophone is found syllable-initially after /s/ in clusters, both in two-member clusters such as "sting" and in three-member clusters such as "string."
- [t̪] voiceless dental plosive. This allophone is found when /t/ is immediately followed by /θ/ or /ð/, in words such as "eighth," or even across word boundaries such as "right then." It clearly reduces articulatory complexity if a single dental articulation is formed for the plosive and then slightly adjusted to provide for the following fricative, instead of starting with an alveolar gesture and having to transform it into a dental one.
- [t̠] voiceless postalveolar plosive. This allophone is found when /t/ is immediately followed by /ɹ/, in words such as "train" and "trim." Many speakers use a postalveolar affricate in this context ([t̠ʃ]), but this is not an allophone of /t/, but the use of a different phoneme (the phoneme /tʃ/ to be described later in this chapter) instead of the phoneme /t/.
- [tʷʰ] labialized aspirated voiceless alveolar plosive. This allophone is found before rounded vowels, when the alveolar closure is accompanied by lip rounding in anticipation of the vowel. Compare "tea" with "two." In fact the former may be characterized as an allophone with marked spread lip shape.
- [t̚] voiceless alveolar plosive with no audible release. This occurs when /t/ is the first member of a two-plosive combination (e.g., "outback"), or as another choice for word final position ("cat").

- [ɾ] voiced alveolar flap (GA). This allophone is used intervocalically when the following syllable is unstressed, e.g., in "letter," but not in "retain." Secondary stress and primary stress both block flapping. Some speakers may maintain the closure long enough to produce a voiced plosive. If this plosive is still basically fortis (for example, when the preceding segment is still shortened), we transcribe it allophonically as [t̬]; if, however, it is exactly the same as the voiced lenis plosive we would use [d] and count it as a phonemic change. Following /n/ (in words such as "international") /t/ may be realized as a flap, or may be omitted altogether.
- [t^{l}] voiceless alveolar plosive with lateral release. Examples include "little" and "at last." The within-word examples such as "little," however, are more likely to have the flap allophone with a following very short schwa vowel in GA.
- [t^{n}] voiceless alveolar plosive with nasal release. Examples include "button" and "at night." Within-word examples such as "button," however, are more likely to have the flap allophone with a following short schwa in GA. Another alternative found in some varieties is glottal stop followed by syllabic nasal ([ʔn̩]), though this sounds virtually the same as a nasally released [t^{n}].
- [t͡ʔ] voiceless alveolar plosive with glottal reinforcement. In syllable-final position some speakers use a plosive reinforced by a simultaneous glottal stop. Especially in British accents, some speakers may use the glottal stop alone.

Despite the wide range of allophones for this sound, when we transcribe phonemically we represent them all by /t/. The only exception to this guideline in this book is that we normally transcribe flapped-t as /ɾ/ because of its markedly different phonetic nature.

Figure 13.4 shows a wideband spectrogram of the word "totter." The most salient feature is the closure phase of the initial stop, shown as an unmarked band roughly at the left of the spectrogram. Also noticeable is the period of aspiration, marked on the spectrogram as pale markings immediately after the unmarked band. Distinctions between plosives at different places of articulation are carried by the formants of the preceding and following sounds. Formant transitions with alveolar sounds are somewhat more complex than with bilabials and velars; alveolar closure causes the second formant of the surrounding vowels to move towards the middle of the frequency range. This means that the formant will bend upward or downward away from this middle range, depending upon whether its normal position is above or below this range. The medial /t/ in this word is realized as a tap ([ɾ]), and this is seen on the spectrogram as a very short unmarked band in the center of the spectrogram.

/d/

This sound is described as a voiced, alveolar plosive, and the name of the symbol is the same as the letter name (/di/). The sound /d/ can occur in word-initial and word-final position, and can be found in initial and final clusters. The sound can also occur word-medially, both as a word-medial syllable-final (e.g., "mid.lands") and as a word-medial syllable-initial ("pre.dict").

Spelling

/d/ The most common spelling is to use <d> or <dd> (this latter is common in the middle and at the end of words but does *not* mean that /d/ is lengthened):

<d>	deem	sad	undo	redo
<dd>	udder	sudden		

The past tense marker <ed> is pronounced /d/ when following a voiced consonant or vowel:

<ed> lugged buzzed wanted

Some exceptional forms are also found in individual words:

<ld> could should would

In a range of words with <d>, no /d/ is pronounced:

handsome handbag grandfather sandwich

The main allophone of /d/ is made with the tongue tip and/or blade (an individual preference) raised until it touches the alveolar ridge, and an air-tight seal formed between the tongue and the alveolar ridge and between the side rims of the tongue and inner surface of the upper side teeth (see Fig. 13.5). The vocal folds are vibrating in the voiced phonation posture throughout all (or most) of the sound. Air from the lungs is pressurized behind the closure, which lasts for around 50–60 ms. At the end of this period, the tongue lowers, and the compressed air rushes out with a popping noise. Throughout the articulation, the lip shape is likely to be influenced by the following segment.

The list of allophones for /d/ is as follows:

- [d] voiced unaspirated alveolar plosive. This is found intervocalically and has voicing lasting throughout the closure and release stages of the stop.
- [d̥] devoiced unaspirated alveolar plosive. This allophone is found word-initially and -finally. In word-initial position the devoicing is found at the beginning of the sound; in word-final position it is found at the end of the sound. This can, if need be, be transcribed as [˳d] and [d˳] respectively.
- [d̪] voiced dental plosive. This allophone is found when /d/ is immediately followed by /θ/ or /ð/, in words such as "width," or even across word boundaries such as "red thing." It clearly reduces articulatory complexity if a single dental articulation is formed for the plosive and then slightly adjusted to provide for the following fricative, instead of starting with an alveolar gesture and having to transform it into a dental one.

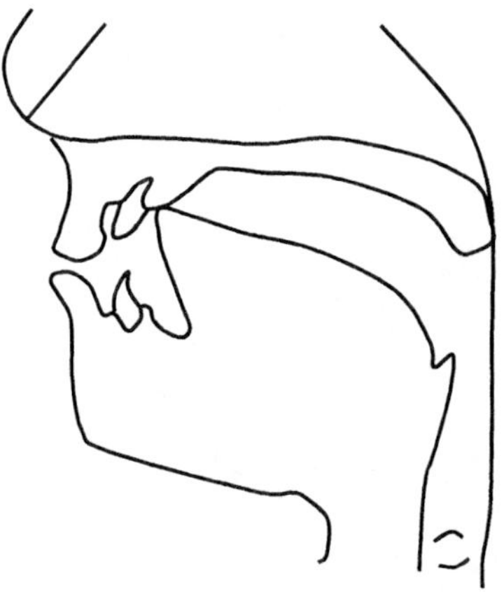

FIG 13.5. Articulator positions for /t, d/.

- [d̠] voiced postalveolar plosive. This allophone is found when /d/ is immediately followed by /ɹ/, in words such as "drain" and "dream." Many speakers use a postalveolar affricate in this context ([d̠ʒ]), but this is not an allophone of /d/, but the use of a different phoneme (the phoneme /dʒ/ to be described later in this chapter) instead of the phoneme /d/.
- [dʷ] labialized voiced alveolar plosive. This allophone is found before rounded vowels, where the alveolar closure is accompanied by lip rounding in anticipation of the vowel. Compare "deem" with "doom." In fact the former may be characterized as an allophone with marked spread lip shape.
- [d̚] voiced alveolar plosive with no audible release. This occurs when /d/ is the first member of a two-plosive combination (e.g., "midtown").
- [ɾ] voiced alveolar flap (GA). This allophone is used intervocalically when the following syllable is unstressed, e.g., in "ladder," but not in "redirect." Many speakers use a fully voiced [d] in this position instead of the flap.
- [dˡ] voiced alveolar plosive with lateral release. Examples include "middle" and "odd lamp." The within-word examples such as "middle," however, may be said with the flap allophone and a following vowel in GA.
- [dⁿ] voiced alveolar plosive with nasal release. Examples include "hidden" and "bad night." Within-word examples such as "hidden," however, may be produced with the flap allophone and a following vowel in GA.

Figure 13.6 shows a wideband spectrogram of the word "redder" (pronounced with a stop rather than a tap realization). The most salient feature is the closure phase of the stop, shown as a mostly unmarked band roughly in the center of the spectrogram, but having the voicing

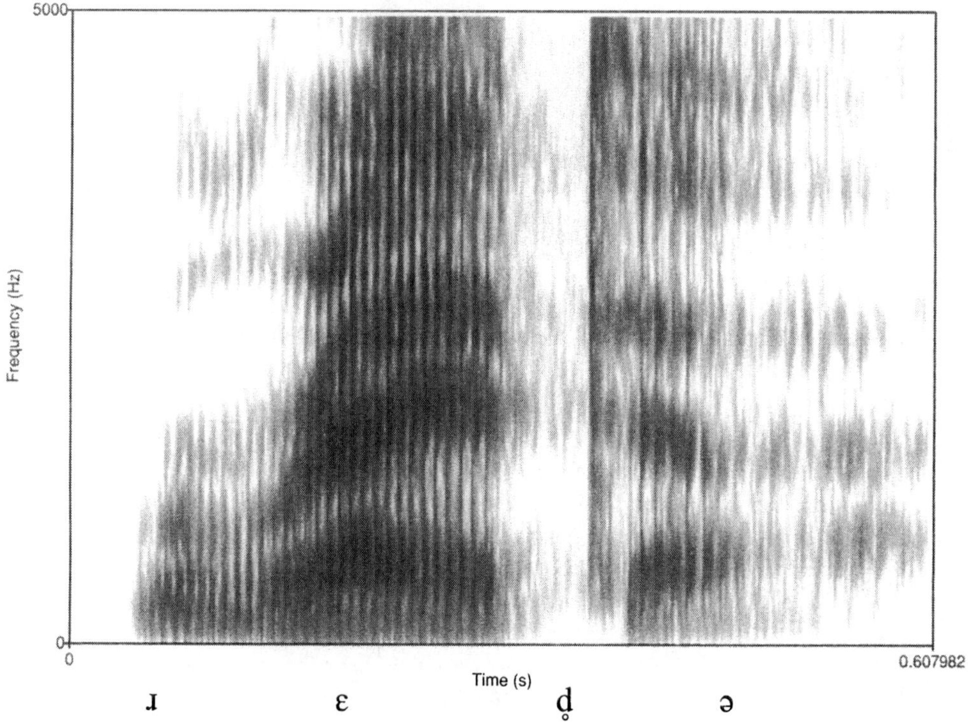

FIG 13.6. Wideband spectrogram of "redder" (RP pronunciation).

bar at the foot of the spectrogram for part of this space (this token was partly devoiced). Notice that there are no aspiration markings on the spectrogram. The same formant transitions we noted for /t/ occur in the surrounding vowels for /d/.

THE VELAR PLOSIVES

/k/

This sound is described as a voiceless, velar plosive, and the name of the symbol is the same as the letter name (/keɪ/). As we saw in chapter 10, /k/ can occur in word-initial and word-final position and can be found in both initial and final clusters. The sound can also occur word-medially, but it should be noted that this term is potentially misleading, because a word-medial consonant is actually either syllable-final for the previous syllable (e.g., "black.board") or syllable-initial for the following syllable ("re.count").

Spelling

/k/ The most common spelling is to use <k>, <ck>, <c>, or <c> (the use of <ck> and <cc> does *not* mean that /k/ is lengthened):

<k>	key	break	turkey	
<ck>	back	lacking		
<c>	cat	maniac		circus
<cc>	account		occur	

Some forms are also found with <q>, <qu>, and <cqu>:

<q>	Qatar	
<qu>	unique	conquer
<cqu>	racquet	

(<qu> and <cqu> usually represent /kw/).
Some exceptional forms are also found in individual words:

<ch>	school	
<lk>	walk	talk

In a range of words with initial <k>, or with <c> no /k/ is pronounced:

knee know muscle

The vocal folds are abducted in the voiceless phonation posture throughout the sound. For the commonest allophone of the phoneme, the back of the tongue dorsum is raised up until it touches the soft palate (the exact position on the velum is determined by the following segment), and an air-tight seal is formed between the tongue and the velum (see Fig. 13.7). Air from the lungs is pressurized behind this closure, which lasts for around 100–140 ms. At the end of this period, the tongue dorsum is lowered, and the compressed air rushes out with a popping noise. After the release of the articulators, some time will pass (perhaps about 60 ms) before vocal fold vibration commences for the following segment, resulting in the aspiration we described earlier. Throughout the articulation, the lip shape will be under the influence of the following sound.

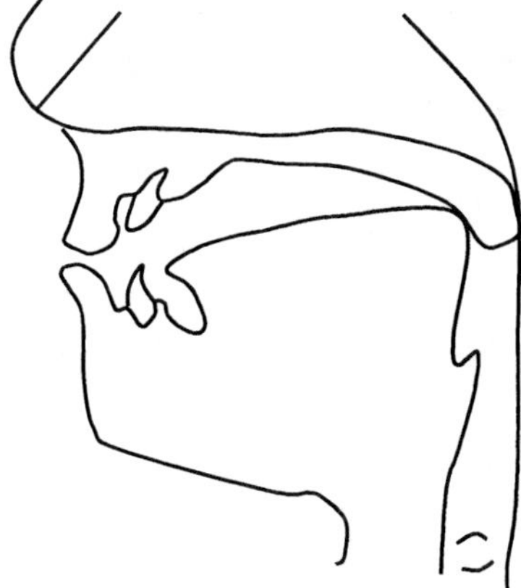

FIG 13.7. Articulator positions for /k, g/.

The main allophones of /k/ are as follows:

- [k^{h}] voiceless aspirated velar plosive. This is found initially in stressed syllables. A less strongly aspirated allophone is found initially in unstressed syllables and is one choice for syllable-final position. This can be shown either by [k^{h}] or [kʿ], but the use of stress marks in a transcription normally tells us the degree of aspiration being used. When /k/ is followed by an approximant, the aspiration takes the form of devoicing of part of the approximant (see also chap. 15).
- [k$^{=}$] voiceless unaspirated velar plosive. This allophone is found syllable-initially after /s/ in clusters, both in two-member clusters such as "skin" and in three-member clusters such as "scream."
- [k̠] voiceless retracted velar plosive (almost as far back as the uvular position). This allophone is found when /k/ is immediately followed by a back vowel in words such as "court" or "car." This reduces articulatory complexity, because the tongue is closer to the position it needs to adopt for the back vowel.
- [k̟] voiceless advanced velar plosive (almost as far forward as the palatal position). This allophone is found when /k/ is immediately followed by a front vowel in words such as "key" or "kept." This reduces articulatory complexity, because the tongue is closer to the position it needs to adopt for the front vowel.
- [k^{wh}] labialized aspirated voiceless velar plosive. This allophone is found before rounded vowels, because the velar closure is accompanied by lip rounding in anticipation of the vowel. Compare "keep" with "coop." In fact the former may be characterized as an allophone with marked spread lip shape.
- [k˺] voiceless velar plosive with no audible release. This occurs when /k/ is the first member of a two-plosive combination (e.g., "act") or as another choice for word-final position ("lack").
- [k^{l}] voiceless velar plosive with lateral release. Examples include "cling" and "buckle."
- [k^{n}] voiceless velar plosive with nasal release. Examples include "bacon" and "dark night."
- [k͡ʔ] voiceless bilabial plosive with glottal reinforcement. In syllable-final position some speakers use a plosive reinforced by a simultaneous glottal stop. Indeed, the glottal stop may occasionally be used alone.

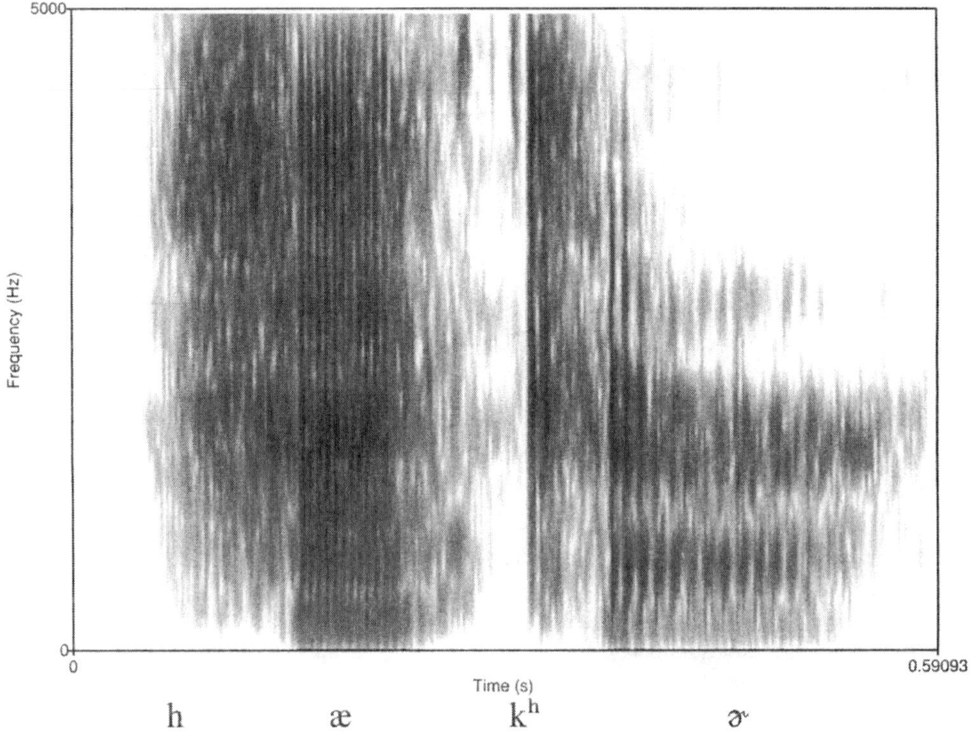

FIG 13.8. Wideband spectrogram of "hacker" (GA pronunciation).

Figure 13.8 shows a wideband spectrogram of the word "hacker." The most salient feature is the closure phase of the stop, shown as an unmarked band roughly in the center of the spectrogram. Also noticeable is the period of aspiration, marked on the spectrogram as pale markings immediately after the unmarked band. Distinctions between plosives at different places of articulation are carried by the formants of the preceding and following sounds. Formant transitions with velar plosives see the second formant of a following vowel move downwards, as in the figure.

/g/

This sound is described as a voiced, velar plosive, and sometimes the symbol is given the same name as the letter (/dʒi/), but, because this name doesn't actually include the sound the symbol represents, some phoneticians prefer to call it /gə/. The sound /g/ can occur in word-initial and word-final position and can be found in initial and final clusters. The sound can also occur word-medially, both as word-medial syllable-final (e.g., "log.jam") and as a word-medial syllable-initial ("re.gain").

Spelling

/g/ The most common spelling is to use <g> or <gg> (this latter is common in the middle and at the end of words but does *not* mean that /g/ is lengthened):

<g>	gum	big	regress
<gg>	bigger	egg	

Some words use a <gu> or <gue> spelling:

<gu>	guilt	guard
<gue>	vague	rogue

Some exceptional forms are also found in a few words:

<gh> ghost

In a range of words with <g>, no /g/ is pronounced:

gnome gnaw gnostic sign reign

The vocal folds are vibrating in the voiced phonation posture throughout all (or most) of the sound. For the most frequent allophone of the phoneme, the back of the tongue dorsum is raised up until it touches the soft palate (the exact position on the velum is determined by the following segment), and an air-tight seal is formed between the tongue and the velum (see Fig. 13.7). Air from the lungs is pressurized behind this closure, which lasts for around 60 ms. At the end of this period, the tongue dorsum is lowered, and the compressed air rushes out with a popping noise. Throughout the articulation, the lip shape will be under the influence of the following sound.

The main allophones of /g/ are as follows:

- [g] voiced unaspirated velar plosive. This is found intervocalically and has voicing lasting throughout the closure and release stages of the stop.
- [g̊] devoiced unaspirated velar plosive. This allophone is found word-initially and -finally. In word-initial position the devoicing is found at the beginning of the sound; in word-final position it is found at the end of the sound. This can, if need be, be transcribed as [˚g] and [g˚] respectively.
- [g̠] voiced retracted velar plosive (almost as far back as the uvular position). This allophone is found when /g/ is immediately followed by a back vowel in words such as "gore" or "garden." This reduces articulatory complexity, because the tongue is closer to the position it needs to adopt for the back vowel.
- [g̟] voiced advanced velar plosive (almost as far forward as the palatal position). This allophone is found when /g/ is immediately followed by a front vowel in words such as "give" or "guess." This reduces articulatory complexity, because the tongue is closer to the position it needs to adopt for the front vowel.
- [g^w] labialized voiced velar plosive. This allophone is found before rounded vowels, because the velar closure is accompanied by lip rounding in anticipation of the vowel. Compare "goose" with "geese." In fact the latter may be characterized as an allophone with marked spread lip shape. The IPA has no diacritic for this, however.
- [g˺] voiced velar plosive with no audible release. This occurs when /g/ is the first member of a two-plosive combination (e.g., "rugby").
- [g^l] voiced velar plosive with lateral release. Examples include "struggle" and "glue."
- [g^n] voiced velar plosive with nasal release. Examples include "ignore" and "dragnet."

Figure 13.9 shows a wideband spectrogram of the word "lugger." The most salient feature is the closure phase of the stop, shown as a mostly unmarked band roughly in the center of the spectrogram, but having the voicing bar at foot of the spectrogram. Notice that there are no aspiration markings on the spectrogram. The same formant transitions we noted for /k/ occur in the surrounding vowels for /g/.

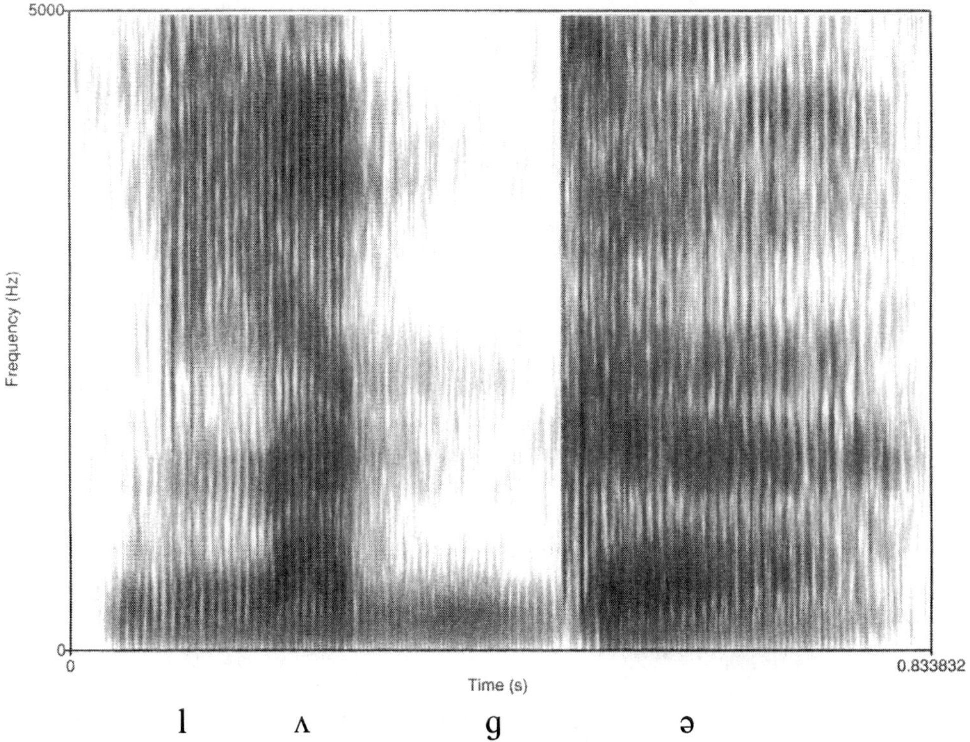

FIG 13.9. Wideband spectrogram of "lugger" (RP pronunciation).

THE POSTALVEOLAR AFFRICATES

/tʃ/

This sound is described as a voiceless, alveolar plosive, and the name of the symbol is either the names of two component parts or (as preferred by some phoneticians) /tʃə/. The sound /tʃ/ can occur in word-initial and word-final position and can be found in final clusters. The sound can also occur word-medially, both as a word-medial syllable-final (e.g., "latch.key") and as a word-medial syllable-initial ("re.charge").

Spelling

/tʃ/ The most common spelling is to use <ch> syllable-initially, and <tch> syllable-finally:

<ch>	chin	chalk	cheese
<tch>	match	butcher; *but also* Tchaikovsky	

Some less common forms are also found:

<ti>	question	
<tu>	virtue	nature
<c>	cellist	

In a range of words with <ch>, /k/ rather than /tʃ/ is pronounced:

mechanic chianti

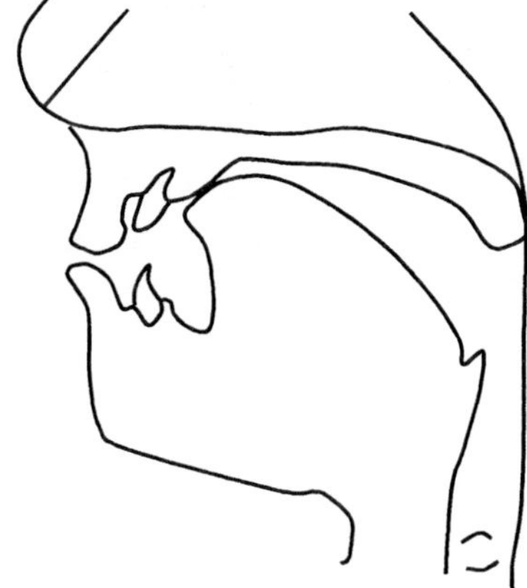

FIG 13.10. Articulator positions for /tʃ, dʒ/.

The main allophone of /tʃ/ is produced in the following way. The vocal folds are abducted in the voiceless phonation posture throughout the sound. The tongue tip and blade are raised up until they touch the rear part of the alveolar ridge, and an air-tight seal is formed between the tongue and the alveolar ridge and between the side rims of the tongue and the inner surface of the upper side teeth. At the same time, the front of the tongue is raised toward the hard palate, leaving only a narrow channel (see Fig. 13.10). Air from the lungs is pressurized behind this closure, which lasts for around 100 ms. At the end of this period, the tongue tip and blade lower slightly, and the compressed air is forced through the narrow channel left between the front of the tongue and the hard palate and between the blade of the tongue and the alveolar ridge. The channel shape is a narrow slit. The duration of the stop part and the fricative part are roughly equal. Throughout the articulation, the lip shape is likely to be influenced by the following segment, although many speakers normally use a rounded lip shape for this sound.

The commonest allophones of /tʃ/ are as follows:

- [t̠ʃ] voiceless postalveolar affricate. This is found in all positions.
- [t̠ʃʷ] labialized voiceless postalveolar affricate. This allophone is found before rounded vowels, because the closure is accompanied by lip rounding in anticipation of the vowel. Compare "cheese" with "choose." This allophone is often the standard pronunciation for many speakers except, perhaps, before lip-spread vowels.
- [t̠ʃ͡ʔ] voiceless postalveolar affricate with glottal reinforcement. In syllable-final position some speakers use an affricate reinforced by a simultaneous glottal stop.

Figure 13.11 shows a wideband spectrogram of the word "wretched." The most salient features are the closure phase of the stop, shown as an unmarked band roughly in the center of the spectrogram, and the fricative release phase, shown as the markings across the frequency range immediately after the unmarked band. Formant transitions are not such important cues with affricates, as the fricative portion carries information on place of articulation in the range of frequencies involved (see more details in chap. 14).

/dʒ/

This sound is described as a voiced, postalveolar affricate, and the name of the symbol is either the names of two component parts or (as preferred by some phoneticians) /dʒə/.

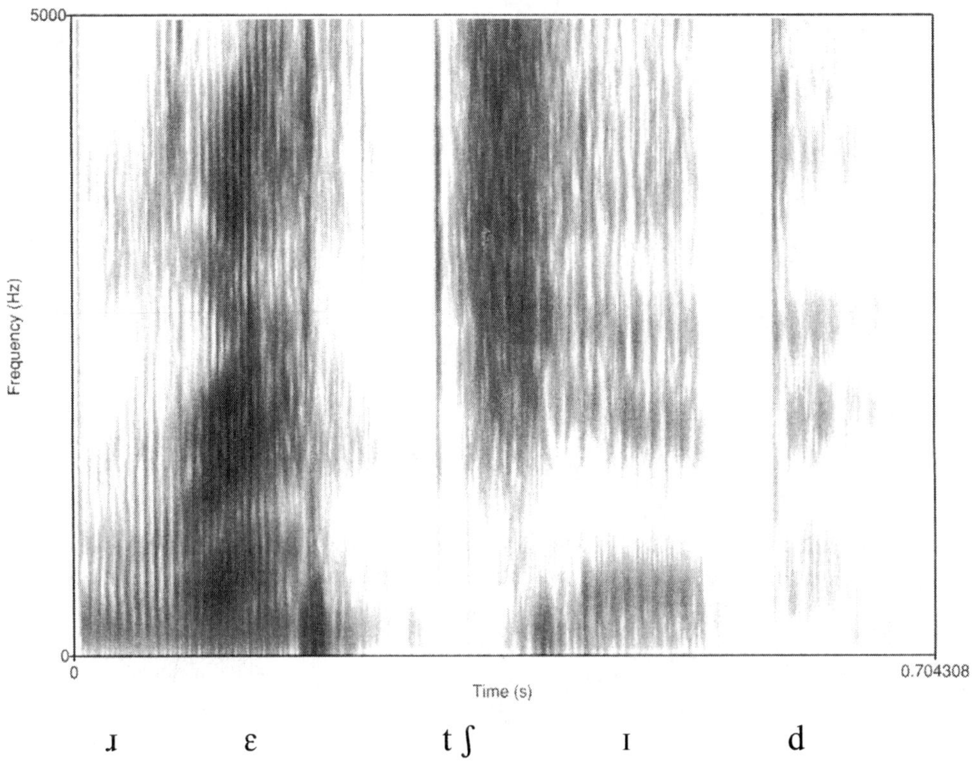

FIG 13.11. Wideband spectrogram of "wretched" (GA pronunciation).

The sound /dʒ/ can occur in word-initial and word-final position and can be found in final clusters. The sound can also occur word-medially, both as a word-medial syllable-final (e.g., "ridge.back") and as a word-medial syllable-initial ("pre.judge").

Spelling

/dʒ/ The most common spelling is to use <j>, <g>, or <dg> (this last is common in the middle and at the end of words):

<j>	jam	rejoice	
<g>	gem	magic	rage
<dg>	ledge	midget	

Some less common forms are also found:

<dj>	adjust adjective	
<gg>	suggest	exaggerate
<gi>	legion religion	

<di>, <de>, <du> soldier grandeur arduous

To make the main allophone of /dʒ/ the tongue tip and blade are raised until they touch the rear part of the alveolar ridge, and an air-tight seal is formed between the tongue and the alveolar ridge and between the side rims of the tongue and inner surface of the upper side teeth. At the same time, the front of the tongue is raised toward the hard palate, leaving only a narrow channel (see Fig. 13.10). Air from the lungs is pressurized behind this closure, which lasts for around 40 ms. At the end of this period, the tongue tip and blade lower slightly, and the compressed air is forced through the narrow channel left between the front of the tongue and the hard palate and the blade of the tongue and the alveolar ridge. The channel shape is a narrow slit. The vocal folds are vibrating in the voiced phonation posture throughout all (or most) of the sound. The durations of the stop part and the fricative part are roughly equal. Throughout the articulation, the lip shape is likely to be influenced by the following segment, although many speakers normally use a rounded lip shape for this sound.

The most common allophones of /dʒ/ are as follows:

- [dʒ] voiced postalveolar affricate. This is found intervocalically, and has voicing lasting throughout the closure and release stages of the stop and fricative portions.
- [d̥ʒ̊] devoiced postalveolar affricate. This allophone is found word-initially and -finally. In word-initial position the devoicing is found at the beginning of the sound; in word-final position it is found at the end of the sound. This can, if need be, be transcribed as [d̥ʒ] and [dʒ̊], respectively.
- [dʒʷ] labialized voiced postalveolar affricate. This allophone is found before rounded vowels, as the closure is accompanied by lip rounding in anticipation of the vowel. Compare "jeans" with "June." This allophone is often the default pronunciation for many speakers except, perhaps, before lip-spread vowels.

Figure 13.12 shows a wideband spectrogram of the word "ledger." The most salient features are the closure phase of the stop, shown as an unmarked band roughly in the center of the

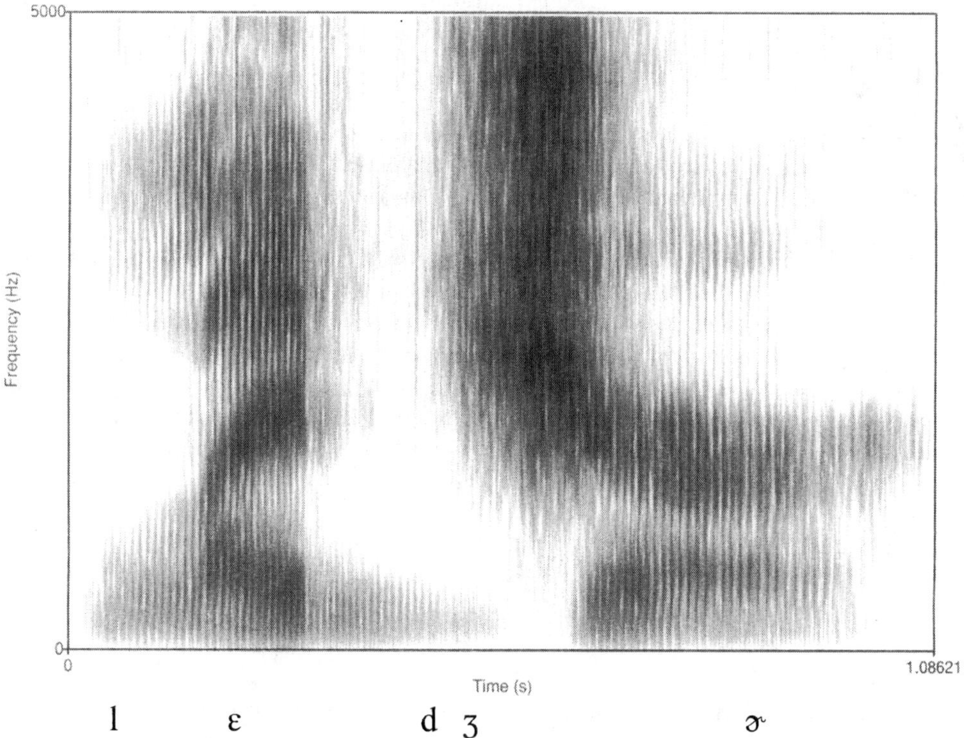

FIG 13.12. Wideband spectrogram of "ledger" (GA pronunciation).

spectrogram but with the voicing bar at that foot; and the fricative release phase, shown as the markings across the frequency range immediately after the unmarked band. Formant transitions are not such important cues with affricates, because the fricative portion carries information on place of articulation in the range of frequencies involved (see more details in chap. 14).

THE GLOTTAL STOP

[ʔ]

This segment does not have phonemic status in English but, despite this, is found relatively frequently in many varieties of the language. Three main uses of the glottal stop are noted here.

- First, as a hiatus blocker. *Hiatus* is the term given to the juxtaposition of two vowels, either within a word, or across a word boundary. Many English speakers avoid the slurring of one vowel into another by inserting a glottal stop between them. Examples include "naʔïve," "reʔact," "we ʔ are here," and "to ʔ a degree." Some speakers may extend this usage to any syllable-initial vowel.
- Second, as an allophone of /t/. In some British English accents intervocalic and word-final /t/ is realized as [ʔ] (as in "better" and "bet"). In American English accents nasally released /t/ may be realized as [ʔ] followed by the nasal segment (e.g., in "button"), although the difference between this realization and [t] followed by nasal release is difficult to perceive.
- Finally, as noted earlier, /p, t, k/ in word-final position may be accompanied by *glottal reinforcement* (the simultaneous use of the plosive and [ʔ]) in many varieties of English.

Because the glottal stop has never been considered a member of the English consonant system, no means of spelling the sound has ever been devised. Hawai'ian, which does use the glottal stop as a full, contrastive, phoneme, employs an apostrophe to mark it, as in the name of the islands, or a word such as *ha'upu* "to recall."

The glottal stop is produced by the adducting of the vocal folds to block the pulmonic egressive airflow. This blockage causes air pressure to build beneath the glottis, and when the folds are released, this compressed air rushes out. Because the glottis is closed, the sound is normally considered to be voiceless (although it might be better to consider a closed glottis as a different glottal state than either voiced or voiceless). No allophones of the glottal stop are generally recognized; however, one could posit a lip-rounded variant before rounded vowels. Acoustically, the glottal stop is characterized by a period of silence with no formant transitions.

BACKGROUND READING

These sounds are also covered in detail in Cruttenden (2001). Other texts also deal with them, such as Small (1999), Edwards (2003), and Shriberg and Kent (2003); however, these texts do not deal with a wide range of allophonic variation and, as noted previously, there may be a tendency to combine allophonic variation with regional and stylistic variation and with phonemic alternation.

EXERCISES

Transcription

(Answers to the transcription exercises are given at the end of the book.)

1. Transcribe the following into phonemic symbols using either GA or RP norms. These words use the consonants from this chapter and the vowels from the previous chapters.
   (a) bead (b) get
   (c) took (d) pipe
   (e) chew (f) deep
   (g) cog (h) jaw
   (i) tube (j) peat
   (k) dead (l) kit
   (m) gap (n) boot
   (o) jab (p) chop
2. Transcribe the following using either GA or RP norms, employing allophonic symbols to mark aspiration, devoicing, and lip-rounding before rounded vowels, where appropriate.
   (a) type (b) spike
   (c) church (d) Bobby
   (e) pike (f) goat
   (g) madder (h) cope
   (i) stew (j) judge
   (k) cat (l) two
   (m) mugger (n) scoot
   (o) deed (p) bike
3. Convert the following GA transcriptions back into ordinary writing. (They all have more than one possible spelling—try to list all these.)
   (a) /taɪd/ (b) /dʒæm/
   (c) /bit/ (d) /ki/
   (e) /gɹeɪz/ (f) /deɪz/
   (g) /tʃuz/ (h) /pliz/
4. Note whether a flap [ɾ] or a plosive [t] would be used in the following words in GA:
   (a) matter (b) retake
   (c) pretend (d) pretty
   (e) citizen (f) detach

Review Questions

1. What are the rules for the use of aspiration with English plosives?
2. Describe the patterns of devoicing in English lenis fricatives and affricates.
3. What place of articulation allophones are found with /t/ and /d/, and what contexts prompt these variants?
4. What is "flapping" in American English, and what are the rules for its use?

Study Topics and Experiments

1. Draw up a list of words with medial /t/ and medial /d/ (e.g., "matter" and "madder"). Choose at least five words of each type. Record yourself and at least nine other people saying these

words in a carrier phrase (e.g., "say X again"). Note whether your speakers flap both /t/ and /d/, and whether they retain the vowel length difference expected (reduced before /t/). Also note whether they are consistent or variable in their realizations.

2. Research the aerodynamic reasons that there is vowel shortening before fortis plosives, and that there is initial and final devoicing with lenis plosives.

CD

The CD has examples of all the consonants covered in this chapter. Do the test examples following the instructions on the CD. Answers to all the exercises on the CD are given at the end of the book.

14

English Fricatives

INTRODUCTION

In this chapter we turn our attention to the fricatives of English. Most varieties of English have nine fricative phonemes. Eight of these consist of pairs of voiceless and voiced fricatives at four different places of articulation; the ninth is the glottal fricative /h/.

The fricatives /f, v, θ, ð, s, z, ʃ, ʒ/ all involve turbulent airflow through a narrow channel between the articulators. They are distinguished from one another by several features, and we will consider these in turn. First, they are produced using four different places of articulation: /f, v/ are both labiodental; /θ, ð/ are dental; /s, z/ are alveolar; and /ʃ, ʒ/ are postalveolar. We can also take channel shape into consideration. /s, z/ are pronounced using a grooved channel for the air to flow out of; /f, v, θ, ð/ require a wide slit channel shape, and /ʃ, ʒ/ a narrow slit channel. Like the plosives, the fricatives fall into two categories in terms of force of articulation. The fortis fricatives (/f, θ, s, ʃ/) are produced with greater muscular effort and stronger airflow and have a longer duration than the lenis fricatives (/v, ð, z, ʒ/). Voicing is also an important distinction within the group of English fricatives. The fortis fricatives /f, θ, s, ʃ/ are always voiceless; the lenis fricatives /v, ð, z, ʒ/ are fully voiced in intervocalic position. In initial and final position, however, the lenis fricatives tend to be devoiced to some extent. In initial position voicing tends to start partway through the fricative; in final position it ends early (indeed, for some speakers, these final fricatives may be almost completely voiceless, but their duration still marks them as lenis). This devoicing may be absent in connected speech, however, if the fricative in question is following or preceding a fully voiced sound. The final feature we need to consider is the length of the preceding segment. Just as we found with the plosives, fortis fricatives shorten preceding vowels and consonants. This can be seen if you say the following pairs of words (and listen very carefully to the length of the segment just before the fricatives): *place* ~ *plays, self* ~ *selves, loath* ~ *loathe.*

For all the consonants described in this chapter the soft palate is in the raised position, thus directing the pulmonic egressive airflow into the oral cavity and blocking off the nasal cavity.

The pairs of fricatives are distinguished in the following ways:

initial position: strength of articulation (mainly duration of frication)
medial position: voicing; also length of preceding segment
final position: length of preceding segment; also strength of articulation

THE LABIODENTAL FRICATIVES

/f/

This sound is described as a voiceless labiodental fricative, and the name of the symbol is the same as the letter name (/ɛf/). As we saw in chapter 10, /f/ can occur in word-initial and word-final position, and can be found in both initial and final clusters. The sound can also occur word-medially, but remember that this term is potentially misleading, because a word-medial consonant is actually either syllable-final for the previous syllable (e.g., "deaf.en") or syllable-initial for the following syllable ("de.fend").

Spelling

/f/ The most common spelling is to use <f>, <ph>, or <ff> (this last is common at the end of words but does *not* mean that /f/ is lengthened):

<f> foot flake refine
<ph> photo graph
<ff> afford off

Some exceptional forms are also found in individual words:

<gh> cough rough

Note <f> for /v/ in:
of

The commonest allophone of /f/ is produced in the following way. The vocal folds are abducted (held apart) in the voiceless phonation posture throughout the sound. The inner surface of the upper lip is brought into close approximation with the undersurface of the upper front teeth, mainly through a closing movement of the lower jaw, and a narrow channel is left between them (see Fig. 14.1). Air from the lungs flows through this channel and becomes turbulent. Throughout the articulation, the tongue is likely to be moving into position for the following segment.

The main allophones of /f/ are as follows:

- [f] voiceless labiodental fricative. This is found in all word positions.
- [f^w] labialized voiceless labiodental fricative. This allophone is found before rounded vowels, because the labiodental closure is characterized by a protruded lip shape. Compare "fool" with "feel."

Figure 14.2 shows a wideband spectrogram of the words "rougher" and "rover" (as with all the other spectrograms in this chapter, the maximum frequency is set at 9000 Hz, to demonstrate more clearly the frequency ranges of the fricatives). The most salient feature is the band of

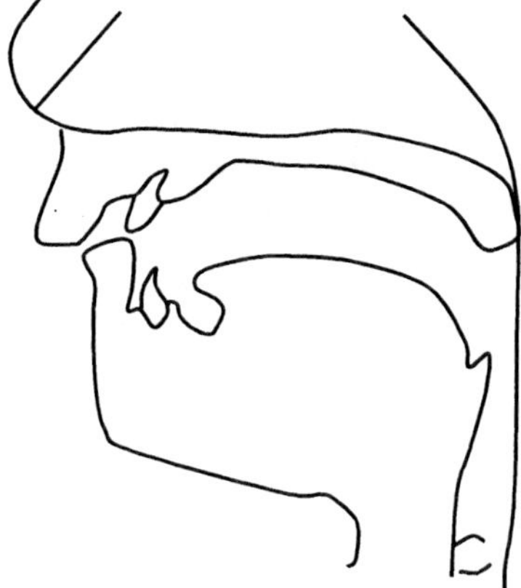

FIG 14.1. Articulator positions for /f, v/.

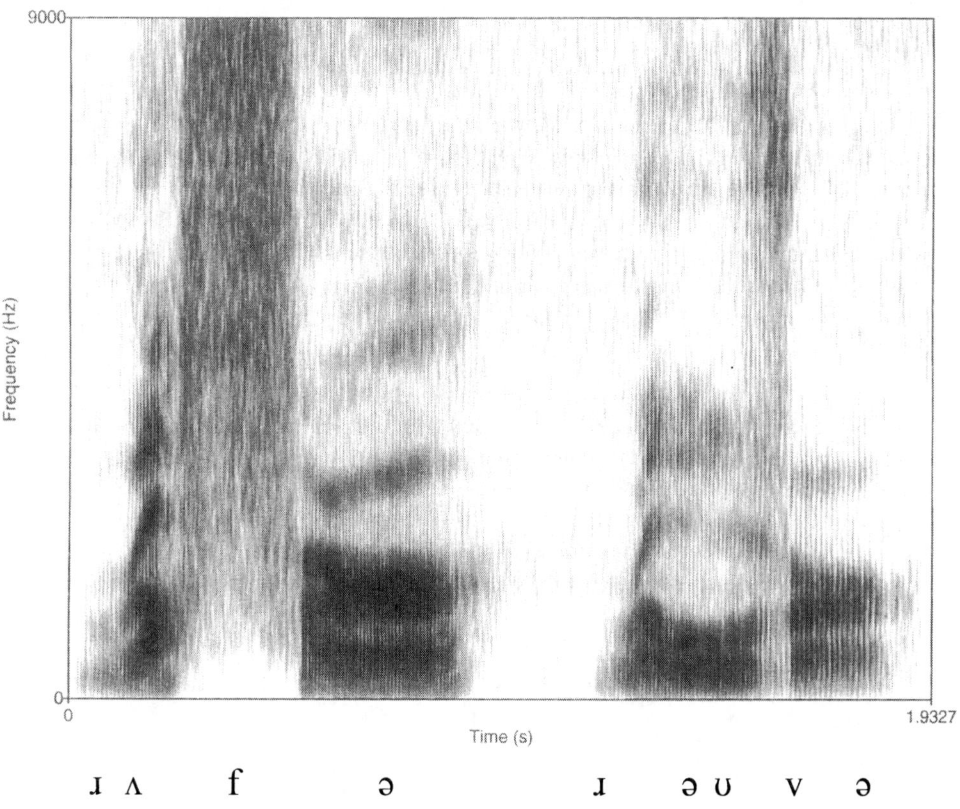

FIG 14.2. Wideband spectrogram of "rougher" and "rover" (RP pronunciation).

markings spreading up the frequency range corresponding to the energy component (i.e., the high-intensity component) of the fricative. For /f/ and /v/, this component is normally situated in the frequency range 1500–7000 Hz. Comparing /f/ with /v/, you will see how much darker (more intense) are the marking for the fortis than the lenis fricative, and that the fortis has a longer duration.

/v/

This sound is described as a voiced labiodental fricative, and the name of the symbol is the same as the letter name (/vi/). As we saw in chapter 10, /v/ can occur in word-initial and word-final position and can be found in both initial and final clusters. The sound can also occur word-medially: either syllable-final for the previous syllable (e.g., "leav.en"), or syllable-initial for the following syllable ("di.vine").

> Spelling
>
> /v/ The most common spelling is <v> (adding a silent <e> in final position):
>
> <v> vat view revisit have
>
> Some exceptional forms are also found in individual words:
>
> <f> of
> <ph> Stephen nephew (in some varieties)
>
> Note <v> for /f/ in:
>
> Tchaikovsky Romanov

To produce the usual allophone of /v/ the inner surface of the upper lip is brought into close approximation with the undersurface of the upper front teeth, mainly through a closing movement of the lower jaw, and a narrow channel is left between them (see Fig. 14.1). Air from the lungs flows through this channel and becomes turbulent. The vocal folds are vibrating in the voiced phonation posture through all (or most) of the sound. Throughout the articulation, the tongue is likely to be moving into position for the following segment.

The main allophones of /v/ are as follows:

- [v] voiced labiodental fricative. This is found in intervocalic position.
- [v̥] devoiced labiodental fricative. This allophone is found word-initially and -finally. In word-initial position the devoicing is found at the beginning of the sound; in word-final position it is found at the end of the sound. This can, if need be, be transcribed as [v̥] and [v̥], respectively.
- [v^w] labialized voiceless labiodental fricative. This allophone is found before rounded vowels, because the labiodental closure is characterized by a protruded lip shape. Compare "voodoo" with "veal."

Figure 14.2 includes spectrographic information on /v/.

THE DENTAL FRICATIVES

/θ/

This sound is a voiceless dental fricative, and the name of the symbol is the same as the name given to the letter of the Greek alphabet from which the symbol was adapted ("theta" /θitə/ or /θeɪtə/). As noted in chapter 10, /θ/ can occur in word-initial and word-final position and can be found in both initial and final clusters. The sound can also occur word-medially: either syllable-final for the previous syllable (e.g., "tooth.paste") or syllable-initial for the following syllable ("de.throne").

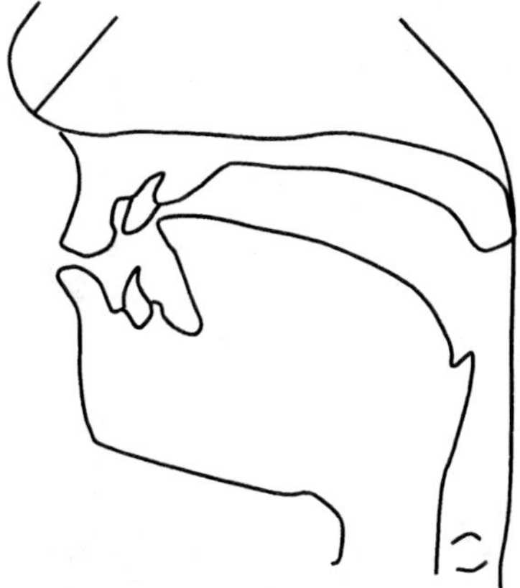

FIG 14.3. Articulator positions for /θ, ð/.

Spelling

/θ/ The spelling for this sound is <th>:

<th> thin method both

See next subsection for examples of <th> representing /ð/.
Note <th> for /t/ in:

Thomas Thames

For /θ/ the vocal folds are abducted in the voiceless phonation posture throughout the sound. The tongue tip is raised to make a close approximation behind the upper front teeth, *or* between the upper and lower front teeth (this depends on individual preference), and a narrow channel is left between them (see Fig. 14.3). The channel has a wide slit shape. Air from the lungs flows through this channel and becomes turbulent. Throughout the articulation, the lip shape will be influenced by the following segment.

The main allophones of /θ/ are as follows:

- [θ] voiceless labiodental fricative. This is found in all word positions.
- [θ^w] labialized voiceless labiodental fricative. This allophone is found before rounded vowels, because the dental closure is accompanied by lip rounding in anticipation of the vowel. Compare "thought" with "thief."

Figure 14.4 shows a wideband spectrogram of the words "author" and "rather." The most salient feature is the band of markings spreading up the frequency range corresponding to the energy component (i.e., the high-intensity component) of the fricatives. For /θ/ and /ð/, this frequency component is normally situated in the frequency range 1400–8000 Hz. As we noted with /f/ and /v/, if you compare the fricative segments in Fig. 14.3, you will see that the fortis is much darker (more intense) than the lenis fricative, and that the fortis has a longer duration.

/ð/

This sound is a voiced, dental fricative, and the name given to the symbol is generally "edh" (/ɛð/). As was described in chapter 10, /ð/ can occur in word-initial and word-final position,

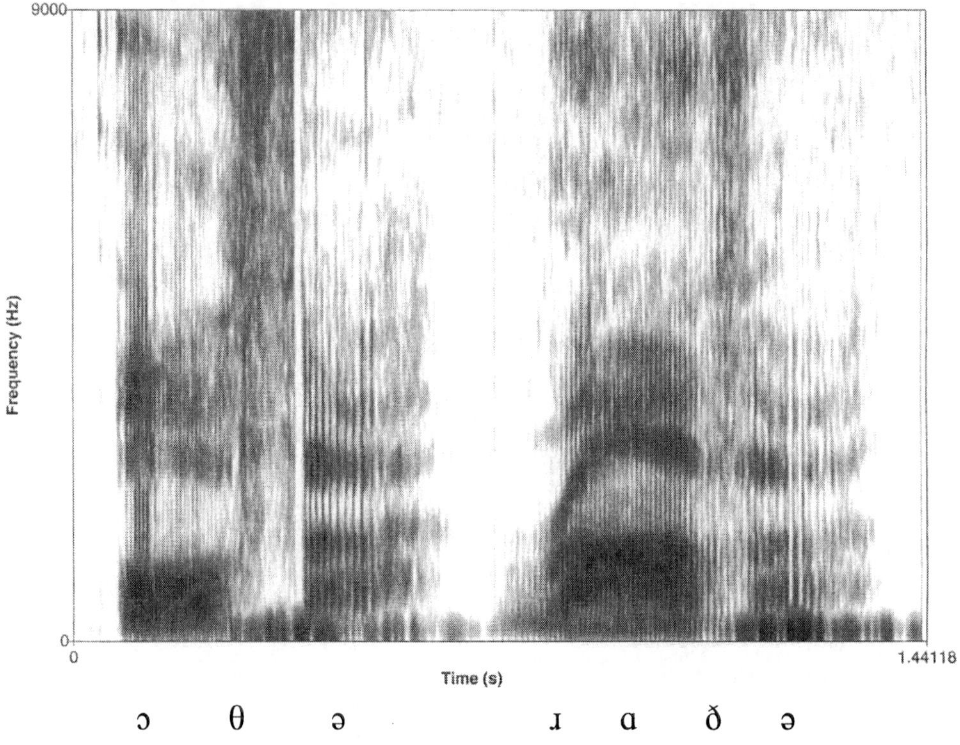

FIG 14.4. Wideband spectrogram of "author" and "rather" (RP pronunciation).

and can be found in final clusters. The sound can also occur word-medially, either syllable-final for the previous syllable (e.g., "smooth.ness"), or syllable-initial for the following syllable ("al.though").

> Spelling
>
> /ð/ The spelling for this sound is <th> (sometimes adding a silent <e> in final position):
>
> <th> that gather seethe
>
> See previous subsection for examples of <th> representing /θ/.

The vocal folds are vibrating in the voiced phonation posture through all (or most) of this sound. The tongue tip is raised to make a close approximation behind the upper front teeth, *or* between the upper and lower front teeth (this depends on individual preference), and a narrow channel is left between them (see Fig. 14.3). The channel has a wide slit shape. Air from the lungs flows through this channel and becomes turbulent. Throughout the articulation, the lip shape will be influenced by the following segment.

The main allophones of /ð/ are as follows:

- [ð] voiced dental fricative. This is found in intervocalic position.
- [ð̥] devoiced dental fricative. This allophone is found word-initially and -finally. In word-initial position the devoicing is found at the beginning of the sound; in word-final position

it is found at the end of the sound. This can, if need be, be transcribed as [̥ð] and [ð̥], respectively.

- [ð^w] labialized voiceless dental fricative. This allophone is found before rounded vowels, because the dental closure is accompanied by lip rounding in anticipation of the vowel. Compare "though" with "thee."

Figure 14.4 includes spectrographic information on /ð/ (see page 220).

THE ALVEOLAR FRICATIVES

/s/

This sound is a voiceless, alveolar fricative, and the name of the symbol is the same as the letter (/ɛs/). As noted in chapter 10, /s/ can occur in word-initial and word-final position and can be found in both initial and final clusters. The sound can also occur word-medially: either syllable-final for the previous syllable (e.g., "pas.time") or syllable-initial for the following syllable ("re.scind").

Spelling

/s/ The most common spellings are <s> and <c> (sometimes with silent <e>), and <ss>:

<s>	seat	gas	goose
<c>	decide	sauce	
<ss>	essential		moss

Less common spellings are:

<sc>	science	descend
<sw>	sword	

Note also <x> representing /ks/:

six oxen

The commonest allophone of /s/ is produced with the vocal folds abducted in the voiceless phonation posture and with the tongue tip and/or blade raised up to make a close approximation with the alveolar ridge; a narrow channel is left between them (see Fig. 14.5). The channel has a narrow grooved shape. Air from the lungs flows through this channel and becomes turbulent. Throughout the articulation, the lip shape will be influenced by the following segment.

The main allophones of /s/ are as follows:

- [s] voiceless alveolar fricative. This is found in all word positions.
- [s^w] labialized voiceless alveolar fricative. This allophone is found before rounded vowels, as the alveolar closure is accompanied by lip rounding in anticipation of the vowel. Compare "seat" with "suit."
- [s̠] retracted voiceless alveolar fricative with a slit channel shape. This allophone is used by some speakers in /stɹ/ clusters (such as "street"), the retraction being the result of the postalveolar nature of the /ɹ/. Some speakers extend this allophone to /spɹ/ and /skɹ/ clusters as well. Indeed, many speakers have a phonemic change in these contexts, using /ʃtɹ/ and some also /ʃpɹ/ and /ʃkɹ/. It is important to listen carefully to these clusters when undertaking a transcription to see whether the first segment is [s], [s̠], or [ʃ].

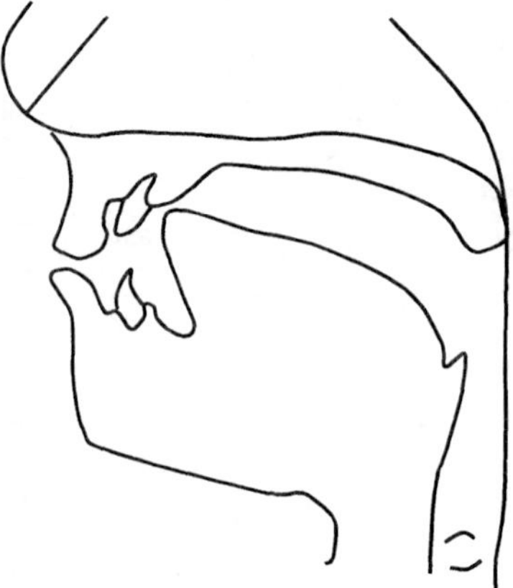

FIG 14.5. Articulator positions for /s, z/.

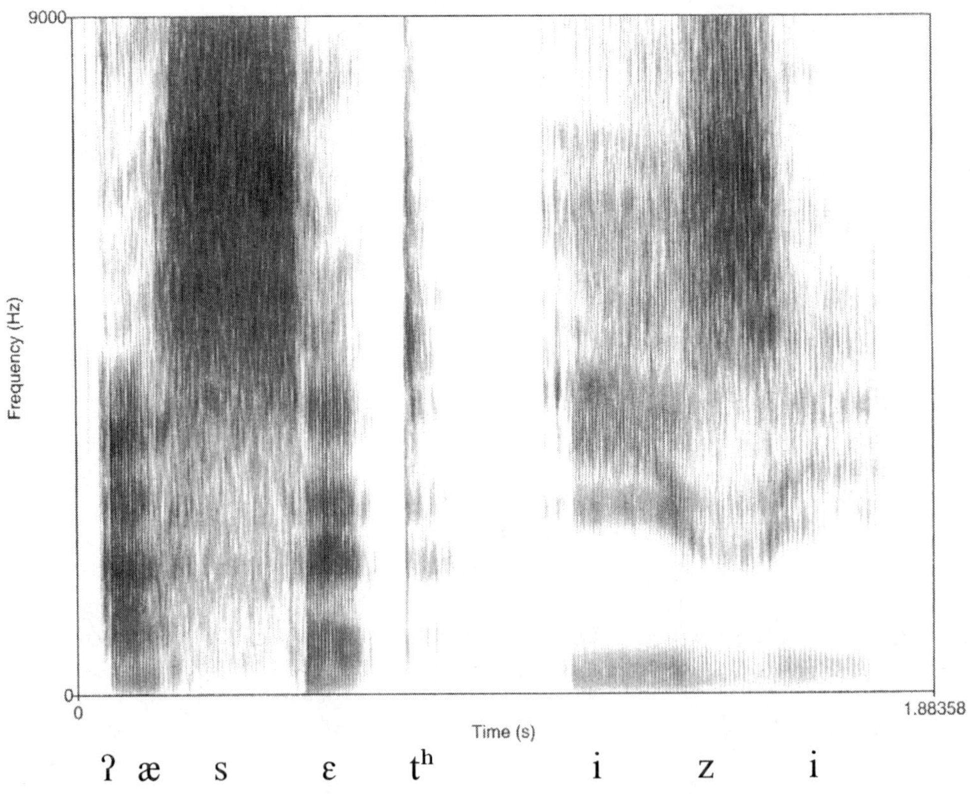

FIG 14.6. Wideband spectrogram of "asset" and "easy" (GA pronunciation).

Figure 14.6 shows a wideband spectrogram of the words "asset" and "easy." The most salient feature is the band of markings spreading up the frequency range corresponding to the energy component (i.e., the high-intensity component) of the fricative. For /s/ and /z/, this component is normally situated in the frequency range 3600–8000 Hz. As we noted with the other fricative pairs, you should compare the intensity and duration of the fricative pair in this figure, which will again show the differences in intensity and duration.

/z/

This sound is a voiced alveolar fricative, and the name given to the symbol is its letter name (United States: /zi/; elsewhere /zɛd/). As was noted in chapter 10, /z/ can occur in word-initial and word-final position and can be found in final clusters. The sound can also occur word-medially, either syllable-final for the previous syllable (e.g., "hus.band"), or syllable-initial for the following syllable ("pal.sy").

Spelling

/z/ The most common spellings are <s> (sometimes with silent <e>), <z> and <ss>:

<s>	news	prison	nose
<z>	zinc	lazy	quiz
<ss>	scissors	dissolve	

Also found are:

<zz>	blizzard	buzz
<es>	dishes	crashes (mostly plurals and third-person present endings)

Note also <x> representing /gz/:

exact anxiety

and <x> representing /z/:

xylophone xeroradiography

For /z/ the vocal folds are vibrating in the voiced phonation posture through all (or most) of the sound. The tongue tip and/or blade is raised up to make a close approximation with the alveolar ridge, and a narrow channel is left between them (see Fig. 14.5). The channel has a narrow grooved shape. Air from the lungs flows through this channel and becomes turbulent. Throughout the articulation, the lip shape will be influenced by the following segment.

The main allophones of /z/ are as follows:

- [z] voiced alveolar fricative. This is found in intervocalic position.
- [z̥] devoiced alveolar fricative. This allophone is found word-initially and -finally. In word-initial position the devoicing is found at the beginning of the sound; in word-final position it is found at the end of the sound. This can, if need be, transcribed as [̥z] and [z̥], respectively.
- [z^w] labialized voiceless alveolar fricative. This allophone is found before rounded vowels, because the alveolar closure is accompanied by lip rounding in anticipation of the vowel. Compare "zoo" with "zeal."

Figure 14.6 includes spectrographic information on /z/ (see page 222).

THE POSTALVEOLAR FRICATIVES

/ʃ/

This sound is a voiceless postalveolar fricative, and the usual name of the symbol is "esh" (/ɛʃ/). In chapter 10 we saw that /ʃ/ can occur in word-initial and word-final position and

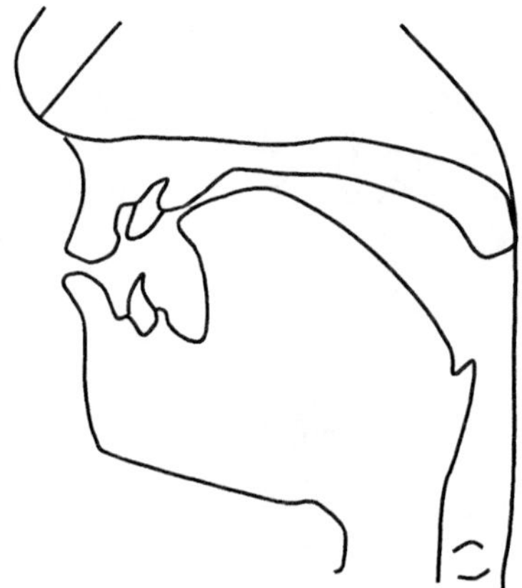

FIG 14.7. Articulator positions for /ʃ, ʒ/.

can be found in both initial and final clusters. The sound can also occur word-medially: either syllable-final for the previous syllable (e.g., "dish.washer"), or syllable-initial for the following syllable ("re.shape").

Spelling

/ʃ/ The most common spellings are <sh> and <ti>:

<sh> shop crash rasher
<ti> station traction

Less common spellings are:

<s>, <ss> sure sugar assure
<si>, <ssi>, <sci>, <ci>, <ce> mansion mission conscience special ocean

Note also <sh> representing /s.h/:

mishap

The vocal folds are abducted in the voiceless phonation posture throughout the production of /ʃ/. The tongue blade is raised to make a close approximation to the rear of the alveolar ridge, and a narrow channel is left between them (see Fig. 14.7), which has a narrow slit shape. At the same time, the front of the tongue body is raised toward the front of the hard palate. Air from the lungs flows through this channel and becomes turbulent. Throughout the articulation, the lip shape will be influenced by the following segment, although many speakers use a rounded lip shape in almost all contexts.

The main allophones of /ʃ/ are as follows:

- [ʃ] voiceless postalveolar fricative. This is found in all word positions.
- [$ʃ^w$] labialized voiceless postalveolar fricative. This allophone is found before rounded vowels, because the postalveolar closure is accompanied by lip rounding in anticipation of the vowel. Many speakers may use this allophone in all contexts except before vowels with lip spreading. Compare "sheet" with "shoot."

Figure 14.8 shows a wideband spectrogram of the words "assure" and "leisure." The most salient feature is the band of markings spreading up the frequency range corresponding to the energy component (i.e., the high-intensity component) of the fricative. For the postalveolar

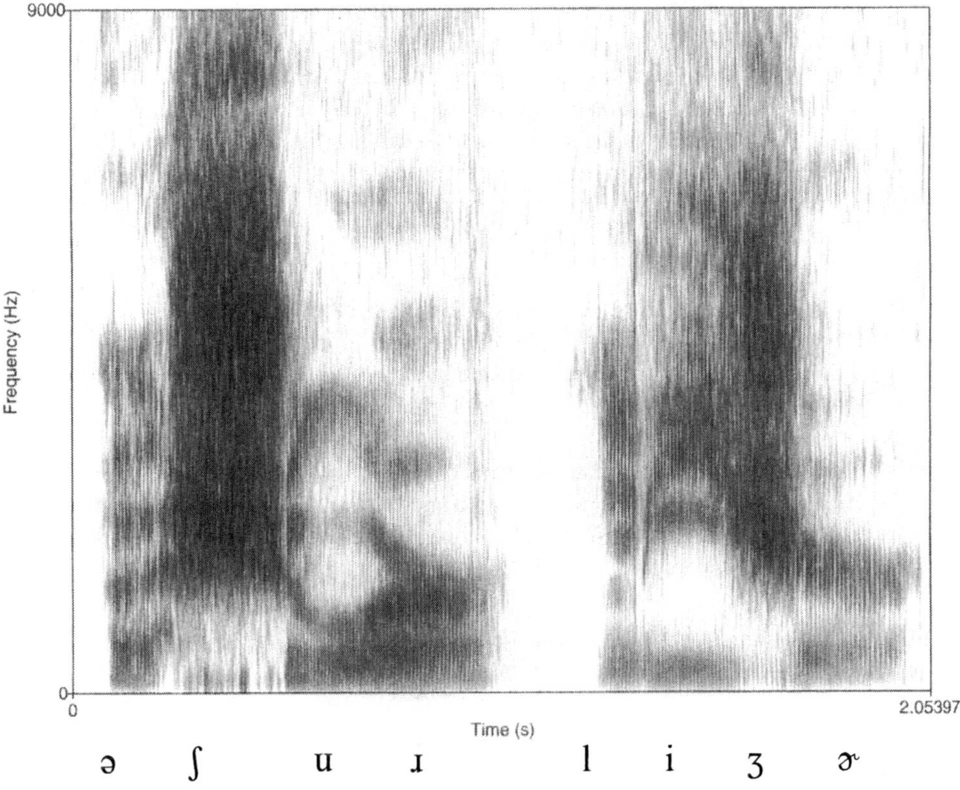

FIG 14.8. Wideband spectrogram of "assure" and "leisure" (GA pronunciation).

fricatives, this component is normally situated in the frequency range 2000–7000 Hz. As we noted with the other fricative pairs, you should compare the intensity and duration of /ʃ/ and /ʒ/ in the spectrogram.

/ʒ/

This sound is a voiced, postalveolar fricative, and the usual name of the symbol is "ezh" (/ɛʒ/). As we saw in chapter 10, /ʒ/ in native words is normally restricted to medial position, although word-initial and -final /ʒ/ can be found in borrowings. /ʒ/ occurs in word-final clusters. Word-final /ʒ/ is replaced by /dʒ/ by many speakers. This sound is the least frequently occurring consonant of English.

Spelling

/ʒ/ The most common spellings are <si> and <s>:

<si>	vision	occasion
<s>	treasure	usual

Also found are:

<z>	seizure		
<ti>	equation		
<ge>	beige	garage	bourgeois
<g>	genre	gigolo	regime

When producing /ʒ/ the vocal folds are vibrating in the voiced phonation posture through all (or most) of the sound. The tongue blade is raised to make a close approximation to the rear of the alveolar ridge, and a narrow channel is left between them (see Fig. 14.7). The channel has a narrow slit shape. At the same time, the front of the tongue body is raised up toward the front of the hard palate. Air from the lungs flows through this channel and becomes turbulent. Throughout the articulation, the lip shape will be influenced by the following segment, although many speakers use a rounded lip shape in almost all contexts.

The main allophones of /ʒ/ are as follows:

- [ʒ] voiced postalveolar fricative. This is found in intervocalic position.
- [ʒ̊] devoiced postalveolar fricative. This allophone is found word-initially and -finally. In word-initial position the devoicing is found at the beginning of the sound; in word-final position it is found at the end of the sound. This can, if need be, be transcribed as [˚ʒ] and [ʒ˚] respectively.
- [ʒʷ] labialized voiceless alveolar fricative. This allophone is found before rounded vowels, because the alveolar closure is accompanied by lip rounding in anticipation of the vowel. Many speakers may use this allophone in all contexts except before vowels with lip spreading. Compare "usual" with "measure."

Figure 14.8 includes spectrographic information on /ʒ/ (see page 225).

THE GLOTTAL FRICATIVE

/h/

This sound is a voiceless, glottal fricative, and the usual name of the symbol is the same as the letter of the alphabet (/eɪtʃ/). In chapter 10 we saw that /h/ can occur only in syllable-initial position, and cannot be found in clusters. The status of /h/ has often been a matter of dispute. Traditionally it is considered to be a fricative, with the two vocal folds acting as articulators. However, as we saw in chapter 4, /h/ can also be thought of as a subtype of voiceless phonation. Because of this, some phoneticians class /h/ as a voiceless onset to the following vowel and may therefore place the segment in the same group as the semivowels. Its acoustic characteristics, on the other hand, show its similarity to the other voiceless fricatives. We class it as similar to the other fortis fricatives (for example, it does shorten preceding segments).

Spelling

/h/ The most common spelling is <h>:

<h> hat happy behave

Also found is:

<wh> who whole

Note that <h> is silent in several instances:

heir hour honest hono(u)r herb (GA) exhaust vehicle shepherd

The commonest allophone of /h/ is produced with the vocal folds abducted. Air from the lungs is forced through the glottis under pressure and becomes turbulent. Throughout the

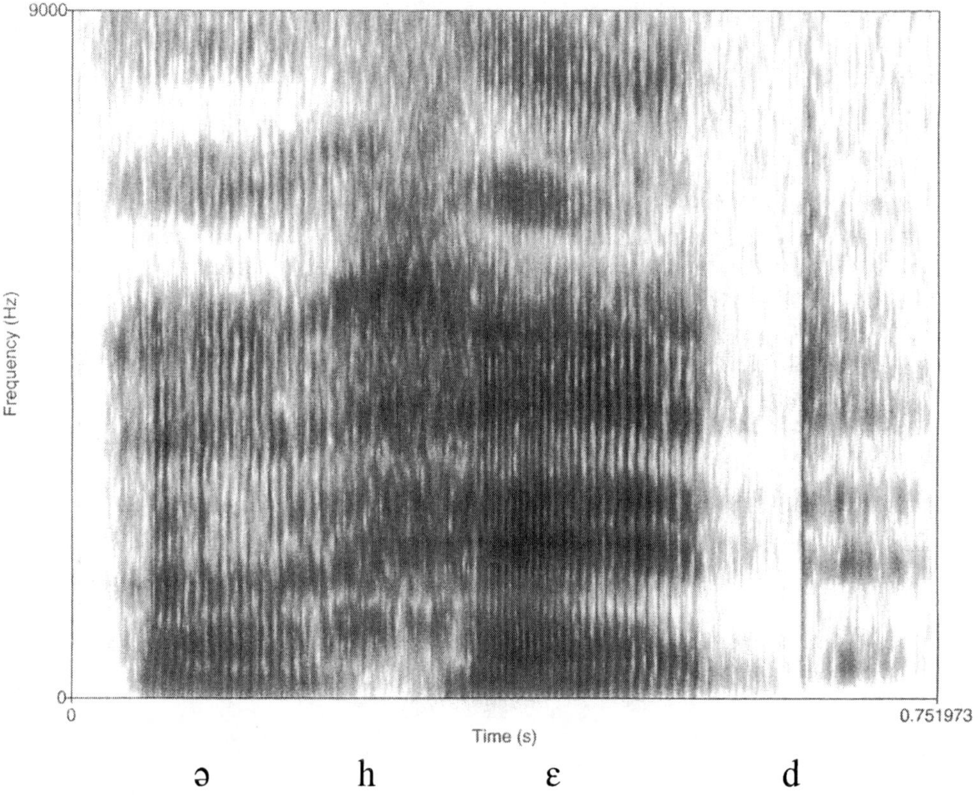

FIG 14.9. Wideband spectrogram of "ahead" (GA pronunciation).

articulation, the position of the articulators in the oral cavity will be influenced by the following segment, so the sound quality of /h/ depends on what vowel follows it.

The main allophones of /h/ are as follows:

- [h] voiceless glottal fricative. This is found in word-initial position.
- [ɦ] voiced glottal fricative (i.e., the murmur phonation type). This allophone is found syllable-initially within words. Only some speakers use this variant, others using the voiceless [h].
- [hʷ] labialized voiceless glottal fricative. This allophone is found before rounded vowels, because the glottal closure is accompanied by lip rounding in anticipation of the vowel. Compare "who" with "he."

Figure 14.9 shows a wideband spectrogram of the word "ahead" (using the [h] allophone). The most salient feature is the band of markings spreading up the frequency range corresponding to the energy component (i.e., the high-intensity component) of the fricative. There is also the voicing bar running across the foot of the spectrogram. For /h/, this component is normally situated in the frequency range 500–6500 Hz.

BACKGROUND READING

The references noted in the previous chapter apply here, too.

EXERCISES

Transcription

(Answers to the transcription exercises are given at the end of the book.)

1. Transcribe the following into phonemic symbols using either GA or RP norms. These words use the consonants from this chapter, and the vowels from the previous chapters.
   (a) fees (b) show
   (c) zoos (d) heave
   (e) these (f) vase
   (g) heath (h) thief
   (i) seizure (j) hush
   (k) shove (l) fuss
   (m) father (n) ether
   (o) seas (p) Asia

2. Transcribe the following using either GA or RP norms, employing allophonic symbols to mark devoicing, and lip-rounding before rounded vowels, where appropriate.
   (a) those (b) seat
   (c) foot (d) that
   (e) whose (f) veal
   (g) dove (h) sore
   (i) zeal (j) beige
   (k) zoos (l) feet
   (m) shoes (n) soothe
   (o) voice (p) thorn

3. Convert the following GA transcriptions back into ordinary writing. (They all have more than one possible spelling—try to list all of these.)
   (a) /faɪl/ (b) /veɪn/
   (c) /ʃu/ (d) /fɹiz/
   (e) /θɹu/ (f) /wɛðɚ/
   (g) /si/ (h) /hiɹ/

Review Questions

1. How are fortis and lenis fricative pairs distinguished by listeners?
2. What air channel differences hold between dental, alveolar, and postalveolar fricatives in English?
3. What are the acoustic differences between the different places of articulation for fricatives?
4. What pattern of distribution generally helps to distinguish the fortis and lenis dental fricatives in word-initial position?

Study Topics and Experiments

1. Draw up a list of words with initial “w” and “wh” (e.g., “witch” and “which”). Choose at least five words of each type. Record yourself and at least nine other people saying these words in a carrier phrase (e.g., “say X again”). Note whether your speakers use /hw/ for the “wh” words. Also note whether they are consistent or variable in their realizations.

2. Draw up a list of words ending with potential /ʒ/ (e.g., "rouge" and "sabotage"). Choose at least 10 words. Record yourself and at least four other people saying these words in a carrier phrase (e.g., "say X again"). Note whether your speakers use /ʒ/ or /dʒ/. Also note whether they are consistent or variable in their realizations.

CD

This section of the CD covers the consonants described in this chapter. As always, we suggest that you undertake the exercises and check the answers at the end of the book.

15

English Sonorant Consonants

INTRODUCTION

The plosives, affricates, and fricatives of the last two chapters compose the class of consonants known as *obstruents*, named because there is always an obstruction of some kind to the free flow of air through the vocal tract. In this chapter we examine the remaining consonants of English, all of which belong to the class of *sonorants*. These consonants all have a relatively free flow of air through the vocal tract, and the airflow remains laminar (smooth). English sonorants are the three nasal stops, one lateral approximant, one central approximant, and two semivowels. (The lateral and central approximants are often grouped together as *liquids*.) Nasals are sonorants because, although air is stopped within the oral cavity, it flows freely through the nasal cavity. Unlike obstruents, where voicelessness is more natural (occurs more commonly in the languages of the world) than voice, sonorants are much more commonly encountered voiced than voiceless. Partly this is due to the fact that voiceless sonorants are not easy to perceive (they are just not very loud). A further point is that voiceless sonorants are normally made with an airflow that is turbulent to some extent. Once we have a turbulent voiceless airflow we have a sound that is very similar to a fricative. Therefore, some phoneticians are of the opinion that voiceless sonorants—if they are audible at all due to a reasonable amount of turbulence in the air—are really better classified as fricatives. We illustrate this point below with the sound used in some English varieties for the <wh> spelling.

The sonorants are distinguished in the following ways:

velic position:	velum lowered for nasal stops; raised for approximants
oral airflow direction:	lateral for /l/; central for other approximants
prolongability:	nonprolongable for semivowels; others prolongable

THE NASAL STOPS

The three nasal stop phonemes of English all share the articulatory feature of a lowered velum. With the velum lowered, of course, the air flowing from the lungs can pass freely through the nasal cavity, although the particular size of the oral cavity (determined by the placement of the articulators) does affect the overall quality of the nasals, allowing us to perceive the difference between them. We need to bear in mind, however, that the lowering of the soft palate to make the nasal stop and its raising after the sound has been completed cannot be instantaneous. It takes a certain amount of time to accomplish velic movement, and speakers therefore start to lower the velum during the preceding segment. This results in a certain degree of nasalization of vowels and consonants that precede nasal stops. Speakers also complete velic raising during any sounds that follow a nasal, so these sounds too will have partial nasalization. We describe these nasalized allophones with the relevant vowel and consonant phonemes.

As we noted earlier, sonorants are generally voiced. The nasal stops are slightly devoiced in some contexts, however. This is especially noticeable after /s/ (e.g., "smile," "snake"), but to a lesser extent after any voiceless consonant ("topmost," "catnip"). Nasals and other sonorants share many characteristics with vowels (the free flow of laminar air and lack of obstructions), and therefore, in some circumstances, they can act as the nuclei of syllables—a role normally assigned to vowels. In English there are many examples of syllabic nasals (e.g., in words such as "prism," "ridden," and "button"), and we include these syllabic nasals as allophones of the relevant phonemes.

Acoustically, nasals share a set of characteristics that we looked at in chapter 7. We can briefly remind ourselves of these. First, they have a lower intensity than other sonorants; second, the addition of the nasal cavity causes certain frequency bands to be suppressed. This *antiresonance* is seen as an *antiformant* at about the 800–2000 Hz level. Finally, the first formant of a nasal sound is usually lower than for nonnasal sonorants, and this is called the *nasal formant*.

The Bilabial Nasal

/m/

The symbol for the voiced bilabial nasal has the same name as the letter name. /m/ can be found word-initially, -medially, and -finally and in initial and final clusters. Medially it can close a syllable, as in "tim.ber," or open a syllable, as in "re.main."

Spelling

/m/ The most common spelling is to use <m> or <mm> (this latter is common in the middle of words but does *not* mean that /m/ is lengthened):

<m>	mat	gum	damage
<mm>	summer		immoral

Some words have a silent <b>:

<mb>	lamb	numb	plumber

See also:

<mn>	autumn	hymn	
<lm>	calm	palm	(Sherlock) Holmes

The main allophone of /m/ is produced in the following way. The vocal folds are vibrating, in the voiced phonation posture, throughout all (or most) of the sound. The upper and lower lips are brought together, mainly through a closing movement of the lower jaw, and form an air-tight seal (see Fig. 15.1). During the articulation, the tongue is likely to be moving into position for the following segment. The lowering of the velum normally precedes the bilabial closure, and its raising again will start after the closure is released, resulting in a degree of nasalization in preceding and following segments.

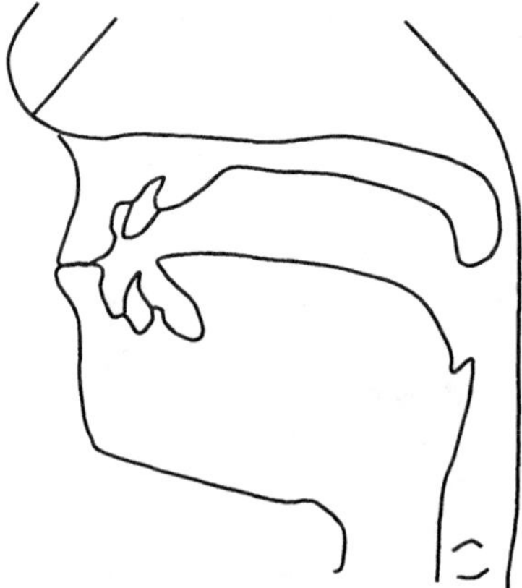

FIG 15.1. Articulator position for /m/.

The commonest allophones of /m/ are as follows:

- [m] voiced bilabial nasal stop. This is found in most contexts.
- [m̥] devoiced bilabial nasal stop. This allophone is found following an /s/ in clusters such as found in "small." A lesser amount of devoicing may be found after any voiceless consonant: "apeman."
- [ɱ] voiced labiodental nasal stop. This allophone is found when /m/ is immediately followed by /f, v/, in words such as "triumph" or "comfy," or even across word boundaries such as "warm van." Although not all speakers will use this context-dependent allophone, it clearly reduces articulatory complexity if a single labiodental articulation is formed for the nasal and then slightly adjusted to provide for the following fricative, instead of starting with a bilabial gesture and having to transform it into a labiodental one.
- [mʷ] labialized voiced bilabial nasal. This allophone is found before rounded vowels, because the bilabial closure is characterized by a protruded lip shape. Compare "moot" with "meat." In fact the latter may be characterized as an allophone with marked spread lip shape, though this lacks an IPA diacritic.
- [m̩] voiced bilabial nasal with syllabic function. There are some instances of /m/ taking on the role of syllable nucleus: "prism," "rhythm," and some pronunciations of "happen" and "seven" ([hæpm̩], [sɛbm̩]). Even in phonemic transcription we tend to mark these syllabic sonorants with the diacritic used in these examples.

Figure 15.2 shows a wideband spectrogram of the word "rummy" (in this chapter, all the spectrograms have a maximum frequency setting of 5000 Hz). The most salient feature is the lowered intensity for the nasal stop, shown as a fainter band roughly in the center of the spectrogram, but having the voicing bar at the foot of the spectrogram. Notice the antiformant and nasal formants described earlier. The same formant transitions we noted for /p, b/ occur in the surrounding vowels for /m/.

The Alveolar Nasal

/n/

The symbol for the voiced alveolar nasal has the same name as that of the letter of the alphabet. The alveolar nasal occurs word-initially, -medially, and -finally and in initial and final clusters. Medially it can close a syllable, as in "ten.der," or open a syllable, as in "de.ny."

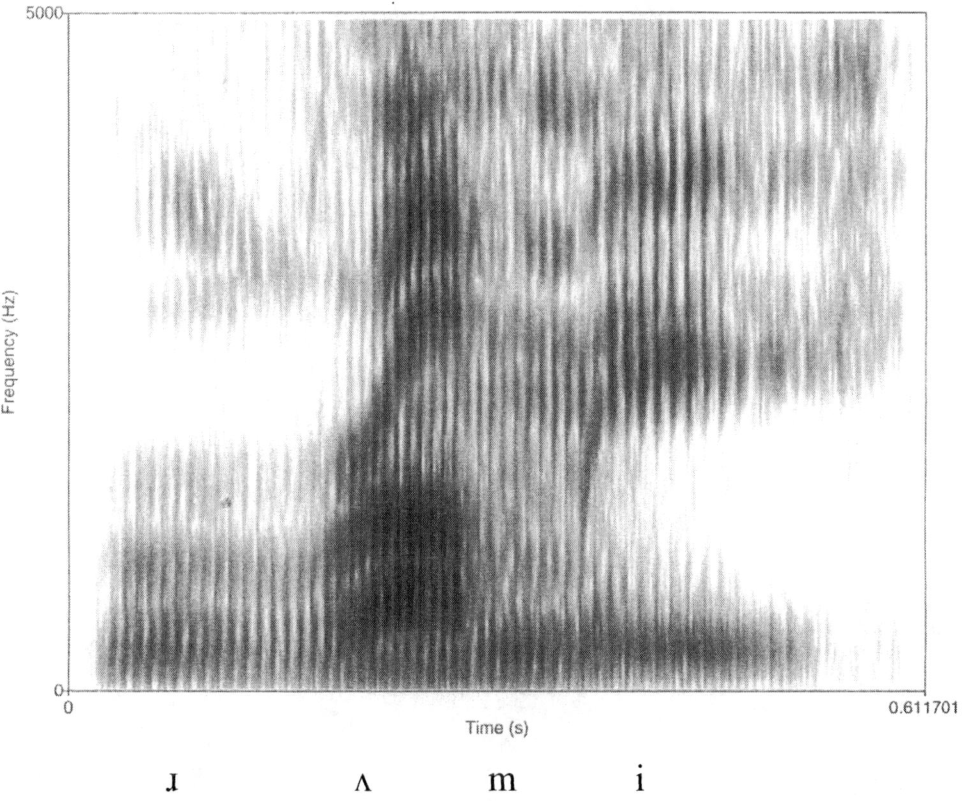

FIG 15.2. Wideband spectrogram of "rummy" (GA pronunciation).

Spelling

/n/ The most common spelling is to use <n> or <nn> (this latter is common in the middle of words but does *not* mean that /n/ is lengthened):

<n>	not	gun	renew
<nn>	dinner	annoy	

Some words have a silent <g> or <k>:

<gn>	gnaw	align	campaigning
<kn>	knight	knowledge	

See also:

<pn>	pneumatic	pneumonia

Note: <n> before <k> or <c> is realized as /ŋ/.

For the main allophone of /n/ the tongue tip and/or blade (an individual preference) is raised until it touches the alveolar ridge, and an air-tight seal is formed between the tongue and the alveolar ridge and between the side rims of the tongue and the inner surface of the upper side teeth (see Fig. 15.3). The vocal folds are vibrating in the voiced phonation posture throughout all (or most) of the sound. Throughout the articulation, the lip shape is likely to be influenced by the following segment. The lowering of the velum normally precedes the alveolar closure, and its raising again will start after the closure is released, resulting in a degree of nasalization in preceding and following segments.

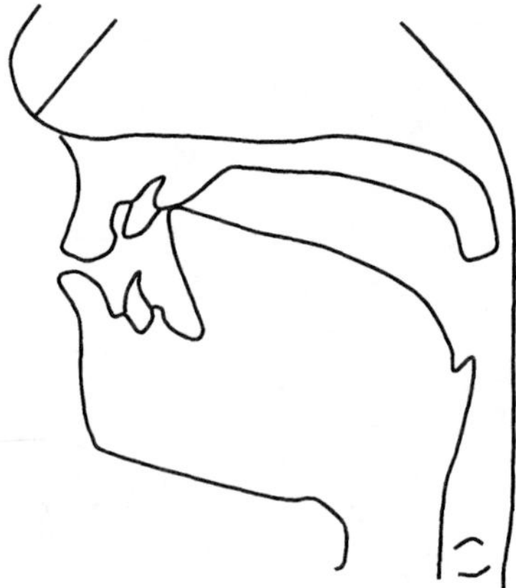

FIG 15.3. Articulator position for /n/.

The most frequent allophones of /n/ are as follows:

- [n] voiced alveolar nasal stop. This is found in most contexts.
- [n̥] devoiced alveolar nasal stop. This allophone is found following an /s/ in clusters such as found in "snail." A lesser amount of devoicing may be found after any voiceless consonant: "catnap."
- [n̪] voiced dental nasal stop. This allophone is found when /n/ is immediately followed by /θ/ or /ð/, in words such as "tenth," or even across word boundaries such as "when that." It clearly reduces articulatory complexity if a single dental articulation is formed for the nasal and then slightly adjusted to provide for the following fricative, instead of starting with an alveolar gesture and having to transform it into a dental one.
- [n̠] voiced postalveolar nasal stop. This allophone is found when /n/ is immediately followed by /ɹ/, in words or phrases such as "unrest," "in reality."
- [n^{w}] labialized voiced alveolar nasal stop. This allophone is found before rounded vowels, because the alveolar closure is accompanied by lip rounding in anticipation of the vowel. Compare "need" with "node." In fact the former may be characterized as an allophone with marked spread lip shape.
- [n̩] voiced alveolar nasal with syllabic function. These are some instances of /n/ taking on the role of syllable nucleus: "cotton," "sudden," "earthen," and some pronunciations of "reason," "vision," and "station." Some word pairs are distinguished by use or otherwise of syllabic-n: "lightening" ~ "lightning" ([laɪtn̩ɪŋ] ~ [laɪtnɪŋ]), where the first has a syllabic-n and the second does not. Even in phonemic transcription we tend to mark these syllabic sonorants with the diacritic used in these examples. GA does not have this full range of syllabic contexts; see chapter 13.

Final /n/ is often affected by the place of articulation of a following consonant; so "ten" may end with an /m/ in the phrase "ten men," and with an /ŋ/ in the phrase "ten girls." These are *not* allophones of /n/, however, but examples of phonemic changes.

Figure 15.4 shows a wideband spectrogram of the word "runner." The most salient feature is the lowered intensity for the nasal stop, shown as a fainter band roughly in the center of the spectrogram, but having the voicing bar at the foot of the spectrogram. Notice the antiformant and nasal formants described earlier. The same formant transitions we noted for /t, d/ occur in the surrounding vowels for /n/.

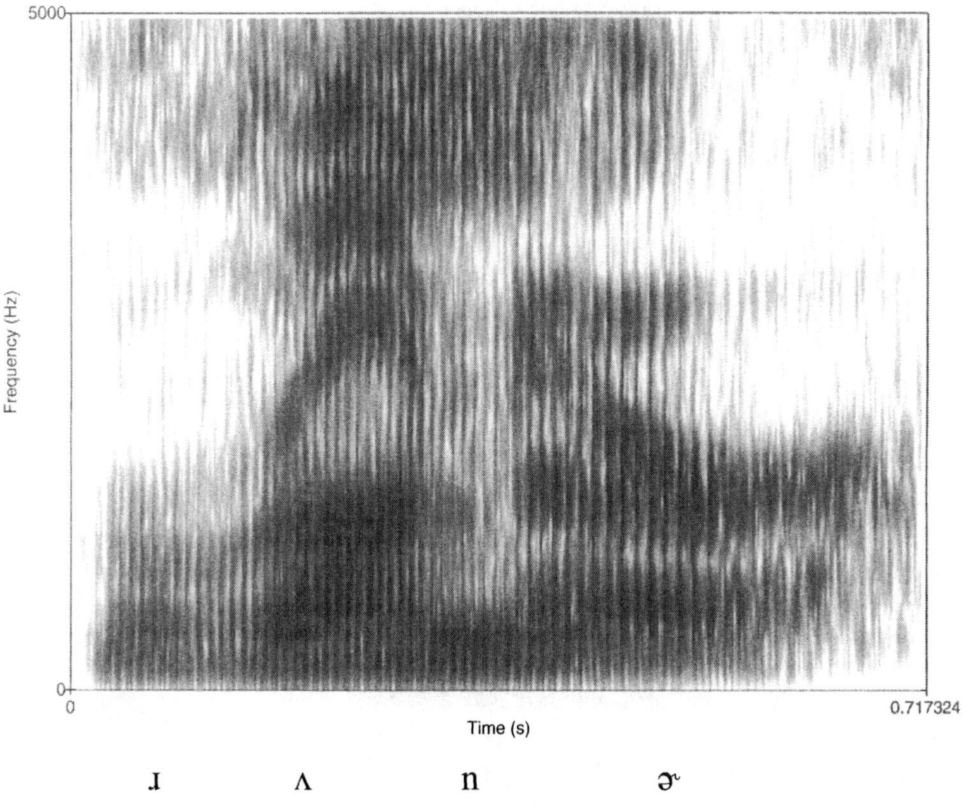

FIG 15.4. Wideband spectrogram of "runner" (GA pronunciation).

The Velar Nasal

/ŋ/

The symbol for the voiced velar nasal is generally given the name "eng" (/ɛŋ/). The velar nasal can only be found in syllable-final position and in final clusters. Therefore, medially it can only close a syllable, as in "sing.ing."

Spelling

/ŋ/ The most common spelling is to use <ng> or <n>:

<ng>	sing	tongue	longing
<n>+<k>	donkey	think	
<n>+<c>	inclement	uncle	
<n>+<x>	anxious		

In some words <ng> represents /ŋ/, in others /ŋg/:

<ng> as /ŋ/	singer
<ng> as /ŋg/	finger

Note that <nge> can also represent /ndʒ/:

<nge>	cringe whinger

See also:

<nd>	handkerchief

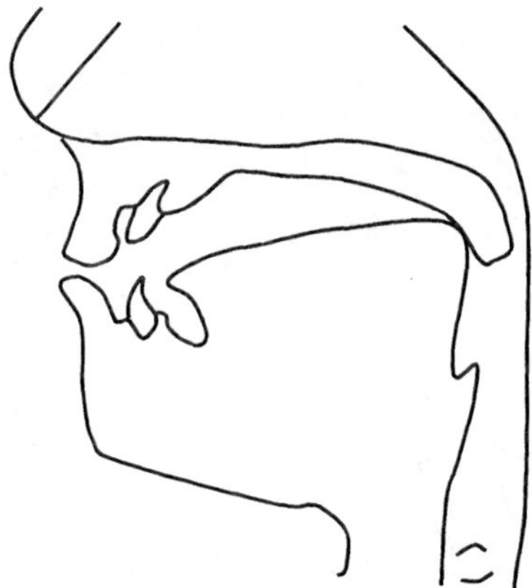

FIG 15.5. Articulator positions for /ŋ/.

The vocal folds are vibrating in the voiced phonation posture throughout all (or most) of /ŋ/. The back of the tongue dorsum is raised until it touches the soft palate (the exact position on the velum is determined by the preceding segment), and an air-tight seal is formed between the tongue and the velum (see Fig. 15.5). Throughout the articulation, the lip shape will be under the influence of the preceding sound. The lowering of the velum normally precedes the velar closure, and its raising again will start after the closure is released, resulting in a degree of nasalization in preceding and following segments.

The main allophones of /ŋ/ are as follows:

- [ŋ] voiced velar nasal stop. This is found in most contexts.
- [ŋ̊] devoiced velar nasal stop. This allophone is rare, as there are few instances where /ŋ/ can occur after a voiceless consonant. Where speakers use a syllabic nasal in the following examples, the nasal will be slightly devoiced: "thicken," "bacon," "lock 'n' key" ([θɪkŋ̩̊], [beɪkŋ̩̊], [lɑkŋ̩̊ki]).
- [ŋ̠] voiced retracted velar nasal stop (almost as far back as the uvular position). This allophone is found when /ŋ/ is immediately preceded by a back vowel in words such as "song." This reduces articulatory complexity, because the tongue is closer to the position it adopted for the back vowel.
- [ŋ̟] voiced advanced velar nasal stop (almost as far forward as the palatal position). This allophone is found when /ŋ/ is immediately preceded by a front vowel in words such as "sing." This reduces articulatory complexity, because the tongue is closer to the position it adopted for the front vowel.
- [ŋ̩] voiced velar nasal with syllabic function. There are just a few instances of /ŋ/ taking on the role of syllable nucleus: "bacon," "taken," "organ," although not all speakers use the syllabic nasal here.

Final /ŋ/, especially in the verb ending "ing," is often pronounced /n/. This is *not* an allophone of /ŋ/, however, but a substitution of one phoneme for another.

Figure 15.6 shows a wideband spectrogram of the word "ringer." The most salient feature is the lowered intensity for the nasal stop, shown as a fainter band roughly in the center of the spectrogram, but having the voicing bar at foot of the spectrogram. Notice the antiformant and nasal formants described earlier. The same formant transitions we noted for /k, g/ occur in the surrounding vowels for /ŋ/.

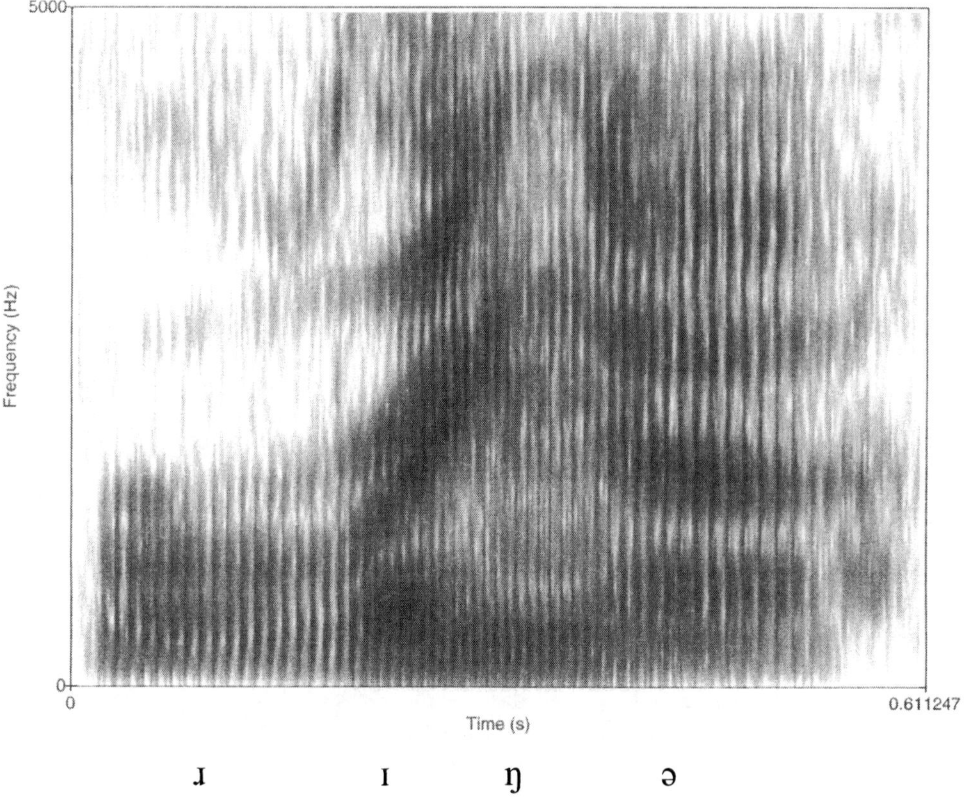

FIG 15.6. Wideband spectrogram of "ringer" (RP pronunciation).

THE LIQUID APPROXIMANTS

The liquids are a group of approximants that are prolongable (unlike the semivowels) and involve a free-flowing airstream without turbulence (an older name of *frictionless continuant* sums up these characteristics). The category liquid includes both lateral approximants and central approximants (although the weak fricative type of approximants described in chapter 6 are not normally included). Lateral approximants normally are made with complete contact between some part of the tongue and some part of the roof of the mouth, but with the tongue rims positioned in such a way as to direct the airflow over the sides of the tongue. Central approximants, on the other hand, have no tongue-palate contact, and the air flows over the median line of the tongue.

For all the liquid approximants the soft palate is in the raised position, thus directing the pulmonic egressive airflow into the oral cavity and blocking off the nasal cavity.

The Alveolar Lateral Approximant

/l/

The alveolar lateral approximant of English is symbolized by /l/, and the name of the symbol is the same as that of the letter of the alphabet. This consonant can be found word-initially, -medially, and -finally and in initial and final clusters. Medially, /l/ can either close a syllable, as in "hall.way," or open one, as in "be.lieve."

Spelling

/l/ The most common spelling is to use <l> or <ll> (the latter is common in medial and final position, but does not mean that /l/ is prolonged):

<l>	lamp	below	rule
<ll>	pull	hollow	

Some exceptional forms include:

<sl>	island	isle
<cl>	muscle	
<tl>	bristle	

Note that <l> can be silent in several words, e.g.:

talk half salmon could folk

There are two distinct variants of /l/ produced in English (together with other allophones, all of which are listed below). Because these two main variants differ in their articulation, we describe each separately together with its contexts of usage. The first main variant is given the name *clear-l*, and the second is termed *dark-l*.

Clear-l is produced in the following way. The vocal folds are vibrating in the voiced phonation posture throughout all (or most) of the sound. The tongue tip and/or blade (an individual preference) is raised up until it touches the alveolar ridge, and the side rims of the tongue are lowered so that the air flows over the side of the tongue (see Fig. 15.7). There may also be a certain amount of raising of the front of the tongue toward the hard palate. The channel shape for the airflow is wide enough so that the air remains laminar without friction. Whereas some speakers have air flowing over both sides of the tongue, others have unilateral airflow; there appears to be no perceptible sound difference between these states. Throughout the articulation, the lip shape is likely to be influenced by the following segment. The clear-l allophone is found in syllable-initial position, before vowels.

Dark-l is produced as follows. As with clear-l the vocal folds are vibrating in the voiced phonation posture throughout all (or most) of the sound. The tongue tip and/or blade (an individual preference) is raised up until it touches the alveolar ridge, and the side rims of the tongue are lowered so that the air flows over the side of the tongue (see Fig. 15.8). The channel shape for the airflow is wide enough that the air remains laminar without friction. What makes dark-l different from clear-l is that at the same time, the back of the tongue dorsum is raised

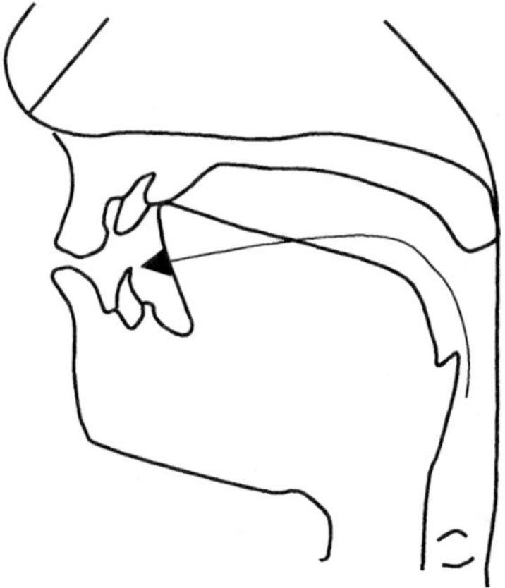

FIG 15.7. Articulator positions for clear-l [l].

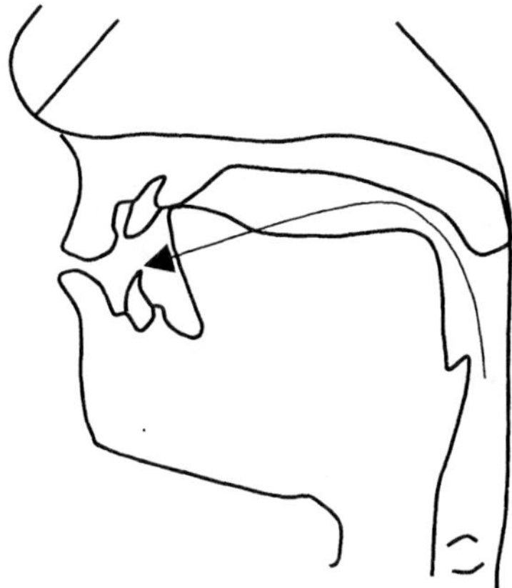

FIG 15.8. Articulator positions for dark-l (ɫ).

up toward the soft palate (though without touching it). Again, some speakers have air flowing over both sides of the tongue, whereas others have unilateral airflow. Some speakers tend to use a rounded lip shape with dark-l, whereas for others rounding only results if the preceding vowel is rounded. The dark-l allophone is found in syllable-final position after vowels and (where present) before consonants.

The allophones listed below are further variants of either a basic clear-l or dark-l, and we list them under these two categories.

Allophones that are Basically Clear-l Variants

- [l] voiced alveolar lateral approximant. This is found in most contexts before vowels. If the /l/ is made with perceptible palatalization (front tongue raised toward the hard palate, giving a front vowel-like resonance), then the transcription [lʲ] may be used.
- [l̥] devoiced alveolar lateral approximant. This allophone occurs when /l/ follows a voiceless plosive, as in "play," "clay." Less devoicing occurs after other voiceless sounds: "slay," "flay," "earthly," and when following voiceless plosives in unstressed syllables.
- [lʷ] labialized voiced alveolar lateral approximant. This allophone is found before rounded vowels, because the alveolar closure is accompanied by lip rounding in anticipation of the vowel. Compare "leap" with "loop." In fact, the former may be characterized as an allophone with marked spread lip shape.

Allophones that are Basically Dark-l Variants

- [ɫ] voiced velarized alveolar lateral approximant. This is found in most contexts following a vowel or before a consonant in syllable-final position. The IPA also allows the transcription [lˠ] for a velarized-l. We choose [ɫ] because this stands for "velarized or pharyngealized," and there is evidence that English dark-l may often have tongue root retraction into the pharynx as well as tongue dorsum raising toward the soft palate.
- [ɫ̪] voiced velarized dental lateral approximant. This allophone occurs when /l/ is found before a dental fricative: "wealth," "will they."
- [ɫ̠] voiced velarized postalveolar lateral approximant. This allophone occurs when /l/ is found before /ɹ/: "already," "all right," or a /tɹ/ or /dɹ/: "ultra," "all dry."
- [ɫ̃] voiced nasalized velarized dental lateral approximant. This allophone occurs when /l/ is found before a nasal consonant: "elm," "kiln," "call me."

- [ɫʷ] voiced labialized and velarized alveolar lateral approximant. This allophone occurs when /l/ is found after a rounded vowel: compare "peel" with "pool." However, some speakers use lip-rounding for all instances of dark-l, except for those following lip-spread vowels.
- [ɫ̩] voiced velarized postalveolar lateral approximant with syllabic function. Dark-l can take on the role of syllable nucleus: "middle," "table," "eagle," "final."
- [ɫ̩̊] devoiced velarized alveolar lateral approximant with syllabic function. This allophone occurs when syllabic /l/ is found after a voiceless consonant. Syllabic laterals in the following examples will be slightly devoiced: "baffle," "rustle." Even in phonemic transcription we tend to mark these syllabic sonorants with the syllabic diacritic.

We also need to consider vocalization. This is a process common in many varieties of English, whereby dark-l is realized as a vowel (or semivowel). This may either be a stylistic variant, or be used most of the time by a speaker. Often, the replacement vowel is /ʊ/, and as this is a phoneme of English, we can consider this as an example of phonemic substitution. Sometimes, however, the vocalization seems to involve back unrounded vowels or semivowels (such as [ɤ], [ɯ], or [ɰ]). It is unclear whether these should be considered allophones of /ʊ/ or of /l/. Finally, some phoneticians (e.g., Shriberg and Kent, 2003) recognize a sound that seems to be partway between a lateral approximant and a vocalization. This is described as having the same tongue posture as for dark-l, except that the tongue tip (although raised) does not contact the alveolar ridge. It is claimed, nevertheless, that air is directed over the side rims of the tongue. It is uncertain whether this should be considered a genuine example of allophonic variation or simply articulatory undershoot that commonly occurs in rapid connected speech. In any case, if there is no central tongue–palate contact, the sound cannot be a lateral, as lateral-only airflow requires a blocking off of the central area. Otherwise, even if the side rims of the tongue are lowered somewhat, the airflow is bound to be mostly central.

Vocalization of /l/ is often reported in the speech disorders literature as a speech error requiring intervention. If clients exhibit l-vocalization, the therapist must ascertain whether this is a feature of their target dialect, or part of a speech disorder.

Some phoneticians describe a voiced velar lateral approximant ([ʟ]) that appears to be a free variant for both clear- and dark-l. This, however, appears to be restricted to certain regional dialects of American English (see chap. 18).

Figure 15.9 shows a wideband spectrogram of the words "alev(iate)" and "all eve(ning)"; the first with a clear-l and the second with a dark-l. Acoustically, /l/ is similar to vowels, with a clearly defined formant structure. The lateral is less intense than surrounding vowels and has a shorter duration. The spectrograms also show that whereas clear-l has a formant pattern similar to those of high front vowels, dark-l is closer to high back vowels.

The Postalveolar Central Approximant

/ɹ/

The postalveolar central approximant of English is symbolized by /ɹ/, and the name of the symbol is "inverted-r." Many books on English phonetics represent this sound with the IPA symbol /r/. However, this symbol should only be used for the alveolar trill (as found for example in Spanish). Very few accents of English have a trilled r (some Scottish English speakers do use it, however), so this symbol is an inappropriate choice. This is reinforced when we consider we may have to record trilled-r in the clinic from multilingual clients whose first language contains this sound. If we have used /r/ for the approximant of English, then we have no symbol left over to transcribe the trill.

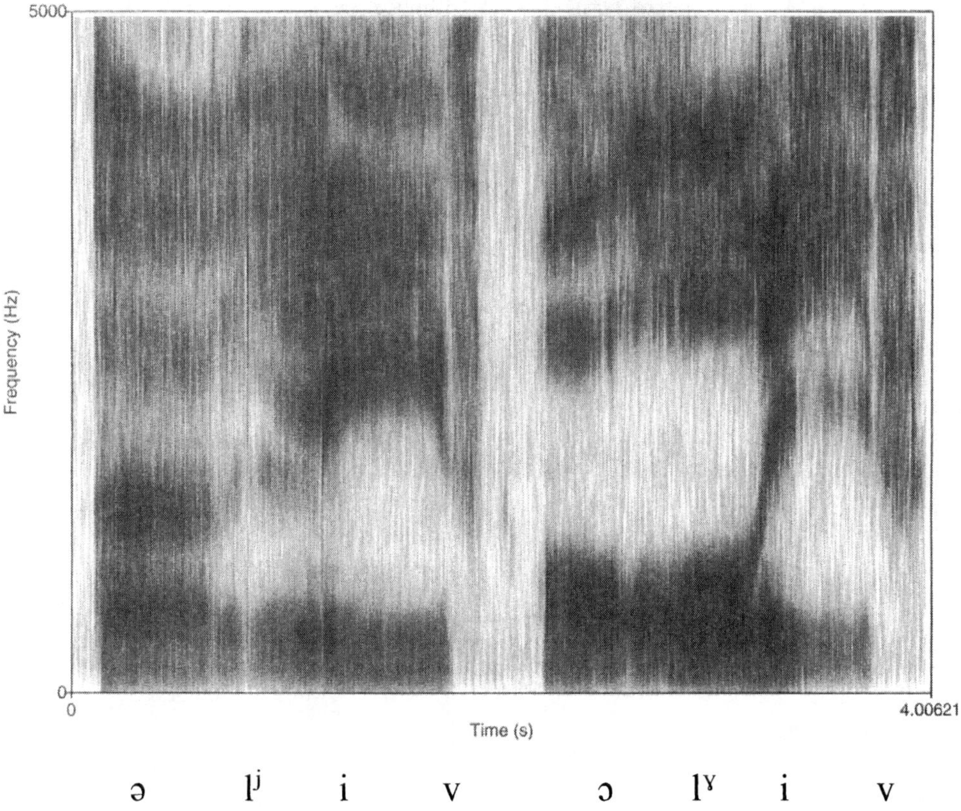

FIG 15.9. Wideband spectrograms of "alev(iate)" and "all eve(ning)" (RP pronunciation).

This consonant can be found word-initially, -medially, and -finally and in initial and final clusters. Medially, /ɹ/ can either close a syllable, as in "car.port," or open one, as in "be.rate." Nonrhotic accents of English do not allow this consonant to close syllables.

Spelling

/ɹ/ The most common spelling is to use <r> or <rr> (this latter is common in medial position, but does not mean that /ɹ/ is prolonged):

<r>	red	derange	bar	share
<rr>	carry	correct		

Some <wr> and <rh> spellings are also found:

<wr>	wretch	rewrite	
<rh>	rhyme	rhythm	rhino

There are two distinct ways of producing the approximant-r. While the two forms both sound the same, the tongue position differs. The version normally described in textbooks on English is the variety we label as a postalveolar approximant (sometimes termed *apical-r*, or *retroflex-r*). The other variety is usually termed a *bunched-r* and could perhaps be labeled as a labial prevelar approximant with tongue tip retraction. It seems that the choice between these forms is one of individual choice, though the bunched-r predominates in western American English. We describe the production of these two variants separately.

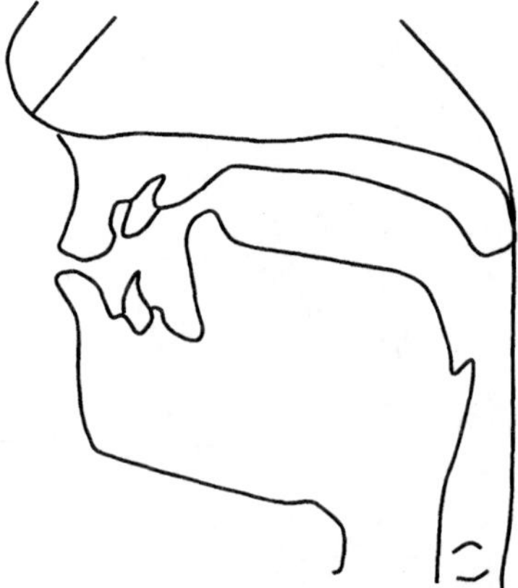

FIG 15.10. Articulator positions for [ɹ].

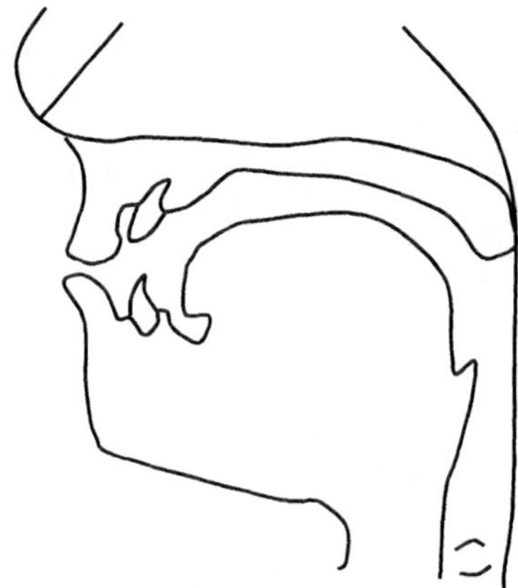

FIG 15.11. Articulator positions for [Ψ] (bunched-r).

Apical-r is produced in the following way. The vocal folds are vibrating in the voiced phonation posture throughout all (or most) of the sound. The tongue tip is curled up toward, but not touching, the alveolar ridge, and the front of the tongue is lowered. The back of the tongue is somewhat higher than the front, so there is a hollow in the body of the tongue. Air flows centrally over the tongue without turbulence (see Fig. 15.10). Throughout the articulation, the lip shape is likely to be influenced by the following segment, although many speakers use lip-rounding always for this sound, or always unless the following vowel is spread. For those speakers who use both the apical-r and the bunched-r, the apical variant may be preferred before vowels. Some speakers may bend the tongue tip back as well as raising it, to produce a retroflex rather than a postalveolar articulation.

We can now consider the production of the bunched-r. The vocal folds are vibrating, in the voiced phonation posture throughout all (or most) of the sound. The tongue dorsum is raised up toward the boundary between the hard and the soft palate and the tongue tip is drawn back into the body of the tongue (see Fig. 15.11). There may be some contact between the side rims of the tongue and the insides of the upper molar teeth, but air is allowed to flow freely over the center of the tongue without turbulence. Many speakers use lip-rounding for this sound in all contexts, or except when a following vowel is spread.

The main allophones of /ɹ/ are as follows:

- [ɹ] voiced postalveolar central approximant. Those speakers who do not use the bunched-r use this allophone in most contexts. If the articulation is retroflex, then the symbol [ɻ] may be used.
- [ɹ̥] devoiced alveolar lateral approximant. This allophone occurs when /ɹ/ follows a /p/ or /k/ in stressed syllables, as in "proud," "crowd." Less devoicing occurs after other voiceless sounds: "threat," "afraid," "shrink," and following voiceless plosives in unstressed syllables.
- [ɹ̝] voiced postalveolar fricative. This allophone occurs when /ɹ/ follows a /d/, as in "drain," "drought."
- [ɹ̝̊] devoiced postalveolar fricative. This allophone occurs when /ɹ/ follows a /t/, as in "train," "trout."
- [ɹʷ] labialized voiced alveolar lateral approximant. This allophone is found before rounded vowels, and many speakers use it in all contexts except before a spread vowel. Compare "read" with "rude." There are some speakers who will use the labialized allophone before spread vowels also.
- [ɻ] voiced retroflex central approximant. As noted earlier, this allophone is a free variant of the postalveolar approximant used by some speakers.
- [Ψ] the bunched-r, as described above. This is another free variant that may be used some or all of the time by speakers. Note that the symbol is not an official IPA one, but was suggested by Laver (1994).

We can at this point reconsider the so-called r-colored or rhotic vowels (see also chap. 12). In American English we normally consider central vowels that are followed by <r> in the spelling to be pronounced with tongue tip retroflexion. In other words, they are not thought of as vowels followed by an /ɹ/, but as retroflex vowels with "the /r/ built in," so to speak. For this reason, we transcribe "word" and "paper" as /wɝd/ and /peɪpɚ/, respectively (long and short rhotic vowels). However, other vowels with following <r> are recognized to be vowel plus consonant combinations; so we transcribe "car" as /kɑɹ/. This probably reflects a difference, in that, for these noncentral vowels, tongue tip raising for the /ɹ/ may well start later than with the central rhotics. It is not altogether certain, though, that this difference is consistent. Further, when the tongue is in position for a central vowel, it is also in roughly the right position for [ɹ]; with other vowels this is not the case, and the tongue will have to move from the vowel position to the [ɹ] position. It is possible that even if a speaker tends to prefer a bunched-r, the central rhotics may still be produced with tongue tip raising; speakers may use tongue bunching with these vowels too, however.

Figure 15.12 shows a spectrogram of the word "hurry." As with the lateral approximant, we see that /ɹ/ has a formant structure and that it is shorter and less intense than the surrounding vowels. Distinguishing it from /l/ is the movement of the third formant. The F3 lowers and then rises again throughout the sound, which is the same pattern we get with other retroflex sounds and with the rhotic vowels.

THE SEMIVOWEL APPROXIMANTS

Semivowels are differentiated from other approximants by the fact that they are not prolongable. A semivowel consists of a gliding tongue movement (hence the alternative name of *glide* that

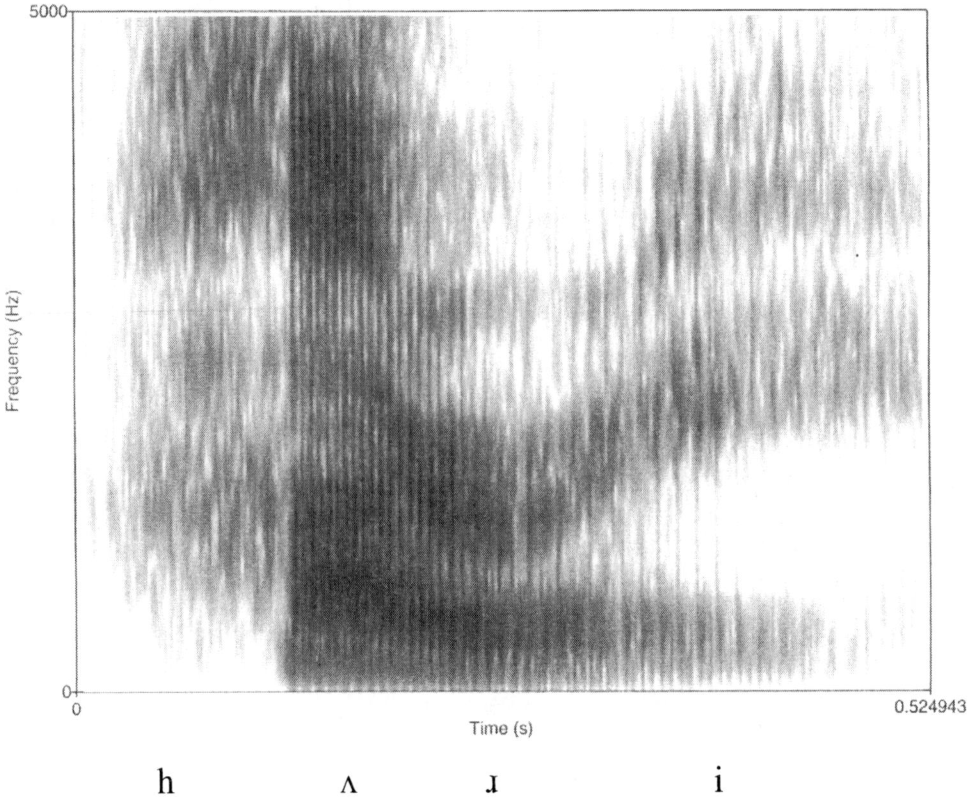

FIG 15.12. Wideband spectrogram of "hurry" (RP pronunciation).

is often given them). This tongue glide starts at the same position as one of the high vowels, but moves immediately away to take up position for the following sound. Therefore, if we prolong the initial tongue position (and so postpone the gliding movement) we end up with a vowel articulation. As we pointed out in chapter 6, all semivowels have a related high vowel, and the two semivowels of English—/w, j/—are related to the vowels /u/ and /i/, respectively. If you try prolonging a /w/, you'll find it turns into an /u/, and if you do the same with /j/, you'll hear an /i/. Semivowels, therefore, are of short duration and, acoustically, will have formant structures similar to those of their related vowels.

For all the semivowel approximants the soft palate is in the raised position, thus directing the pulmonic egressive airflow into the oral cavity and blocking off the nasal cavity.

The Labial-Velar Semivowel Approximant

/w/

The labial-velar semivowel approximant of English is symbolized by /w/, and the name of the symbol is the same as that of the letter of the alphabet. However, as this name doesn't actually contain the sound, some prefer to use the name /wə/. This consonant can be found syllable-initially and in initial clusters only. Medially, /w/ can only open a syllable, as in "be.ware."

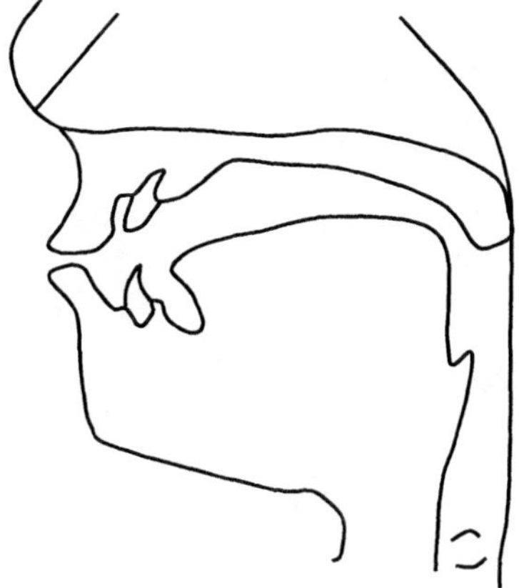

FIG 15.13. Articulator positions for /w/.

Spelling

/w/ The most common spelling is to use <w>:

<w> win unwind twig

For those who do not have a voiceless labial-velar, <wh> also represents /w/:

<wh> when which whether

After <q>, <g> and <s>, the <u> usually represents /w/:

<u> quick requite penguin suede

Some exceptional forms with <o> occur:

<o> one once choir

See below for more on <wh>.

The labial-velar approximant consists of a double articulation (see chapter 8) and is produced as follows. The vocal folds are vibrating in the voiced phonation posture throughout all (or most) of the sound. The two lips are in close approximation and assume a rounded shape with some lip protrusion. The back of the tongue dorsum is raised up toward the soft palate (but does not touch it). Air flows centrally over the tongue without turbulence (see Fig. 15.13).

The main allophones of /w/ are as follows:

- [w] voiced labial-velar semivowel approximant. This is found in most contexts.
- [w̥] devoiced labial-velar semivowel approximant. This allophone occurs when /w/ follows a /t/ or /k/ in stressed syllables, as in "twin," "queen." Less devoicing occurs after other voiceless sounds: "swim," "thwart," "squeamish," and following voiceless plosives in unstressed syllables.

Figure 15.14 shows a spectrogram of the word "rewire." As with the other approximants, we see that /w/ has a formant structure (in this case similar to that of /u/), and that it is shorter and less intense than the surrounding vowels.

The Labial-Velar Fricative

/ʍ/~/hw/

Some speakers of American and British English varieties still distinguish words spelled with <w> from words spelled with <wh>: "witch" ~ "which," "weather" ~ "whether," "watt" ~

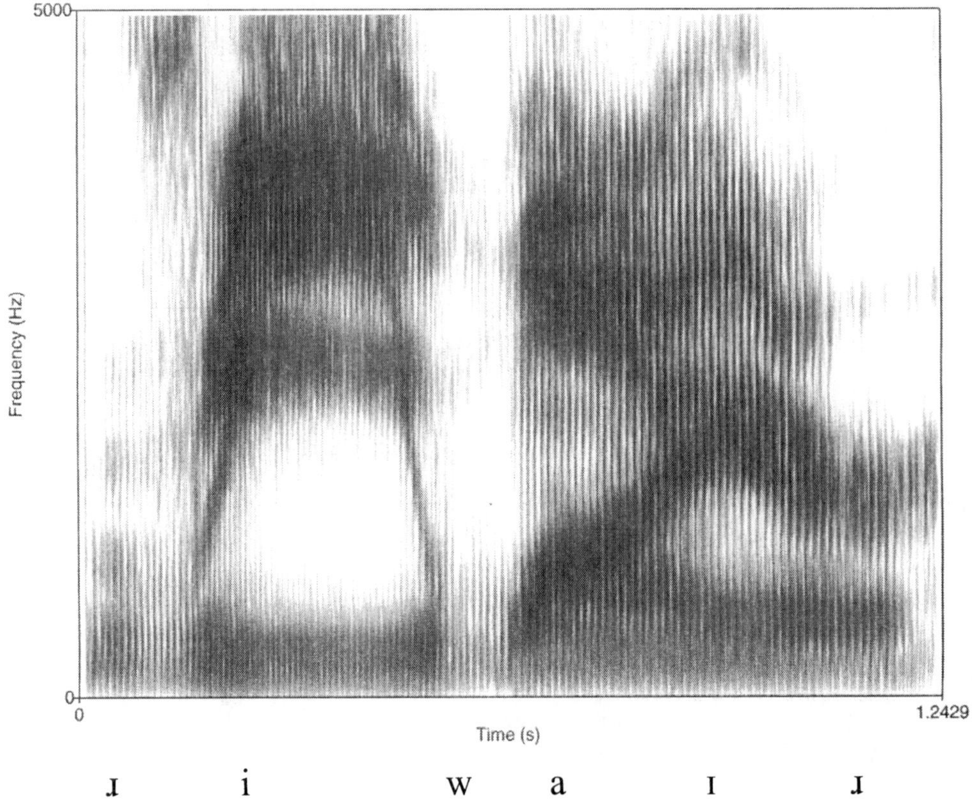

FIG 15.14. Wideband spectrogram of "rewire" (GA pronunciation).

"what," and so on (in Scottish and Irish English this distinction is more consistently found). For those speakers, <wh> represents a voiceless equivalent of /w/, but because the airflow is strongly turbulent, this sound is normally considered to be a fricative. The only recorded spelling for this sound is <wh>. The production of the labial-velar fricative is as follows. The vocal folds are apart, in the voiceless phonation posture throughout all of the sound. The two lips are in close approximation (closer than for /w/) and assume a rounded shape with some lip protrusion. The back of the tongue dorsum is raised up toward the soft palate (but does not touch it). Air flows centrally over the tongue and through the lips with considerable turbulence. No allophones are reported for this sound.

Phoneticians debate whether this sound (when used by speakers) should be considered a separate phoneme. Because there are minimal pairs (see the ones listed earlier), the voiceless labial-velar cannot be considered an allophone of /w/. However, because few speakers use it, and there are not a large number of words that contain it, one solution proposed is to consider the sound as a cluster of /h/ + /w/. This reflects the fact that the turbulent airflow seems strongest at the beginning of the sound, but that a degree of voicing and smooth airflow may return at the end of the sound. This proposal means we don't have to add an extra phoneme—/ʍ/—to the list of consonants for speakers using this sound, especially because speakers may shift between /w/ and /hw/ stylistically. We suggest that the decision whether to consider the sound as a single phoneme or as a sequence is one the clinician should take, considering the overall phonological system of the client.

The Palatal Semivowel Approximant

/j/

The palatal semivowel approximant of English is symbolized by /j/. The name of this symbol is "jod" or "jot" (/jɑd/, /jɑt/). This consonant can be found syllable-initially and in initial clusters only. Medially, /j/ can only open a syllable, as in "be.yond."

Spelling

/j/ The most common spellings are <y> and <i>:

<y>	yes	yellow	twig	lawyer
<i>	senior	million	view	spaniel

Combinations of /j/ + /u/ often have no letter for /j/:

<u>	use	opulent	congratulate
<ue>	barbecue	argue	

This combination may have <e> representing /j/:

<eu>	feud
<ew>	spew

Some exceptional forms occur:

<ll>	bouillon
<e>	azalea (in some varieties)

The palatal approximant is produced as follows. The vocal folds are vibrating in the voiced phonation posture throughout all (or most) of the sound. The front of the tongue dorsum is raised toward the hard palate (but does not touch it). Air flows centrally over the tongue without turbulence (see Fig. 15.15). Lip shape is determined by the following sound.

The main allophones of /j/ are as follows:

- [j] voiced palatal semivowel approximant. This is found in most contexts.
- [ç] voiceless palatal fricative. This allophone occurs when /j/ follows a voiceless plosive or glottal fricative in stressed syllables, as in "pure," "cure," or "hue."
- [j̊] Devoiced palatal semivowel approximant. Less devoicing occurs after other voiceless sounds: "few," "spurious," and following voiceless plosives in unstressed syllables.

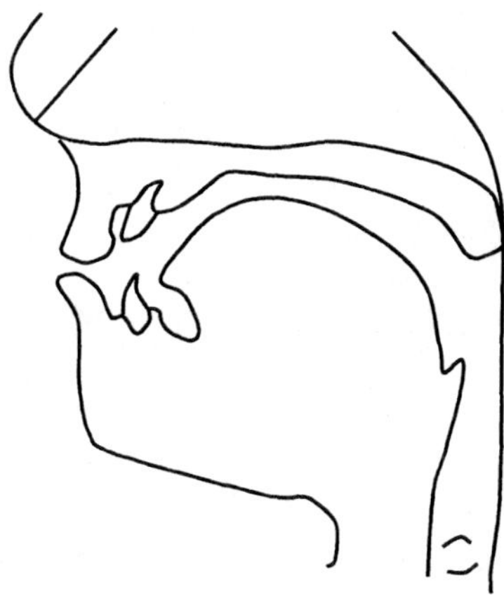

FIG 15.15. Articulator positions for /j/.

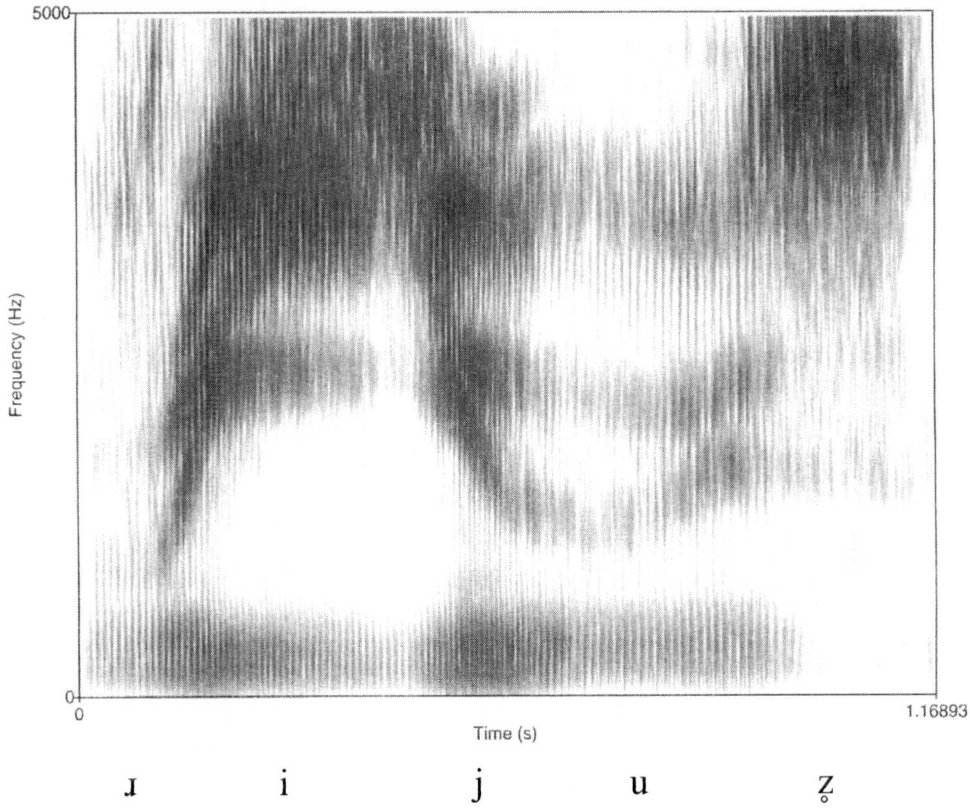

FIG 15.16. Wideband spectrogram of "reuse" (GA pronunciation).

Although /j/ can follow bilabial and velar plosives and nasals, it usually does not follow alveolar ones in American English. However, some speakers do produce "tune," "dune," and "news" as /tjun/, /djun/, and /njuz/, respectively, and these are the norm pronunciations for most varieties of British English. Speakers who do use these clusters may also convert /t+j/ and /d+j/ to /tʃ/ and /dʒ/ in rapid speech (/tʃun/, /dʒun/). Likewise, clusters of /s+j/ and /z+j/ are often realized as /ʃ/ and /ʒ/, as in "assume" and "presume."

Figure 15.16 shows a spectrogram of the word "reuse." As with the other approximants, we see that /j/ has a formant structure (in this case similar to that of /i/) and that it is shorter and less intense than the surrounding vowels.

BACKGROUND READING

The references noted in the previous chapter apply here, too.

EXERCISES

Transcription

(Answers to the transcription exercises are given at the end of the book.)

1. Transcribe the following into phonemic symbols using either GA or RP norms. These words use the consonants from this chapter, and the vowels from the previous chapters.
   (a) among (b) wall
   (c) kneel (d) wing
   (e) year (f) wrung
   (g) numb (h) leer
   (i) young (j) real
   (k) maul (l) yellow
   (m) runner (n) lung
   (o) limb (p) near
2. Transcribe the following using either GA or RP norms, employing allophonic symbols to mark devoicing, clear-, dark-, and syllabic-l, and lip-rounding before rounded vowels, where appropriate.
   (a) slow (b) goal
   (c) pool (d) twice
   (e) snail (f) riddle
   (g) clay (h) loom
   (i) smile (j) fuel
   (k) noodle (l) lean
   (m) pure (n) news
   (o) rude (p) crane
3. Convert the following GA transcriptions back into ordinary writing. (They all have more than one possible spelling—try to list all these).
   (a) /læm/ (b) /naɪt/
   (c) /mid/ (d) /ɹɛtʃ/
   (e) /bɪld/ (f) /wʌn/
   (g) /plʌm/ (h) /hju/

Review Questions

1. What distinguishes the consonants /m, n, ŋ/ from all other English consonant sounds?
2. What are the main differences between sonorant and obstruent consonants?
3. In what ways does the allophonic variation of /n/ remind you of other alveolar consonants?
4. What phonetic features are used to distinguish the approximants of English from one another?

Study Topics and Experiments

1. Undertake a survey among family or friends (at least 15 people) on the use of apical-r and bunched-r. Explain the different types of /ɹ/, and ask them to tell you their use of these variants in word-initial, -medial, and -final position and in initial and final clusters. Also ask about how they make the rhotic vowels if these are part of their dialect. Discuss the distribution of variants in terms of the age, sex, and regional/social background of the speakers.
2. What are syllabic nasals and laterals? Describe how they are made (include diagrams) and exemplify their use with typical examples. Research information on normal patterns of acquisition of these sounds in English and discuss possible errors with syllabic consonants.

CD

The final set of English consonants is exemplified on the CD, with exercises to test your ability to transcribe phonemically and phonetically.

16

Words and Connected Speech

INTRODUCTION

The vowels and consonants of English are used to make the words of the language, so we need to know about the sound structure of words as well as that of individual sounds. In turn, words go to make up utterances, so we need to know about the sound patterns of connected speech as well as that of words. In this and the following chapter we look at these aspects, concentrating on word stress patterns and boundary effects between words in this chapter, and on intonation in chapter 17. Most of the examples given in this chapter are transcribed into General American; however, Received Pronunciation equivalents can be worked out by using the information in chapters 10–15.

ENGLISH WORD STRESS

As we noted in chapter 9, word stress patterns in English are not predictable. In other words, we do not always stress the first, or the next to last syllable of a word. Indeed, words with similar structure may have different stress patterns (e.g., "sedate" and "rebate" /səˈdeɪt /~/ˈɹibeɪt/, where main stress is shown by [ˈ] before the stressed syllable). Furthermore, different regional varieties of English may differ in stress placement for some words (e.g., "debris" in General American is /dəˈbɹi/, whereas in British English it is /ˈdɛbɹi/).

> Remember that stress is manifested in various ways phonetically:
>
> stressed syllables are louder than unstressed ones
> stressed syllables may be longer than unstressed syllables
> stressed syllables may contain tenser vowels than unstressed ones
> stressed syllables may contain a pitch movement.

It is possible to distinguish various degrees of syllable stress, although for transcription purposes we normally deal with only two: stressed and unstressed. However, it is often useful to recognize an intermediate level, giving us primary stress, secondary stress, and unstressed, as this can explain certain patterns of vowel reduction seen in English (see below). For this reason,

TABLE 16.1
Stress Patterns for English Words of 1–5 Syllables

Syllable Type	*Example*	*Transcription*
ˈΣ	cat, and	ˈkæt ˈænd
ˌΣˈΣ	unlike, eighteen	ˌʌnˈlaɪk ˌeɪˈtin
ΣˈΣ	obey, beneath	əˈbeɪ bəˈniθ
ˈΣˌΣ	prolog, window	ˈpɹoʊˌlɑg ˈwɪnˌdou
ˈΣΣ	hinder, prism	ˈhɪndɚ ˈpɹɪzm̩
ˌΣΣˈΣ	interpose, seventeen	ˌɪnɾɚˈpoʊz ˌsɛvənˈtin
ˈΣΣΣ	quality, traveler	ˈkwɑləɾi ˈtɹævəlɚ
ˈΣΣˌΣ	spectrogram, telegraph	ˈspɛktɹəˌgɹæm ˈtɛləˌgɹæf
ΣˈΣΣ	debating, endeavor	dəˈbeɪɾɪŋ ɪnˈdɛvɚ
ˌΣˈΣΣ	unhappy, retaken	ˌʌnˈhæpi ˌɹiˈteɪkən
ΣˈΣˌΣ	potato, risotto	pəˈteɪˌɾoʊ ɹɪˈzɑˌɾoʊ
ΣˈΣΣΣ	impassable	ɪmˈpæsəbəl
ˌΣˈΣΣΣ	ungenerous	ˌʌnˈdʒɛnəɹəs
ΣˈΣΣˌΣ	acclimatize	əˈklaɪməˌtaɪz
ˌΣΣˈΣΣ	telegraphic	ˌtɛləˈgɹæfɪk
ˈΣΣΣΣ	witticism	ˈwɪɾɪsɪzm̩
ˈΣΣˌΣΣ	educated	ˈɛdʒəˌkeɪɾəd
ˈΣΣΣˌΣ	counterattack	ˈkaʊnɾəɹəˌtæk
ˌΣΣΣˈΣ	aquamarine	ˌækwəməˈɹin
ΣˌΣΣˈΣ	misunderstand	mɪsˌʌndɚˈstænd
ΣˌΣΣˈΣΣ	consideration	kənˌsɪdəˈɹeɪʃn̩
ˌΣΣΣˈΣΣ	interdependence	ˌɪnɾɚdɪˈpɛndəns
ˌΣΣˈΣΣΣ	subjectivity	ˌsʌbdʒɛkˈtɪvəɾi
ˌΣΣˈΣΣˌΣ	incapacitate	ˌɪŋkəˈpæsɪˌteɪt
ΣˈΣΣΣΣ	catholicism	kəˈθɑlɪsɪzm̩

we will mark secondary as well as primary stress in the examples used in this section. We also have to bear in mind that the stress patterns of words spoken in isolation (or emphasized) may differ from the patterns used when those same words are part of a complete utterance. In English, these differences are especially marked in *function words* (that is, grammatical words such as determiners, prepositions, and conjunctions), and we look in detail at such differences in the next section.

We will examine the stress patterns of English by looking at words of different length (in terms of numbers of syllables). Even words of one syllable may receive stress, whether they are *content words* (such as nouns, verbs, and adjectives) or function words (although, as we will see, these latter tend to lose stress in connected speech). Naturally, it is only when we reach words of two or more syllables that we can see a contrast between different degrees of stress. In the examples, in Table 16.1, we use the symbol Σ to stand for syllable, with ˈΣ denoting a primary stressed syllable, ˌΣ a secondary stressed one, and plain Σ an unstressed one. The example words are given in normal orthography and in General American phonemic transcription with stress marks (following our practice described in chapter 13, we transcribe the flapped-t allophone separately).

Words in English can be even longer than five syllables, of course. Different patterns hold for six-syllable words (compare "imˌpossiˈbility" with "iˌdentifiˈcation," for example) and seven-syllable words (compare "ˌunreˌliaˈbility" with "inˌdustrialiˈzation"), and for even longer words. Compound words—that is, words constructed out of two independent words—also have their own distinctive patterns of stress assignment. Often, two-syllable compounds will have primary

TABLE 16.2
Word Stress Patterns in Nouns/Adjectives and Verbs

Word	*Noun/Adjective*	*Verb*
export	ˈɛkˌspɔɹt	ˌɪkˈspɔɹt
object	ˈɑbˌdʒɛkt	əbˈdʒɛkt
conflict	ˈkɑnˌflɪkt	kənˈflɪkt
permit	ˈpɝˌmɪt	pɚˈmɪt
protest	ˈpɹoʊˌtɛst	pɹəˈtɛst
contest	ˈkɑnˌtɛst	kənˈtɛst
conduct	ˈkɑnˌdʌkt	kənˈdʌkt
transport	ˈtɹænˌspɔɹt	ˌtɹænˈspɔɹt
accent	ˈækˌsɛnt	ˌækˈsɛnt

stress on the first syllable and secondary on the second. Examples include "ˈbookˌcase," "ˈblueˌjay," and "ˈteaˌcup." The alternative pattern of secondary stress followed by primary can also be found: "ˌupˈstairs," "ˌsouthˈeast," "ˌlong-ˈterm." Compounds of more than two syllables also occur, and these mostly fall into two categories in most varieties of English: those with first-syllable primary stress ("ˈdog-ˌcollar," "ˈbooby-ˌtrap'), and those with first-syllable secondary stress ("ˌcold-ˈblooded," "ˌsecondˈhand," "ˌpost-ˈgraduate").

Interestingly, English has a set of word pairs with identical or very similar pronunciations, where one of the pair has first-syllable primary stress and the other has second-syllable primary stress. It turns out that the first-syllable primary stress words in these pairs are nouns or adjectives, whereas the second-syllable primary stress equivalents are verbs. We can illustrate some of these in the Table 16.2 and will deal with some more of them in the exercises at the end of the chapter.

Identifying word stress patterns is an important skill for the speech-language pathologist. Transcribing ability at the segmental level is clearly necessary for the identification of segmental level errors, but errors with suprasegmentals, including word stress, also occur. You should, therefore, practice your ability to assign primary stress, and if possible also secondary stress, with the exercises at the end of the chapter, on the audio CD, and with words chosen at random from your reading.

STRESS IN CONNECTED SPEECH

Content Words

Word stress in connected speech is not necessarily the same as when the words are said in isolation (often termed the *citation* form). This is especially true of function words (which normally lose stress completely), but content words may also be affected to some degree. For example, in the phrase, "keep off the grass!" we may assign full stress to the first second and fourth words (/ˈkip ˈɑf ðə ˈɡɹæs/), or we may downgrade the stress on the first word to emphasize the second (/ˌkip ˈɑf ðə ˈɡɹæs/). Many researchers are of the opinion that there is a whole range of subtly differing stress levels in connected speech, and they have designed tree-diagrams to show the relations between different syllables in an utterance and their respective levels of stress. We can look here at the notion of the *foot* as used to illustrate the stress-timed nature of English rhythm (see chap. 9). The following utterance is used to exemplify feet: "Mr. Rogers drew a picture," /ˈmɪstɚ ˈɹɑdʒɚʒ ˈdɹu ə ˈpɪktʃɚ/. When we divide this utterance into feet we get

/ˈmɪs tɚ | ˈɹɑ dʒɚʒ | ˈdɹu ə | ˈpɪk tʃɚ/

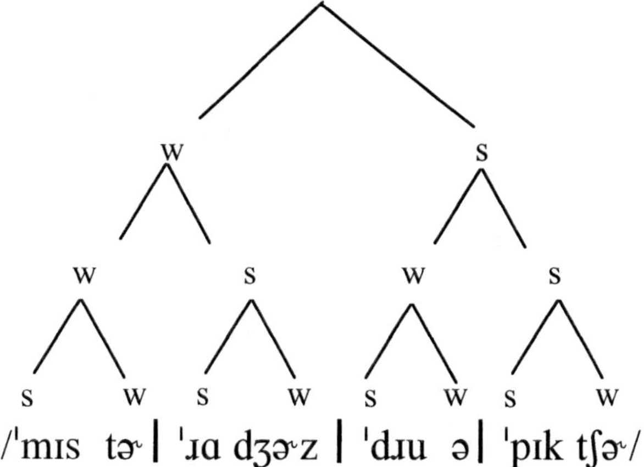

FIG 16.1. Stress tree for "Mister Rogers drew a picture."

The tree-diagram in Fig. 16.1 shows that this utterance may be thought of as having varying degrees of primary stress and varying degrees of lack of stress depending upon where in the utterance the syllable occurs. In the diagram, "w" stands for *weak*, and "s" stands for *strong*.

This diagram shows that although the individual syllables are stressed and unstressed as we would expect from their citation forms, the strongest of all the stressed syllables is that in "picture" (dominated by three strong nodes in the tree), whereas the weakest is that in "Mister" (dominated by only one strong node). Of course, not all utterances fall into such symmetrical trees as we see in Fig. 16.1, and not all feet conveniently have a strong and a weak syllable. In the following example (repeated from chap. 9), we have an utterance with a string of adjectives before a final noun and several feet of one syllable only. In this latter case it is easiest to assume empty weak syllables following the strong one, and we show this in the tree by using the zero sign: ø. The utterance is, "Pat has got a bright red coat," /ˈpæt əz ˈgɑɾ ə ˈbɹaɪt ˈɹɛd ˈkoʊt/. When we divide this into feet we get

/ˈpæt əz | ˈgɑɾ ə | ˈbɹaɪt | ˈɹɛd | ˈkoʊt/

The tree diagram in Fig. 16.2 shows this utterance and the stress strength relations between the feet.

Again, we can see that, in this case, "coat" is the strongest stressed syllable (dominated by five strong nodes), whereas "Pat" is the least strong stressed syllable (dominated by only one strong node).

> The rhythmic patterns seen in these two trees also reflect the nature of English intonation. As we will see in chapter 17, English intonation tends to place the most marked pitch change toward the end of an utterance. It is for this reason that these two tree diagrams have the strongest stressed syllables in the final feet.

Function Words

We can now turn our attention to what happens to function words in connected speech. As we saw in the two example utterances above, function words usually do not receive stress in connected speech. Furthermore, they are often subject to varying degrees of reduction. So, in

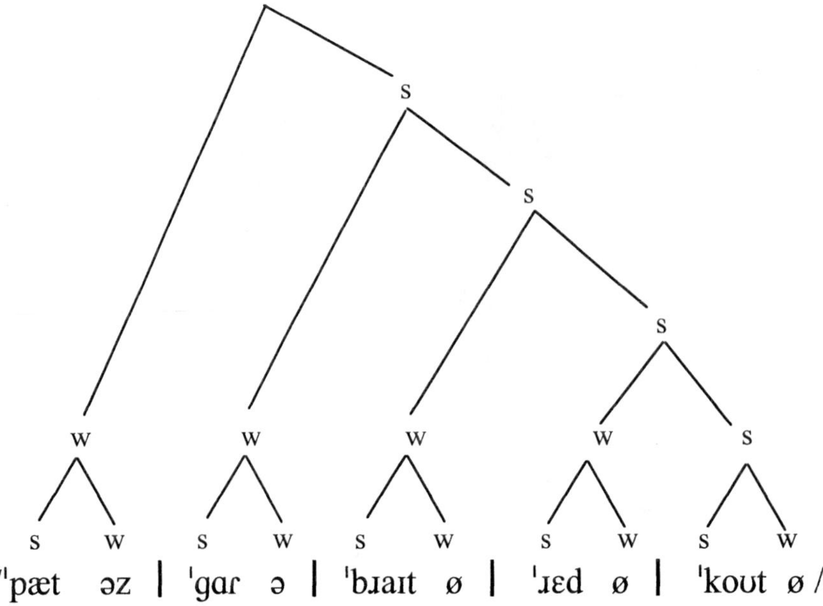

FIG 16.2. Stress tree for "Pat has got a bright red coat."

Fig. 16.1, we see that the indefinite determiner "a," with a citation pronunciation of /ˈeɪ/, is reduced in connected speech to /ə/. In Fig. 16.2, the auxiliary verb "has," with a citation form of /ˈhæz/, is reduced to /əz/. This reduction gives rise to what are called *weak forms* of function words, and we give a list of the commonest of these in Table 16.3. Weak forms generally show vowel reduction (usually to schwa), loss of consonants and simplification of consonant clusters to singletons, and an overall reduction in length. This reduction

TABLE 16.3
Citation and Weak Forms of Function Words

Function word	*Citation form*	*Weak form*
a	ˈeɪ	ə
and	ˈænd	ən, n̩ (/d/ retained before vowels)
as	ˈæz	əz
at	ˈæt	ət
but	ˈbʌt	bət
can	ˈkæn	kən
could	ˈkʊd	kəd
does (aux)	ˈdʌz	dəz, z, s
for	ˈfɔɹ	fɚ
from	ˈfɹɑm	fɹəm
his	ˈhɪz	ɪz
not	ˈnɑt	nt, n
of	ˈɑv	əv
shall	ˈʃæl	ʃəl, ʃl̩
than	ˈðæn	ðən, ðn̩
them	ˈðɛm	ðəm, əm, m̩
was	ˈwʌz	wəz
will	ˈwɪl	l, l̩

of function words in connected speech is a natural consequence of the strong rhythmic differential between stressed and unstressed syllables in a stress-timed language like English.

> Remember that function words are not always reduced in connected speech. If we wish to emphasize a function word—perhaps when we are contrasting two options—then the full, stressed, pronunciation is used,
>
> I need coffee *and* tea /ˌaɪˈnid ˈkɑfi ˈænd ˈti/
>
> as opposed to a version of the same sentence when the "and" is not emphasized':
>
> I need coffee and tea /ˌaɪˈ nid ˈkɑfi ən ˈti/

It is important that we know the weak forms of the common function words because, in assessing speech clients, it is vital that we distinguish a genuine problem with vowel reduction or consonant deletion from the normal application of connected speech realizations of function words. Table 16.3 lists many of these together with their citation pronunciations; again, we'll return to some more examples in the exercises at the end of the chapter.

The following examples show the use of these weak forms in connected speech:

1. I'll be seeing James and Tom but only at the weekend
   /ˌaɪl bi ˈsiɪŋ ˈdʒeɪmz ən ˈtɑm bət ˈoʊnli ət ðə ˈwikˌɛnd/
2. This is for Angela from all of us
   /ˌðɪs ɪz fɚ ˈændʒələ fɹəm ˈɔl əv əs/
3. We shall meet them at the house
   /ˌwe ʃəl ˈmit ðəm ət ðə ˈhaʊs/
4. Kiri can sing better than you
   /ˈkɪɹi kən ˈsiŋ ˈbɛrɚ ðən ˈju/

> Even some nouns can have weak forms—but only when they act as titles.
>
> For example, "saint," when used before a saint's name, is weakened by reduction of the vowel to schwa and loss of the final /t/ (unless the saint's name starts with a vowel, when the /t/ is retained). For example:
>
> "he has the patience of a saint" /ˌhi əz ðə ˈpeɪʃəns əv ə ˈseɪnt/
> "Saint Joan," "Saint Andrew" /sən ˈdʒoʊn/, /sn̩t ˈændɹu/

ASSIMILATION

Whenever we put sounds together to make syllables (and then words and utterances), some aspects of the pronunciation of these sounds are likely to be due to the influence of neighboring sounds (even across word boundaries). These changes are usually called *assimilations*. Many of the changes brought about through the influence of a neighboring sound are allophonic, and we have encountered these in our descriptions of the individual consonants and vowels of English. For example, the lip-rounding in certain consonants before rounded vowels is an allophonic assimilation (often termed a *similitude*). When a syllable has a rounded vowel in it, the lip-rounding acts as an independent articulatory gesture that normally starts at the beginning of the syllable (thus making any onset consonant lip-rounded) and may remain through the vowel and continue on to any following consonant. Other examples of allophonic assimilation include the nasalization of preceding (and to some extent following) vowels in the context of a nasal consonant; the dental placement of /t, d, n/ before dental fricatives; the advanced velar placement of /k, g/ before front vowels; the devoicing of /m, n, l/ after voiceless /s/; and the labiodental placement of /m/ before labiodental fricatives.

Of course, these allophonic changes are automatic, and make articulation easier (for example, by reducing a series of two different places of articulation, e.g., alveolar followed by dental, to a single place, dental). There are other assimilatory changes that involve the change of one phoneme to another, and these changes are normally studied under the heading of *juxtapositional assimilation.* We are most interested in these changes when they take place across word boundaries, but there are also some phonemic changes that take place within words, for example, when a prefix is added to a word stem. We can look at what happens when we add the negative prefix "un-" to a variety of different stems. In "unhappy" the /n/ of the prefix remains an alveolar nasal (/ˌʌnˈhæpi/); however, when we add "un" to "convincing" then the /n/ of the prefix usually changes to /ŋ/ (it assimilates to the velar place of the first sound of "convincing") to give /ˌʌŋkənˈvɪnsɪŋ/. Finally, the /n/ is usually realized as bilabial in words such as "unbounded"; it assimilates to the bilabial place of the /b/: /ˌʌmˈbaʊndɪd/. Note that not all speakers make these changes, and they appear to be more common in British than American English.

Note that we recognize in spelling the bilabial assimilation with the prefix "in-" but not the velar assimilation:

intolerant	/ˌɪnˈtɑləɹənt/
impossible	/ˌɪmˈpɑsəbəl/
inclement	/ˌɪŋˈklɛmənt/

We don't recognize in spelling any assimilations with the "un-" prefix, however.

Juxtapositional assimilations across word boundaries are more pervasive and therefore more important in the study of English pronunciation. Even when we transcribe phonemically, we have to listen for these changes and record them. Phonemic assimilations across word boundaries can, in principle, operate in two distinct ways. First, the final consonant of the first word under consideration could affect the initial consonant of the second word, changing it phonemically to become a different sound phonetically closer to the first sound. This direction of influence is called *progressive assimilation.* Alternatively, the converse can occur: The initial sound of the second word can affect the pronunciation of the last consonant of the first word, changing it into a phoneme that is phonetically closer to the influencing sound. This is called *regressive assimilation*, and is what is found in English.

Assimilation of both types can produce a variety of changes. For example, assimilation can result in changes to voicing, so that both sounds become voiced or voiceless (e.g., "have to" /hæv tə/ changing to /hæf tə/ in English). Another possible change is in manner of articulation (for example, a stop becoming an affricate under the influence of a fricative). Finally, we can consider changes to the place of articulation, and this is the type of assimilatory change most common in English. We can also classify assimilations according to whether they involve a *total assimilation* (both sounds end up identical) or a *partial assimilation* (the affected sound becomes more like the influencing sound, but they are not identical). In English, assimilations are usually only partial, because the place changes, but the manner and voicing normally do not. Total assimilation only occurs if the two sounds concerned already share identical voicing and manner of articulation.

In English only certain final consonants are susceptible to assimilation: the alveolar plosives, nasals, and fricatives. The plosives and nasals behave in much the same way, so we will deal with them first. Word-final /t, d, n/ can assimilate to bilabial /p, b, m/ if the initial consonant of the following word is a bilabial *and* if the two words form a close syntactic group (e.g., a determiner and noun, adjective and noun, etc.). Word-final /t, d, n/ can assimilate to velar /k, g, ŋ/ if the initial consonant of the following word is a velar *and* if the two words form a close syntactic group. We can show how these assimilations work with the following examples:

word-final /t/		
that dog	/ˌðæt ˈdɑg/	no assimilation; second word starts with alveolar
that person	/ˌðæp ˈpɝsən/	bilabial assimilation under influence of /p/
that book	/ˌðæp ˈbʊk/	bilabial assimilation under influence of /b/
that machine	/ˌðæp məˈʃin/	bilabial assimilation under influence of /m/
that card	/ˌðæk ˈkɑɹd/	velar assimilation under influence of /k/
that game	/ˌðæk ˈgeɪm/	velar assimilation under influence of /g/
word-final /d/		
bad dog	/ˈbæd ˈdɑg/	no assimilation; second word starts with alveolar
bad person	/ˈbæb ˈpɝsən/	bilabial assimilation under influence of /p/
bad book	/ˈbæb ˈbʊk/	bilabial assimilation under influence of /b/
bad machine	/ˈbæb məˈʃin/	bilabial assimilation under influence of /m/
bad card	/ˈbæg ˈkɑɹd/	velar assimilation under influence of /k/
bad game	/ˈbæg ˈgeɪm/	velar assimilation under influence of /g/
word-final /n/		
one dog	/ˈwʌn ˈdɑg/	no assimilation; second word starts with alveolar
one person	/ˈwʌm ˈpɝsən/	bilabial assimilation under influence of /p/
one book	/ˈwʌm ˈbʊk/	bilabial assimilation under influence of /b/
one machine	/ˈwʌm məˈʃin/	bilabial assimilation under influence of /m/
one card	/ˈwʌŋ ˈkɑɹd/	velar assimilation under influence of /k/
one game	/ˈwʌŋ ˈgeɪm/	velar assimilation under influence of /g/

Note that final alveolar clusters can also undergo assimilation to both members of the cluster:

word-final /nt/		
don't drink	/ˈdoʊnt ˈdɹɪŋk/	no assimilation; second word starts with alveolar
don't play	/ˈdoʊmp ˈpleɪ/	bilabial assimilation under influence of /p/
don't blink	/ˈdoʊmp ˈblɪŋk/	bilabial assimilation under influence of /b/
don't munch	/ˈdoʊmp ˈmʌntʃ/	bilabial assimilation under influence of /m/
don't cry	/ˈdoʊŋk ˈkɹaɪ/	velar assimilation under influence of /k/
don't go	/ˈdoʊŋk ˈgoʊ/	velar assimilation under influence of /g/

Assimilations with /s, z/ are somewhat different. These only involve a change from alveolar to postalveolar and are triggered by only two contexts: word-initial /ʃ/ or /j/.

word-final /s/		
this suit	/ˌðɪs ˈsut/	no assimilation; second word starts with alveolar
this shirt	/ˌðɪʃ ˈʃɝt/	postalveolar assimilation under influence of /ʃ/
this yacht	/ˌðɪʃ ˈjɑt/	postalveolar assimilation under influence of /j/
word-final /z/		
these suits	/ˌðiz ˈsuts/	no assimilation; second word starts with alveolar
these shirts	/ˌðiʒ ˈʃɝts/	postalveolar assimilation under influence of /ʃ/
these yachts	/ˌðiʒ ˈjɑts/	postalveolar assimilation under influence of /j/

Linked to these last assimilations is a process usually termed *coalescence*, where word-final /t, d, s, z/ merge with following word-initial /j/ to produce /tʃ, dʒ, ʃ, ʒ/ respectively (though the fricative finals may show extra length). Examples can be seen in

what you . . .	/ˈwʌt ju/	→	/ˈwʌtʃu/
would you . . .	/ˈwʊd ju/	→	/ˈwʊdʒu/
. . . miss you	/ˈmɪs ju/	→	/ˈmɪʃu/ or /ˈmɪʃʃu/
as you . . .	/ˈæz ju/	→	/ˈæʒu/ or /ˈæʒʒu/

These phonemic-level assimilations (unlike the allophonic-level similitudes) are to some extent under speaker control. In rapid, casual speech most of us use these assimilations. However, in slower, more formal, or more careful speech, we may avoid them. As with the weak forms of function words, we need to know about these assimilations to ensure that we do not characterize normal connected speech processes as speech errors. It is also useful to know about them, because they may explain why some clients with acquired neurological speech disorders sound stilted when they speak: it may be because they are not using these assimilations and other connected speech phenomena.

Assimilations may result in utterances that differ in slower, formal speech being pronounced the same in connected speech:

he rang quickly ~ he ran quickly	/ˌhi ɹæŋ ˈkwɪkli/
it's light cream ~ it's like cream	/ɪts ˈlaɪk ˈkɹim/
a right pair ~ a ripe pear	/ə ˈɹaɪp ˈpɛɹ/

Weak forms of function words can also produce similar examples:

two of them ~ two have them /ˈtu əv ðəm/
what's he like (= what does he like ~ what is he like) /ˈwɑts i ˈlaik/
I'd put it here (= I had put it here ~ I would put it here) /ˌaɪd ˈpʊɾ ɪt ˈhiɹ/

ELISION AND LIAISON

Another characteristic of connected speech in English is *elision*. Elision is the loss of sounds. English demonstrates two main types of elision: vowel elision and consonant elision.

Vowel Elision

The unstressed vowel schwa is especially prone to deletion (along with the entire syllable in which it is situated) in various contexts. Particularly common is the deletion of schwa when it is followed by a liquid (/l, ɹ/) or by a nasal, and then when there is another weak vowel after that. A good example is "camera," where the middle syllable is often elided in connected speech so that /ˈkæməɹə/ is realized as /ˈkæmɹə/ (in fact, in some varieties of English, such as British, this is the only possible pronunciation, and the full form sounds artificial). We'll look at some more examples of words of this type in the exercises at the end of the chapter.

Schwa may also be deleted at word boundaries, with the syllable absorbed as a syllabic lateral or nasal. The following examples illustrate this:

"run along"	/ˈɹʌn əˈlɑŋ/	→	/ˈɹʌn̩ ˈlɑŋ/
"not alone"	/ˈnɑɾ əˈloʊn/	→	/ˈnɑɾl̩ ˈloʊn/

If there is an /r/ after the schwa, then complete elision may occur in some accents:

"after a while"	/ˈæftɚ əˈwaɪl/	→	/ˈæftɹə ˈwaɪl/
"over and over"	/ˈoʊvɚ ənd ˈoʊvɚ/	→	/ˈoʊv ɹənd ˈoʊvɚ/

Consonant Elision

The consonants most susceptible to elision in English are the alveolar plosives /t, d/, and this occurs most often in word-final two-consonant clusters, especially when the following word starts with a consonant, or if the plosive is the middle consonant in a three-consonant cluster. We can look at examples, starting with the most common types and working through to those subject to elision less often.

voiceless nonplosive + /t/ + consonant or voiced nonplosive + /d/ + consonant

passed by	/ˈpæs ˌbaɪ/	found them	/ˈfaʊn ðəm/
next week	/ˈnɛks ˈwik/	cold night	/ˈkoʊl ˈnaɪt/
last night	/ˈlæs ˈnaɪt/	raised them	/ˈɹeɪz ðəm/
east Texas	/ˈis ˈtɛksəs/	refused them	/ˈɹəfjuz ðəm/
soft cushion	/ˈsɑf ˈkʊʃən/	old car	/ˈoʊl ˈkɑɹ/
finished work	/ˈfɪnɪʃ ˈwɝk/	moved through	/ˈmuv ˈθɹu/
facts	/fæks/	friendship	/ˈfɹɛnʃɪp/
mostly	/ˈmoʊsli/	handsome	/ˈhænsəm/

voiceless plosive/affricate + /t/ + consonant or voiced plosive/affricate + /d/ + consonant

helped Jane	/ˈhɛlp ˈdʒeɪn/	robbed them	/ˈɹɑb ðəm/
looked sick	/ˈlʊk ˈsɪk/	nagged me	/ˈnæg ˈmi/
reached back	/ˈɹitʃ ˈbæk/	nudged Fred	/ˈnʌdʒ ˈfɹɛd/
prompts	/pɹɑmps/		

/nt/ and /lt/+ consonant (less prone to elision; hardly ever in single words)

went through	/ˈwɛn(t) ˈθɹu/	melt down	/ˈmɛl(t) ˈdaʊn/
mints	/mɪnts̩/	belts	/bɛlts/

consonant + /t/ or /d/ + /h/ (elision rare)

kept hope	/ˈkɛpt ˈhoʊp/	changed house	/ˈtʃeɪndʒd ˈhaʊs/
left home	/ˈlɛft ˈhoʊm/	loved Harry	/ˈlʌvd ˈhæɹi/

consonant + /t/ or /d/ + /j/ (usually coalescence)

helped you	/ˈhɛlptʃu/	sold you	/ˈsoʊldʒu/
liked you	/ˈlaɪktʃu/	robbed you	/ˈɹɑbdʒu/

> Some of these elisions result in the collapse of the distinction between present and past tense. For example, /ˌaɪ ˈwɔk ˌðɛɹ/ could be "I walk there" or "I walked there." The context has to help us disambiguate such utterances. Note that elision doesn't take place if the second word is vowel-initial: /ˌaɪ ˈwɔkt ˌɪn/ "I walked in."

negative /nt/ + consonant (often elided in two-syllable words)

mustn't go	/ˈmʌsn̩ ˈgoʊ/	couldn't see	/ˈkʊdn̩ ˈsi/
doesn't Jim	/ˈdʌzn̩ ˈdʒɪm/	shouldn't they	/ˈʃʊdn̩ ˈðeɪ/

/t/ + /t/ or /d/ (elision occurs in some common phrases)

got to go /ˈgɑɾə ˈgoʊ/ what do you want /ˈwɑdʒə ˈwɑnt/

miscellaneous (a few commonly occurring phrases)

want to go	/ˈwɑnə ˈgoʊ/	give me	/ˈgɪmi/
let me go	/ˈlɛmi ˈgoʊ/	get me	/ˈgɛmi/

I'm going to /ˈaɪm gənə/~/ˈaɪŋənə/~/ ˈaɪŋnə/~/ˈaɪmə/~/ˈamə/

> Often, initial /h/ in function words is elided in casual speech, even in accents that normally retain /h/:
> /wi ˈsɔ ɪm ˈoʊpən ɪz ˈdɔɹ/ "we saw him open his door"

Liaison

Liaison is the term given to the insertion of a consonant to avoid a sequence of word-final vowel followed by word-initial vowel. In French, for example, this vowel–vowel hiatus (as it is sometimes called) can be avoided through the insertion of a [t] ("y a-*t*-il personne?" = "is anyone there") or by the pronunciation of a final consonant that is normally left silent ("le peti[t] animal" ~ "le peti[Ø] garçon" = "the little animal" ~ "the little boy").

In English, we tend to avoid such hiatus through using the glottal stop, for example, in a sequence such as "Tony [ʔ] is away [ʔ] at the moment." However, a different form of liaison operates in those varieties of English called *nonrhotic*. Nonrhotic accents of English are those that do not normally pronounce postvocalic /ɹ/ (i.e., /ɹ/ that follows a vowel and either precedes a consonant or is word-final). We can illustrate rhotic and nonrhotic realizations of some words in the following table.

TABLE 16.4
Rhotic and Nonrhotic Pronunciations

	Rhotic accent	*Nonrhotic accent*
better	/ˈbɛɾɚ/	/ˈbɛtə/
card	/kɑɹd/	/kɑd/
air	/ɛɹ/	/ɛə/
ear	/ɪɹ/	/ɪə/
tour	/tʊɹ/	/tʊə/

Table 16.4 demonstrates that in nonrhotic accents the /ɹ/ is sometimes simply omitted, and in other cases is replaced by /ə/, giving rise to a set of centering diphthongs (see chap. 18). Although most North American accents are rhotic, some southern and African American varieties are nonrhotic, as well as some northeastern accents. Also, the English of England (apart from the west and southwest and parts of the northwest), Australia, New Zealand, and South Africa is nonrhotic. Scottish English is rhotic, although both trills and taps may be used in addition to the approximant /ɹ/ in Scotland. Irish English is also rhotic, using an approximant /ɹ/.

TABLE 16.5
/ɹ/ Liaison in Nonrhotic Accents

Hiatus	*/ɹ/ Liaison*	*Nonhiatus*	*No Liaison*
better off	/ˈbɛtɚ ˈɒf/	better job	/ˈbɛtə ˈdʒɒb/
far away	/ˈfɑɹ əˈweɪ/	far back	/ˈfɑ ˈbæk/
answer Ann	/ˈɑnsɚ ˈæn/	answer Jack	/ˈɑnsə ˈdʒæk/
tour Ireland	/ˈtuɹ ˈaɪələnd/	tour Wales	/ˈtʊə ˈweɪlz/
here it is	/ˈhiɹ ɪt ɪz/	here they come	/ˈhɪə ðeɪ ˈkʌm/

Nonrhotic accents, then, have more vowel-final words than rhotic ones, due to the loss of word-final /ɹ/. This means there is more opportunity for hiatus to arise, in phrases such as "better off," "far away," "answer Ann," "tour Ireland," "here it is," and so on. Rather than use the glottal stop in these instances, most nonrhotic speakers pronounce the /ɹ/ in these circumstances. In Table 16.5 we can see the use of /ɹ/ liaison in sample cases compared to the normal nonrhotic pronunciation before consonant initial words.

Speakers of some nonrhotic accents often extend the use of /ɹ/ as a hiatus breaker even to forms that never historically had /ɹ/ pronounced (this is especially the case with schwa-final words). This is sometimes referred to as *intrusive-r*, and has been castigated as historically incorrect. Of course, it is not the history of a pronunciation that is important, so there is no reason to consider intrusive-r as a speech error. Examples of this usage can be seen in "law and order" /ˈlɔɹ ən ˈɔdə/, "India is" /ˈɪndɪɚ ɪz/, "idea of" /ˈaɪdɪɚ əv/, "area of" /ˈɛɹɪɚ əv/, and "awe-inspiring" /ˈɔɹ ɪnˈspaɪɹɪŋ/. It can even occur word-internally, as in "drawing" /ˈdɹɔɹɪŋ/.

If the client you're dealing with speaks a nonrhotic variety of English, remember the nonpronunciation of /ɹ/ after vowels and before consonants or word-finally is not an error. Further, if the client then uses an intrusive-r, that is not an error for that client either. This underlines again the necessity of having information on the client's target accent before you assess his or her speech.

Epenthesis

Interestingly, while there is a strong tendency to elide /t/ in final clusters (as we saw on page 259), there is the opposite tendency to insert /t/ in some final clusters—especially final /-ns/ clusters. Examples include "dance," "fence," "sense," and "mince," which may be pronounced either /dæns/, /fɛns/, /sens/, /mɪns, or /dænts/, /fɛnts/, /sents/, /mɪnts/. Sometimes, this process of epenthesis is extended to bilabials and velars. This can give examples such as "warmth" and "Kingston"; either /wɔɹmθ/, /ˈkɪŋstən/, or /wɔɹmpθ/, /ˈkɪŋkstən/.

Epenthesis can lead to the collapse of phonological distinction between word pairs. For example, the following pairs of words will have the same pronunciation when epenthetic /t/ is inserted into the first of each pair:

mince	mints	/mɪnts/
prince	prints	/pɹɪnts/
sense	cents	/sɛnts/
tense	tents	/tɛnts/

JUNCTURE

Many of the connected speech processes we have examined have taken place at word boundaries. The juncture between two words has also been studied to see what phonetic cues are available for the listener to help him or her perceive the boundary. More often than not, we do not pause between words (clearly sometimes we do, especially between major intonation groups, which we look at in detail in the next chapter). Therefore, if there is no pause between words corresponding to the white space on the printed page, how can we tell that one word has ended and another begun?

Usually, the segmenting of words from the stream of speech is not a problem for an experienced speaker of the language, because there is seldom any doubt as to the intended string of words. However, there are occasions where two possible segmentations of the phonemes can be made, which would lead to two different strings of words and, thus, potential confusion. A common example used to illustrate this point is the string of phonemes /ˈpistɑks/. If we segment this string into two words after the /s/ we have "peace talks"; if we segment it before the /s/ we have "pea stalks." However, we never actually have any trouble interpreting the intended segmentation. Why is this? If we examine the allophonic transcription of this phrase, we see that there are significant differences that we can hear clearly, and that allow us to perceive the intended meaning. For "peace talks" [ˈpʰi·s tʰɑ·ks] we have a reduced-length vowel in "peace" because of the fortis consonant following the vowel and an aspirated plosive at the beginning of the second syllable. For "pea stalks" [ˈpʰiː st⁼ɑ·ks], on the other hand, we have the full-length vowel in "pea," because it is in an open syllable, and we have no aspiration on the /t/ because it is in an /s/ cluster. Below we have some more examples of junctural similarity, with an explanation of the allophonic differences between the two possible segmentations. All these examples come from Cruttenden (2001).

It has to be admitted, however, that in rapid speech some of these allophonic differences may be so slight that listeners cannot actually perceive them clearly. The influence of the semantic context is such, though, that we rarely encounter any difficulties in decoding the intended message.

BACKGROUND READING

Cruttenden (2001) deals with all these areas in detail, whereas Fudge (1984) provides a thorough investigation of word-stress in English.

TABLE 16.6
Juncture Differences

	Transcription	*Allophonic Features*
I scream	/ˈaɪ ˈskɹim/	full length /aɪ/; voiced /ɹ/
ice cream	/ˈaɪs ˈkɹim/	reduced /aɪ/; devoiced /ɹ/
why choose	/ˈwaɪ ˈtʃuz/	long /aɪ/; short /ʃ/
white shoes	/ˈwaɪt ˈʃuz/	reduced /aɪ/; long /ʃ/
a name	/ə ˈneɪm/	long /n/, opening stressed syllable
an aim	/ən ˈeɪm/	reduced /n/, coda of unstressed syllable
nitrate	/ˈnaɪˌtɹeɪt/	devoiced /ɹ/ in /t/ cluster
night rate	/ˈnaɪt ˈɹeɪt/	/ɹ/ not devoiced; also stress difference
illegal	/ɪˈligəl/	clear /l/ as syllable initial
ill eagle	/ˈɪl ˈigəl/	dark /l/ as syllable final; also stress difference

EXERCISES

Transcription

(*Answers to the transcription exercises are given at the end of the book.*)

1. Stress assignment. Add the primary (and if you can, secondary) stress marks to the following words (not all words will have secondary stress).
   (a) grasshopper (b) bachelor
   (c) personification (d) indistinguishable
   (e) internationalization (f) relation
   (g) photography (h) program
   (i) incapacitate (j) borderline
   (k) objectivity (l) diplomatic

2. Stress pairs. Some of the following words have stress pairs (one noun/adjective the other verb) with stress on different syllables. Transcribe all the words that have stress pairs (remember, vowel qualities may differ as well as the stress assignment) and show the correct stress with each transcription. Note which member of the pair is a verb, and which a noun/adjective.
   (a) abstract (b) digest
   (c) torment (d) require
   (e) transfer (f) absent
   (g) defend (h) segment
   (i) subject (j) produce

3. Transcribe the strong and weak forms of the following function words.
   (a) would (b) am
   (c) have (d) had
   (e) is (f) must
   (g) to (h) should
   (i) has (j) some (unspecified quantity)

4. Connected speech. The following sentences could all contain examples of assimilations, weak forms, and possibly also elisions in casual speech. Transcribe each sentence using either GA or RP norms showing all possible such features.
   (a) Joan and Cathy wouldn't be walking in this weather.
   (b) She put her handbag on the brown box.
   (c) He walked back to his car to fetch his coat.
   (d) Last month Vicky had a good many customers in the store.
   (e) They couldn't go any faster than they were.
   (f) Fred gulped down seven bottles of beer and a ham sandwich.

Review Questions

1. What does the term *weak forms* refer to? Illustrate your answer with examples in transcription.
2. Describe *elision* in English, giving examples from the various categories of elidable combinations. Use phonemic transcription for all your examples.
3. Illustrate all the possible word stress patterns for four-syllable words. Use examples different from those given in the chapter, and put all examples into phonemic symbols with stress marks for primary and secondary stress.
4. Explain how junctural ambiguities in connected speech may be resolved.

Study Topics and Experiments

1. Describe the variety of possible assimilation types, and note which ones occur in English. Give examples of all possible English juxtapositional assimilation types, using phonemic transcription. What might be an explanation for assimilation?
2. Record 10 minutes of natural connected speech (either from friends or from the radio or television). Briefly describe the sample and the speakers involved. Ignore the first 5 minutes; then take any 3-minute section and listen to this numerous times. Make a list of the weak forms, assimilations, and elisions you hear in this section, and note down each example in transcription. If more than one speaker is involved in the section, note which speaker uses which of these features.

CD

The CD gives examples of stress placement and various connected speech processes. It is important for clinicians to be able to identify these, so you are encouraged to undertake the exercises.

17

Intonation of English

INTRODUCTION

In chapter 9 we briefly introduced the use of pitch as intonation, and in this chapter we will take the topic further, looking at the main units of intonation in English and how they correspond to different syntactic forms and semantic functions. The main purpose of intonation is not simply to avoid sounding monotonous (though, of course, that is at least part of the story). Intonation highlights new and important information. In any utterance there may be quite a lot of material that the listener need not concentrate on fully. This is because some words have purely grammatical functions (the function words we referred to in chap. 16) and so lack full semantic content, and because some information will be already known to the listener. For example, if in reply to the question, "Where are you going?" a speaker replies, "I'm going to town," then the only new (and so important) piece of information in that reply is the word "town." This is because the question already established the other main pieces of information ("you/I" and "going"), and the auxiliary "(a)m" and the preposition "to" are function words not needing to be emphasized. This means that we will wish the listener to concentrate mainly on "town," and we will use an intonation pattern designed to highlight that particular piece of information. In the following sections of this chapter we will show just how this can be done. The broad patterns of intonation that we give are applicable to both GA and RP. Where specific differences do occur, we note this in the text.

Stress, Accent, and Information Structure

The domain of intonation (that is to say, the stretch of speech over which intonation units operate) is called here the *intonation group* (though a number of different terms have been employed, including *word group, breath group,* and *intonational phrase*). We use a neutral term such as this because intonation groups may be very short (e.g., "yes"), or relatively long ("I like that new coat you're wearing") and do not necessarily correlate to syntactic boundaries. The examples given in this chapter will illustrate a range of different length and different types of intonation group, but we can give some idea of the possibilities here. We mark intonation group boundaries in this chapter by slants (/) and use double slants (//) to denote a major boundary coinciding with a pause, end of semantically linked groups, or end of turn.

1. ("Is it raining outside") "Yes //" one-syllable intonation group
2. "That unpleasant-looking old horse in the corner of the field /" multiword group
3a. "My uncle was born in California //" single intonation group
3b. "My uncle, / was born in California //" two intonation groups
4a. "My brother who lives in Pittsburgh / has a new job //" two intonation groups
4b. "My brother, / who lives in Pittsbugh, / has a new job //" three intonation groups

Note that the difference between 3a and 3b is purely one of style, whereas the difference between 4a and 4b reflects different meanings. With 4a the information about Pittsburgh helps us determine which brother is being referred to (i.e., the one in Pittsburgh, not the one in Philadelphia), whereas in 4b the reference to Pittsburgh is just extra information, but not actually needed to identify the correct referent.

As we saw in the previous chapter, syllables can take various levels of stress. We also pointed out that stress is manifested in several ways: extra volume, extra duration, and some kind of pitch prominence. In intonation studies, we normally distinguish *stress* (extra volume/duration only) from *accent* (which has extra pitch prominence as well). Pitch prominence can be realized in several ways. First, there may be a pitch glide on the relevant syllable: that is to say, the pitch of the voice may rise or fall (and sometimes rise and fall, or fall and rise) during the syllable. Alternatively, there may be step up in pitch to and from the accented syllable, or a step down. Often, these steps involve a considerable change in pitch, but sometimes they are only slight.

In the pitch diagrams we employ later in the chapter, we show accented syllables by a filled circle (●), and stressed but not accented syllables by an unfilled circle (○); unstressed syllables are shown by a small filled circle (•). Pitch glides are shown by a rising, falling, or level line leading from the filled circle (●⟍).

Accent is the device we use in English intonation to highlight new over given information. Words that need to be highlighted have their main syllables realized as accented syllables (i.e., with pitch prominence), whereas words expressing given information will have their stressed syllables produced without pitch prominence (i.e., stress without accent). Of course, function words will normally remain unstressed. Attention is thus directed to the new, or highlighted, information through the use of pitch prominence on accented syllables. However, there may be several pieces of new information in any one intonation group. In English, it is the last accented word that is most prominent. The last accented word has the major pitch movement of the group, with pitch gliding on the relevant syllable, or stepping up or down over any unstressed syllables that may follow. We will see below the types of pitch changes we find in these cases.

Accent allows us to identify the major constituents of an intonation group. The stressed syllable of the last accented word is termed the *nucleus* (or in some accounts, the *tonic*). Any syllables that come after the nucleus are called the *tail*, and the behavior of the tail syllables is predictable from the choice of pitch movement for the nucleus. Of course, an intonation group may have accented words preceding the nucleus (though an utterance such as "yes" has a nucleus only). The syllables stretching from the accented syllable of the first accented word up to the nucleus are termed the *head* (or the *pretonic*), and these head syllables tend to be either fairly high and level, or fairly low and level, although some stepping up and stepping down varieties can be used in some circumstances. Finally, any unstressed syllables before the head (or before the nucleus if there is no head) are termed the *prehead* (or *proclitic*).

This gives us an overall structure of (prehead) + (head) + nucleus + (tail) constituting the intonation group. In the following sections we will look at the options for each of these units, and how they can combine with each other, but we can conclude here with some examples of intonation groups of different structure. In these examples, accented syllables are in italics.

5. "*Please* //"			nucleus
6. "*Thank* you //"			nucleus + tail
7. "*Don't* be a *fool* //"		head +	nucleus
8. "*Don't* be *stu*pid //"		head +	nucleus + tail
9. "He's a *fool* //"	pre-head +		nucleus
10. "He's a *stupid* *fool* //"	pre-head +	head +	nucleus
11. "He's *real* *stu*pid //"	pre-head +	head +	nucleus + tail

NUCLEAR TONES AND POSTNUCLEAR PATTERNS

Most nuclear tones involve some kind of pitch movement, as we noted earlier. The two basic pitch movements are rising and falling, but of course the amount of pitch fall or rise is important, as well as the direction. When we describe intonation, however, we normally only need to note amount of pitch change when it has a contrastive function (i.e., telling one type of meaning from another). We know, for example, that over an entire utterance, most speakers' pitch gradually gets lower (this is known as *declination*, because the pitch level declines). That means a pitch rise or fall at the beginning of an utterance might involve quite different absolute values in Hz than at the end. Because this sort of difference is predictable, and not meaningful, we ignore it in this account.

Further, we can all chose to speak in a set *key*, or overall pitch setting, and may use different keys from time to time. If our key is a high one, then any falls may be of a different extent and cover different values in Hz than if our key had been low. Again, we ignore this difference when describing the pitch movements in intonation groups, although we may refer to the speaker's key separately, as it may help illuminate factors such as emotional state or attitude. Emphatic speech may also result in greater pitch movements than nonemphatic speech, but other factors also play a part in emphatic intonation usage, in particular the pitch levels and directions of the various combinations of prenuclear patterns with the nuclear tone in question.

Many dialects of English appear to share basic similarities in the way their intonation is structured. Common, therefore, to most North American and some British English varieties is the use of seven nuclear tones. Three fall types are identified: Low Fall (LF), High Fall (HF), and Rise–Fall (RF); there are also three rises: Low Rise (LR), High Rise (HR), and Fall–Rise (FR); finally there is one nuclear tone where the pitch neither rises nor falls: the Mid–Level (ML). We can illustrate these seven types with the following examples, where we've kept the utterance the same (the word "yes"), but given it seven different nuclear tones relevant to the seven different contexts provided. We also show the diacritics that are used to mark nuclear tones (these are placed immediately before the relevant accented syllable).

12. ("Are you going out tonight?") "ˎYes //"	LF
13. ("Are you *really* going out tonight?") "ˋYes //"	HF
14. ("He said yes to the proposal") "ˆYes //"	RF
15. ("So, have you agreed at last. . . ?") "ˏYes //"	LR
16. ("Well, 'yes' I think is the answer") "ˊYes //"	HR
17. ("Don't you like it?") "ˇYes //"	FR
18. ("Is this the right decision to take?") "˃Yes / (and then again / no //)"	ML

Considering these examples, we can see that (12) demonstrates a typical neutral statement; (13) a more emphatic agreement; (14) expresses surprise; (15) an encouragement to continue; (16) a questioning response requiring reaffirmation; (17) a contrasting response; and (18) a sense of incompleteness, requiring a further utterance. It should be noted, however, that these senses are not the only ones conveyed by these nuclear tones, and neither are these nuclear tones the only ones usable in the contexts given—simply typical usages.

> There are alternative ways of characterizing English intonation. For example, Bolinger in his work recognizes three main pitch movements, A (movement to and from a high fall), B (movement to and from a high rise), and C (movement to and from a low rise), and describes all other pitch types as combinations of these. Therefore, for example, a fall–rise will be AC. Halliday in his work adopts five "primary" tones, which he numbers 1 (falling), 2 (high rising or falling-rising), 3 (low rising), 4 (falling-rising), 5 (rising-falling). Pike treated intonation as a series of pitch levels (numbered 1 to 4), and any pitch movement was deemed to be a series of different pitch levels — from lower to higher, higher to lower, and so forth. See *Background Reading* for references.

The single syllable examples in (12) through (18) cannot illustrate what happens to any syllables following the nucleus: the tail syllables. So we give here expanded versions of our seven utterances, each with a nucleus and tail. We also give each of these an intonation diagram. These diagrams are modeled on musical scores. The upper line represents the top of the speaker's pitch range, and the lower line represents the bottom. All syllables are marked onto the diagram as dots (small filled dots are unstressed syllables, large filled dots are accented syllables, and unfilled dots are stressed but not accented syllables). The location of the dots on the vertical axis denotes their pitch height. Lines leading from large filled dots (looking somewhat like the tails of musical notes) represent any glide in pitch height that is accomplished during the production of the syllable in question. If successive dots are of different levels with no glide marks, this represents stepping up or down between the syllables. We will use these *stave* diagrams for longer utterances later in the chapter.

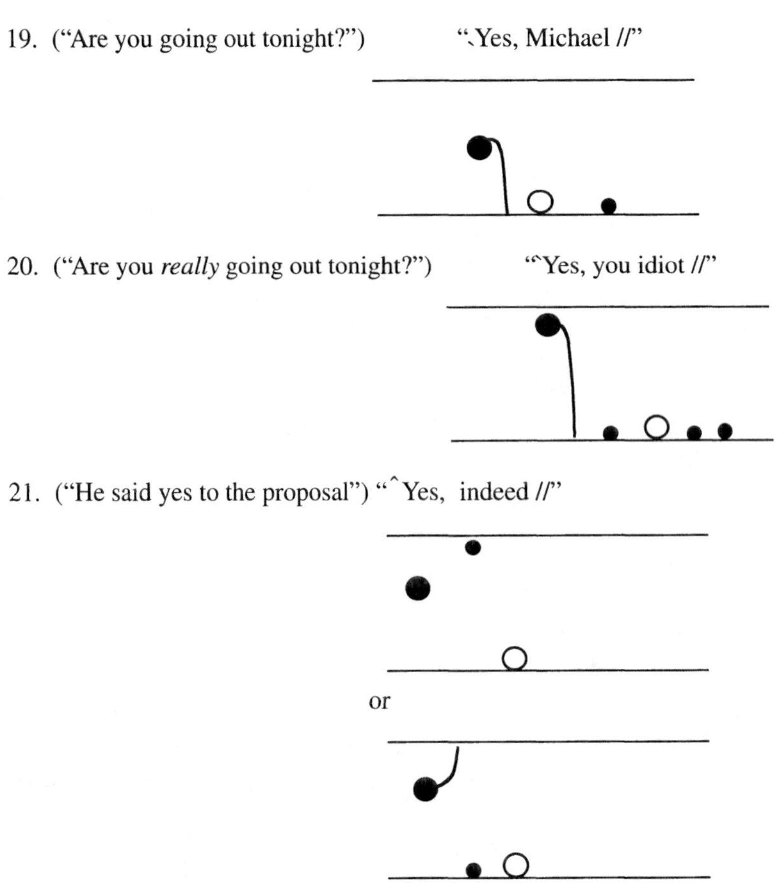

19. ("Are you going out tonight?") "ˎYes, Michael //"
20. ("Are you *really* going out tonight?") "ˋYes, you idiot //"
21. ("He said yes to the proposal") "ˆYes, indeed //"
or

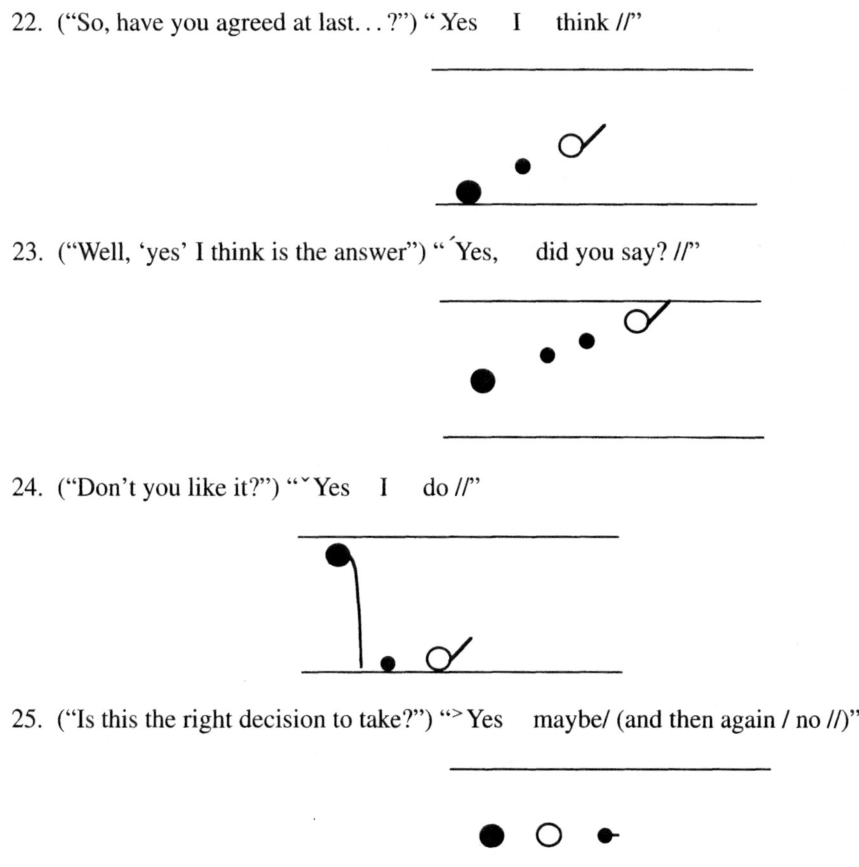

22. ("So, have you agreed at last. . . ?") "ˏYes I think //"
23. ("Well, 'yes' I think is the answer") "ˊYes, did you say? //"
24. ("Don't you like it?") "ˇYes I do //"
25. ("Is this the right decision to take?") ">Yes maybe/ (and then again / no //)"

From these diagrams it becomes clear that tail syllables after falling nuclear tones remain low in pitch, whereas with rising nuclear tones the tail syllables continue to step up in pitch one by one after the nucleus. The exceptional pattern is the fall–rise, where the fall takes place on the nucleus, but the rise is postponed until the end of the tail. Some phoneticians (such as O'Connor and Arnold) distinguish the fall–rise from a similar "compound tune" of a fall followed by a rise. They note that there are several ways of distinguishing these two tunes. If there is a head preceding the nucleus, the fall–rise will always have a falling head, and the fall plus rise will always have the high head (see the next section for a description of head types). If the nucleus is followed by a tail with no stressed syllables in it, then the tune is a fall–rise, as fall plus rise always needs a stressed tail syllable to host the rise. If there is no tail at all, then the pattern is fall–rise (the fall plus rise always needs to operate over different syllables). A problem arises when there is no head, and when the tail has stressed and unstressed syllables. In these circumstances, both a fall–rise and a fall plus rise will see the fall on the nucleus and the rise on the final stressed syllable of the tail. In such cases the difference between the two patterns is signalled by a greater fall in the fall plus rise pattern, and by the fact that in this pattern all the syllables of the tail stay very low until the rise occurs, unlike with the fall–rise where the tail syllables may well climb slightly between the fall part and the rise part. O'Connor and Arnold justify making this distinction due to the meaning differences signaled by these patterns. Examples (26) and (27) illustrate the difference between these two patterns.

26. "↘Jonathan and ˇJack were born in Kansas //" Fall–Rise

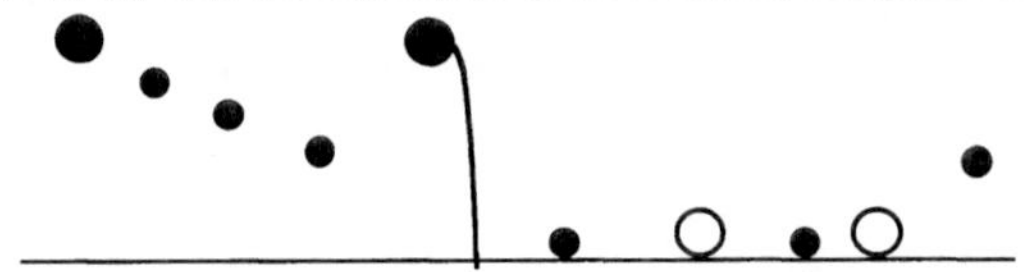

27. "ˈJonathan and ˋJack were born in ˏKansas //" Fall plus Rise

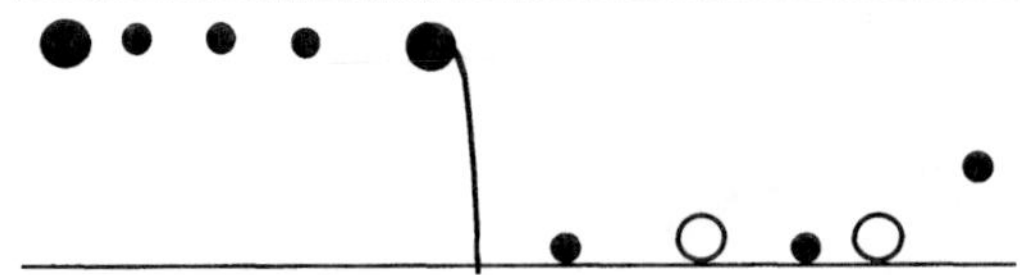

> Different ways of diagramming intonation are also found in the literature. Bolinger, for example, types his syllables on different levels to show their pitch movements,
>
> Y
> e o
> s I d
>
> for the fall-rise on "Yes I do."
>
> Many publications on American English intonation draw lines through the text to show pitch movements (though these lines cannot show pitch steps as opposed to glides, and often are not very accurate at portraying different pitch heights):
>
> Yes I do
>
> We feel that the stave model is clearer than these other approaches.

PRENUCLEAR PATTERNS

As we noted earlier, all syllables before the nucleus are grouped into two possible units: the head (from the first accented syllable up to the nucleus) and the prehead (any syllables before the first accented syllable). Clearly, if there is only one accented word, this contains the nucleus and there is no head.

Head Patterns

We recognize four head types. The most common head pattern is the *high head*, where all the syllables are fairly high. They are not, however, right at the top of the speaker's range, so there is a slight stepping up from head syllables to the beginning of a high fall nuclear tone. It is possibly this slight step up before high falls that has been interpreted in some text-books as a rise–fall pattern in statements in English. This interpretation is clearly erroneous; rise–fall nuclear tones are actually comparatively rare, and when they do occur the rise is on the nucleus, not before, as shown in these texts. Such a stepping up does not occur, of course, when the high head is used before a low fall (the other common statement nuclear tone), so the characterization of statements as having a rising–falling overall pattern seems even less accurate here. It is possible that a slightly lower variant of the high head is used before low falls by some speakers giving the impression of rising to reach the accented syllable of the subsequent fall. The high head can occur before all nuclear tones with the exception of the fall–rise. We illustrate the high head in various combinations in the following examples. (We give stave diagrams for only some of the examples from now on.)

28. ˈMake her get you a ˋnew one // HH+HF

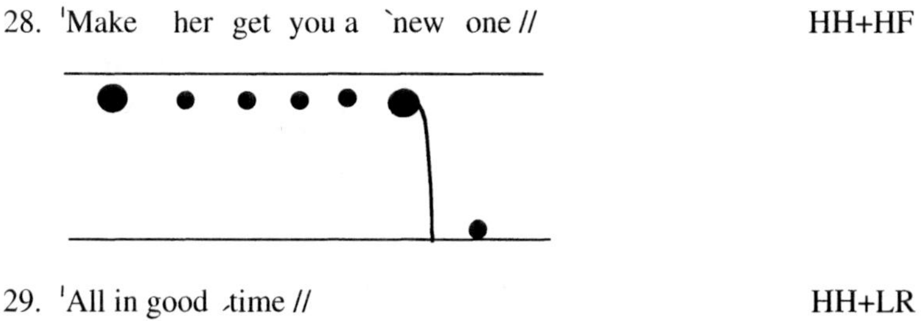

29. ˈAll in good ˏtime // HH+LR
30. ˈWelcome back to New ˎOrleans! // HH+LF

The *low head* contains syllables that are all at the bottom of the speaker's range. This is found only before the low rise nuclear tone, as in the following example. As the low head is not found before any falls, it cannot be appealed to to account for the rising-falling claims mentioned above.

31. ˌWhich do ˏyou prefer, then? // LH+LR

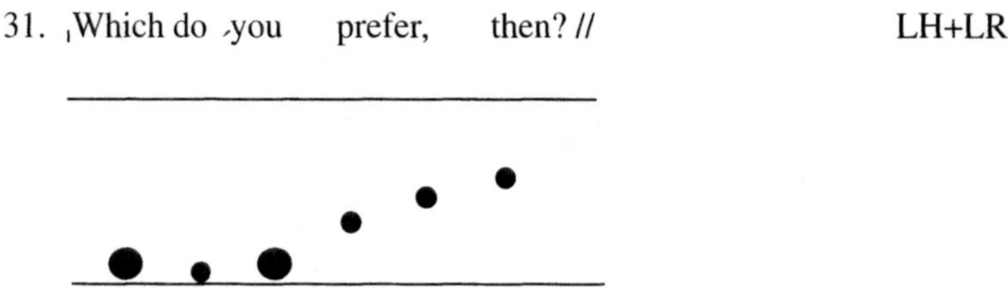

The *falling head*, as the name implies, has syllables that start relatively high and step down one by one to a comparatively low pitch level. This head is found only before the fall–rise nuclear tone, and the last syllable of the head is always somewhat lower than the accented syllable of the nucleus. The following example utterance illustrates this point.

32. ↘Quarter past ˇfour it was // FH+FR

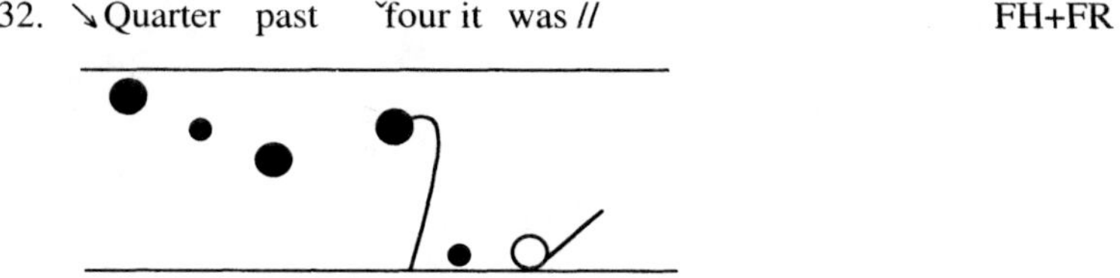

The final head type is the *rising head.* In this head, the first syllable is low and subsequent syllables step up toward the top of the pitch range. This head type is found only before the high fall nuclear tone, and the final syllable of the head is always slightly lower than the accented syllable of the nucleus. The following diagram illustrates the use of this head.

33. ↗How on earth did you manage to ˋeat that? // RH+HF

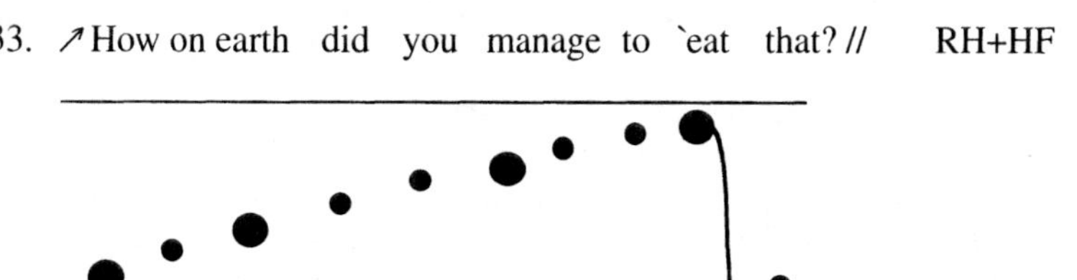

The symbols we use for heads are as follows:

ˈHigh Head:	ˈLots of them don't really ˆknow //	HH+RF
ˌLow Head:	ˌNot if they don't ˏneed to //	LH+LR
↘Falling Head:	↘Everybody's going to go there ˇsometime //	FH+FR
↗Rising Head:	↗Why did you decide to do ˋthat? //	RH+HF

To mark the emphatic heads, the relevant diacritics are repeated for each stressed syllable in the head:

Stepping Head:	I ˈreally ˈdon't know ˈwhere he ˎis //	StH+LF
Sliding Head:	He ↘can't ↘expect her to ↘do his ˇwork //	SlH+FR
Climbing Head:	He ↗never ↗really ↗gives us a ˋthing! //	CH+HF

There are also emphatic versions of the high head, the falling head, and the rising head. To add emphasis when using a high head, each stressed syllable of the high head can be lowered slightly in pitch compared to the previous stressed syllables (any unstressed syllables remain on the same level as the previous stressed syllable). This gives the impression of stepping downward and, indeed, this head is called the *stepping head.*

To add emphasis to a falling head a series of short falls is used, each series starting on a stressed syllable with the following unstressed syllables falling one after another. This is termed the *sliding head.* The converse occurs when we add emphasis to a rising head: a series of short rises is used, each series starting on a stressed syllable with the following unstressed syllables rising one after another. This is called the *climbing head.* All three of these emphatic heads are illustrated in the following examples.

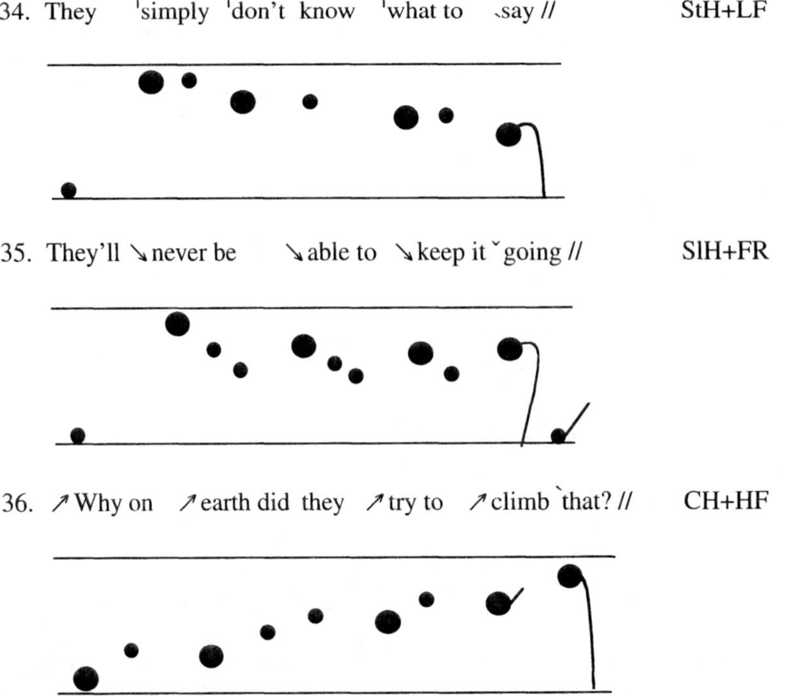

34. They ˈsimply ˈdon't know ˈwhat to ˎsay // StH+LF
35. They'll ↘never be ↘able to ↘keep it ˇgoing // SlH+FR
36. ↗Why on ↗earth did they ↗try to ↗climb ˋthat? // CH+HF

Prehead Patterns

There are only two prehead patterns: the *low prehead*, and the *high prehead*. The low prehead is the commonest and can occur before all the head types and, if there is no head, can occur directly before all the nuclear tones described earlier. The syllables in the low prehead are all comparatively low in pitch, and if followed by a rise they are fully low. The following examples show the low prehead before a variety of head patterns and nuclear tones.

37. I was at ˋhome // LPH+HF
38. Did you ˊmeet them? // LPH+HR
39. The writing is ↘reasonably ˇneat // LPH+FH+FR
40. It was a ˈperfectly clear ˎday // LPH+HH+LF

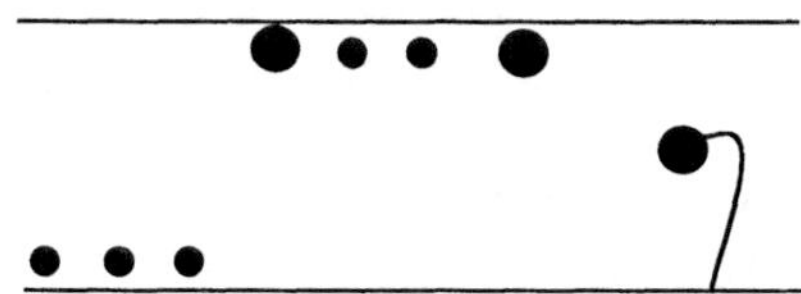

> In the system of diacritics used in this book, low preheads are unmarked (i.e., any syllables before a head diacritic that have no diacritic of their own are deemed to constitute a low prehead). A high prehead is marked with a horizontal line:
>
> | | | |
> |---|---|---|
> | Low prehead: | I was at ˋhome | LPH + HF |
> | High prehead: | ˉYou ˋwouldn't! | HPH + HF |

The high prehead is found less often than the low one, and its use often expresses more emphasis. The syllables in the high prehead are all relatively high, and before a high fall they are at the same pitch height as the beginning of the fall. Some combinations of the high prehead with different head types and nuclear tones are shown in the following examples.

41. ˉI said ˈno such ˎthing // HPH+HH+LF
42. ˉIt's got ˌnothing to do with ˏthem // HPH+LH+LR
43. ˉNo matter ˈwhat she >says /. . . // HPH+HH+ML
44. ˉThey ˈdon't really ˋlike it // HPH+HH+HF

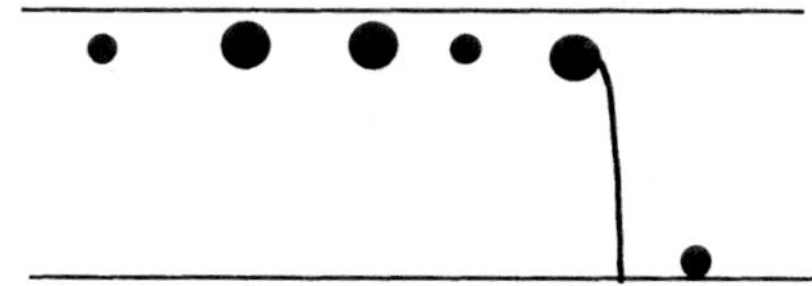

INTONATION TUNES

As we saw earlier, an intonation group can consist (as a maximum) of a prehead, head, nucleus, and tail. At first sight, therefore, it might appear that a vast number of possible combinations between these elements is possible. We should recall, however, that certain of the head patterns were restricted to certain nuclear tones, and that tail syllables are always predictable from the choice of nuclear tone. It turns out that there are relatively few *intonation tunes* (that is, the entire pattern of intonation units stretching over the intonation group). In this section we describe 10 different tunes, and note that any one of these tunes may consist of a nucleus alone, a nucleus plus a tail, or either of these types with head and/or prehead units. These tunes are all found with a variety of utterance types (statement, question, command) and in both nonemphatic and emphatic varieties. The tunes are the meaning-bearing units of intonation. Although we can associate meanings with the seven nuclear tones, it seems to be easier to do this with the 10 tunes, as they take into account different head+nucleus combinations, differences due to emphasis, and the compound fall plus rise pattern referred to earlier.

We will sketch these 10 tunes out briefly in this section and note some of the basic meanings often associated with them. For a more detailed account of meaning in intonation, the reader is referred to the background reading section at the end of the chapter. The examples are shown with diacritics but no stave diagrams. The terms *statements*, *questions*, and *commands* refer to syntactic form (i.e., a statement with a rising intonation may be meant semantically as a question, or at least may be so interpreted).

Tune 1: Low Fall Ending. This tune has the following constituents: an optional low prehead, an optional high head, and a low fall nuclear tone. When it is emphatic, a high prehead may be used, or a stepping head. Statements used with this tune sound definite and complete, whereas questions sound urgent, and commands serious. Examples are in (30) and (40) among others.

Tune 2: High Fall Ending. This tune has an optional low prehead, an optional high head, and a high fall nuclear tone. When it is emphatic a high prehead can be used, and a stepping head may be employed. Statements said with this tune sound definite and complete but also involved and not too serious. Questions sound businesslike but not urgent, and commands act like suggestions rather than orders. Examples include (28) and (44).

Tune 3: Low Rise Ending. This tune contains an optional low prehead, and an optional low head followed by a low rise. When it is emphatic there are a high prehead, a low head, and a low rise. Statements invite further comment from the listener and may give the impression of grumbling, whereas wh-questions sound wondering, and yes–no questions show disapproval and skepticism. Commands are rarely used with this tune, and express an appeal to the listener. Examples are in (22) and (31).

Tune 4: High Low Rise Ending. The constituents of this tune are an optional low prehead followed by a compulsory high head and a low rise, or a compulsory high prehead followed by a low rise. The emphatic pattern is a high prehead plus a high head plus a low rise, or a stepping head plus a low rise with an optional prehead. Statements with this tune sound reassuring, while questions suggest genuine interest. Commands may seem encouraging or maybe patronizing. An example of this tune is given in (29).

Tune 5: Fall–Rise Ending. This tune has an optional low prehead, an optional falling head, and a fall–rise nuclear tone. The emphatic form uses a high prehead and/or a sliding head. Statements with this tune express contrast, questions express astonishment, and commands express urgent warning. Examples are found in (24), (26), and (32).

Tune 6: Rising High Fall Ending. As the name suggests, this tune has a compulsory rising head followed by a high fall nuclear tone, with an optional low prehead. In emphasis a high prehead is employed, or the head is changed to a climbing head. Statements express definiteness and involvement and sometimes also protest. Questions also show protest, whereas commands are recommendations, possibly also with surprise and criticism. See the examples in (33) and (36).

Tune 7: High Rise Ending. The pattern here is an optional low prehead and an optional high head followed by the high rise nucleus. Emphatic patterns use either a high prehead or a stepping head. Statements with this tune often are interpreted as questions, or nonfinally suggest continuation. Commands also sound like questions, whereas questions said on this tune may sometimes be "echo" questions, repeating the other speaker's words, although many speakers use this tune as their standard one for questions. Examples can be found in (23) and (38).

Tune 8: Rise–Fall Ending. The structure of this tune is an optional low prehead, an optional high head, and a rise–fall, with a high prehead or a stepping head used when emphatic. Statements sound definite, with the speaker being impressed; yes–no questions also sound impressed, but wh-questions sound antagonistic. Commands give an impression of lack of involvement. An example of tune 8 is given in (21).

Tune 9: Fall plus Rise Compound Tune. This compound tune has a high fall preceded by an optional low prehead and high head, with a low rise on the final stressed syllable. When emphatic, this tune employs a high prehead or a stepping head. In statements, this tune points out two important ideas, one toward the beginning and a subsidiary one toward the end; it gives an impression of definiteness without reservations. This tune is rare with questions, but with commands it has an effect of pleading. The tune is illustrated in (27).

Tune 10: Mid-Level Ending. The mid-level nuclear tone is preceded by an optional low prehead and an optional high head, with a high prehead or stepping head employed to show emphasis. It expresses nonfinality for all utterance types and is normally only employed when another intonation group follows, in which the nonfinality can be resolved by the speaker. Often, however, speakers may be interrupted after this tune (especially if they pause to search for words to finish their initial thoughts), so this tune may be utterance-final in such circumstances. Examples are in (25) and (43).

> In many English-speaking areas various sorts of rises have recently become popular with statements. This feature (often characteristic of younger speakers) may make statements sound less secure, but the use of these rises should not be considered disordered prosody.

The description of the meanings associated with particular tunes requires much more detail than we are able to provide here, but the outline given in this section does provide a starting point for further investigation of the background readings.

BACKGROUND READING

An excellent survey of intonation is found in Cruttenden (1986). A more detailed exposition of the model presented here can also be found in O'Connor and Arnold (1973), whereas Halliday's alternative approach is outlined in Halliday (1970). The classic text on American English is Pike (1945); also important are Bolinger (1986, 1989), although these authors adopt approaches different from that taken here.

EXERCISES

Transcription

(Answers to the transcription exercises are given at the end of the book.)

1. Draw stave diagrams for the following intonation groups, using the diacritics to guide you. (In these examples, accented syllables that neither start a head nor are a nucleus are marked with •; stressed, but unaccented, syllables are marked with ○). State which tune is being used.

(a) I ˎloathe •driving at ˏnight //
(b) ˈNo one •heard the ˋslightest •noise //
(c) How ↗ absolutely ˋterrible! //
(d) It's ↘ nothing to be ˇproud ∘ of //
(e) ˈNow don't disˏcourage him //

2. Add the correct diacritics to the following intonation groups, using the stave diagrams to help you. State which tune is being used.
   (a) Who does he need to speak to? //

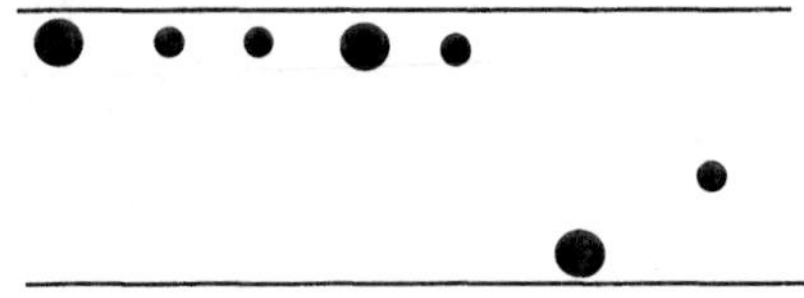

   (b) I've never seen anything like them //

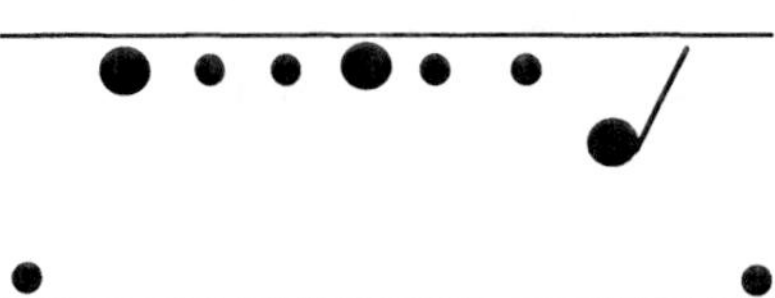

   (c) I'm only too happy to do it //

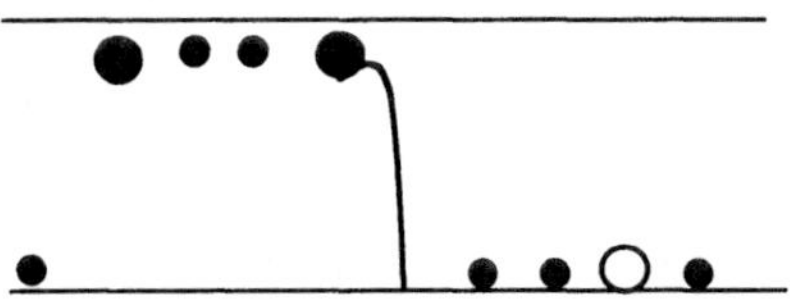

   (d) Somewhere in Oregon would be nice this year //

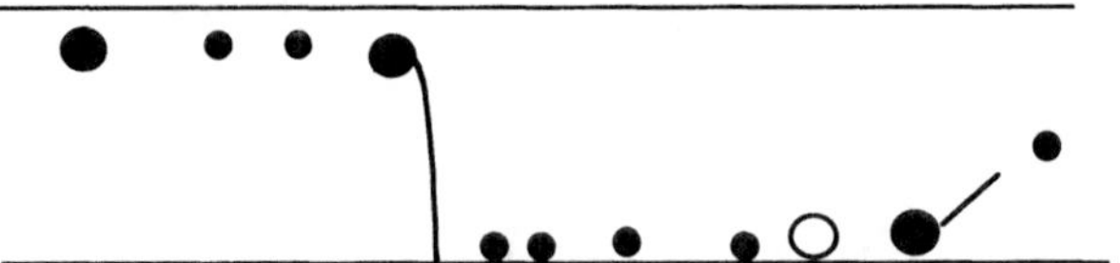

   (e) Well give him a dollar / (and send him off to the mall) //

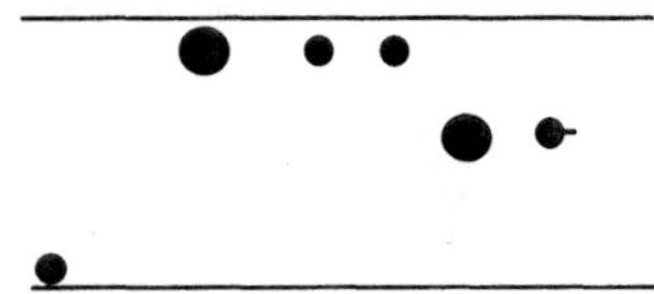

Review Questions

1. What is the difference between *accent* and *stress* when used in intonation studies?
2. How could we define the *nucleus* in intonation?
3. What are the seven nuclear tones of English?
4. What are the prenuclear patterns of English, and where are their boundaries?
5. In what ways can a nonemphatic tune be made emphatic?

Study Topics and Experiments

1. Devise one utterance each for the 10 tunes listed in this chapter. Make sure the utterance sounds natural for the tune chosen. Record yourself speaking the utterances using the tunes you chose. Get a colleague to listen to your recording and to give judgments as to how accurate you were and how naturalistic your utterances sound. Then you do the listening for your colleague's choices.
2. Working in pairs, record some natural speech, or some speech off the radio or television. Take just a few minutes of the recording and transcribe the utterances using ordinary writing. Then each of you separately should attempt to annotate these with intonation diacritics. Compare your transcriptions with your colleague and see what features you disagree on, and what features you agree on. Was there a pattern to the disagreements?

CD

Listen to the examples of different intonation units, and see if you can identify the test examples following the instructions on the CD. Answers to all the exercises on the CD are given at the end of the book.

18

Varieties of English

INTRODUCTION

So far, in this part of the book, we have been describing the phonology and phonetics of General American English (GA) and Received Pronunciation (RP). We all know, of course, that in terms of pronunciation there are many different varieties of English. Some of these varieties are geographically based, some are linked to particular social groupings, and others to the ethnic background of the speaker, and of course all these factors may interact.

Looking at the geographical spread of English, we can start by considering the major national territories that have English as the majority language (or one of several). These include the United States, Canada, Great Britain, Ireland, Australia, New Zealand, and many Caribbean countries, all of which have English as the mother tongue of many of the inhabitants, and the second language of many immigrants. In addition, there are a large number of countries where English is an official language even if not the mother tongue of a majority (e.g., South Africa, Ghana, and Nigeria). For example, there are distinctive national varieties of English in India, Singapore, countries in West and East Africa, the Hong Kong Special Administrative Area of China, and many countries in the Pacific.

Within any one country, of course, there are typically also regional varieties. We all know that a speaker from Georgia is likely to sound different from a speaker from New York, who in turn may differ from a Californian. The speech of a Londoner differs in many respects from that of a Liverpudlian, which in turn will differ from that of a Glaswegian speaker in Scotland. However, the study of regional differences in language does not stop at units the size of a state, or even a city. Dialectologists have come to realize that differences (although often slight differences) exist between neighboring villages, or boroughs, and even between streets in the same neighborhood. In fact, because we all have our own way of speaking (or to be precise our own repertoire of speech styles), it is not actually possible to specify the smallest unit of interest for those that study language variation. Individual speakers, therefore, can be the subject of study and, because we all have our range of styles from formal to casual, a speaker's idiolect can be quite a complex set of varieties. Nevertheless, workable units (of varying sizes) have been proposed to account for broad geographical tendencies in English in North America (and of course in other English-speaking countries as well). We return to these later in the chapter.

Some notes on terms:

variety: a nonspecific term referring to any variant of a language
accent: a variety with specific pronunciation patterns
dialect: a variety with specific grammatical, lexical, and pronunciation patterns
standard: a variety officially recognized for a geographical/national area; often a variety not linked to any one region
vernacular: a nonstandard variety linked to a region or socioeconomic group (or both)
idiolect: repertoire of styles used by a specified individual
interference: influence of a speaker's first language on his or her second language, or the other way around

We noted above that factors other than geographical distribution are also important in accounting for language variation. Studies of social class and language suggest that working class speakers retain more localized language features than upper class speakers; that women have a tendency to use more nonregional features than men; that certain speech characteristics are likely to differ between younger and older speakers; and that the ethnic background of a speaker may be linked to a particular variety of a language. Finally we must recognize that speakers of English as a second language may demonstrate pronunciation patterns that differ from those of standard English, and may derive from the phonological and phonetic patterns of their first languages. Speech language pathologists need to be aware of these factors influencing pronunciation; they need to distinguish between pronunciation patterns due to a speech disorder of some type, and those that derive from one of the factors noted earlier: region, class, ethnic background, and so on.

WAYS IN WHICH ACCENTS CAN DIFFER

Before we can look at specific varieties of English and how they compare to the patterns outlined for GA in the preceding chapters, we need to know the different ways in which pronunciation varieties (i.e., accents) can differ from each other. These differences can operate at the phonemic level and at the allophonic level, and at the system level and at the structure level.

Systemic Differences

Differences between phonological systems are seen when one accent has more (or fewer) phonemic units than the other. For example, some New England varieties have an extra low back rounded vowel (/ɒ/ as in "hot") not found in GA, and this same vowel is also found in British English. The dental fricatives /θ, ð/ may be missing in African American English and in the local variety of London, England (though for both varieties they may be used in formal styles). Finally, we can note that nonrhotic accents of English (found in many regions) often have three or four extra diphthongs compared to rhotic accents (see more later in this chapter).

Structural Differences

Accents can also differ in terms of their structure. We use this category to refer only to syllable structure (the overall syllable shape, including the number of consonants found in clusters). Examples can be found in southern U.S. varieties, where the simplification of final clusters may be found even in slow, careful speech (see chap. 16 for a discussion of elision in clusters in fast connected speech), and African American English, where open syllables are often preferred over syllables closed by a consonant or a cluster of consonants.

Realizational Differences

Two accents may share exactly the same system of phonemes, and exactly the same structural properties, but still sound different. This is because the way in which the phonemes are *realized* (that is to say, their precise pronunciation and allophonic patterning) may differ. This category of differences is often very large between accents of English, and we will point to only a few examples. In Southern Hemisphere English (e.g., Australia, New Zealand, South Africa) the realization of the front vowels differs from that of GA, even though the same number of vowel phonemes are employed. Thus, there is a general shift of the vowels upward, such that South African /æ/ sounds like GA /ɛ/, and so forth. In Irish English, /θ, ð/ are often realized as [t̪, d̪], and final /t/ may be realized as an alveolar slit fricative. Finally, we can note the so-called northern cities chain shift in an area from western New England to the northern Midwest, where the values of a whole range of vowels have been shifted (this is discussed further below).

> There are relatively few systemic differences between English varieties; the bulk of the differences we find are realizational, and affect vowels more than consonants.

Distributional Differences

Accents can also differ in terms of their phonotactics (for example, the specific consonants allowed in a cluster or in a syllable position). A variety of phonotactic differences have been described in different accents of English. These include the exclusion of /s/ from initial clusters when followed by /tɹ/, and its replacement by /ʃ/ (such that /stɹ-/ becomes /ʃtɹ-/), in the speech of younger people throughout the English-speaking world, and the disappearance of /ɹ/ in postvocalic position in many varieties including African American English, US southern English, and Australian, among others. Another commonly cited example is the choice of /æ/ versus /ɑ/ before voiceless fricatives and nasal–consonant clusters (i.e., in words such as "bath," "laugh," "pass," "dance," "aunt"). In GA the former vowel is used, but in parts of New England and the Atlantic coast the latter is favored. Interestingly this same distinction is found in England, where southern varieties use /ɑ/ and northern /æ/ (though in this variety /æ/ is a lower vowel, closer to [a]—a realizational difference as well).

Selectional Differences

Selectional differences are nonpredictable phoneme choices in specific words. The example we gave under distributional differences of the /æ/—/ɑ/ choice was predictable, in that it occurs in all words of the specific structure noted. With selectional differences, on the other hand, some words will have a different choice of phoneme but other, phonologically similar words, will not. For example, the word "catch" may in several areas be pronounced as /kɛtʃ/, and the word "get" as /gɪt/, even though other /æ/ and /ɛ/ vowels are unaffected in similar words such as "scratch" and "bet."

> Differences affect suprasegmental as well as segmental aspects of speech. This is particularly noticeable in English spoken by those with other languages as their mother tongues; however accurate they are segmentally, aspects of the rhythm and intonation systems of their first language often persist when they speak English.

NATIONAL VARIETIES OF ENGLISH

We only have space here for very brief sketches of the phonological characteristics of national varieties of English outside the United States. Readers should consult the relevant texts listed in the *Background Reading* section for fuller details.

English in the Americas

English is one of the official languages of Canada, and is the official language of many of the Caribbean islands, including Jamaica, Trinidad and Tobago, Barbados, the Bahamas, and islands in the Windward and Leeward groups, Guyana on the mainland of South America, and Belize on the mainland of Central America.

Canadian English is similar in many respects to General American; there are, however, some realizational, distributional, and selectional differences. The most salient of these is called *Canadian raising* and refers to the realization of the diphthongs /eɪ/ and /oʊ/ when these sounds are followed by a fortis consonant. In these circumstances the diphthongs are realized as [ɐi] and [ʌʊ], respectively. This feature has spread to some states bordering Canada, especially in the northeast of the United States of America. Examples include "write" ~ "ride" ([ɹɐit] ~ [ɹaɪd]) and "out" ~ "loud" ([ʌʊt] ~ [laʊd]). We can also note that in Canadian English the usual realization of /l/ is dark in all positions.

Distributional differences include the retention of /j/ before high back vowels after alveolars by many Canadians. Thus, "tune," "due," and "news" may be pronounced /tjun/, /dju/, and /njuz/. Selectional differences include the retention of British English versions of many lexical items (though younger speakers may prefer American English pronunciations). So "lever" may be /ˈlivɚ/ rather than /ˈlɛvɚ/, "schedule" may be /ˈʃɛdjul/ rather than /ˈskɛdjul/, and the letter "z" is still more commonly called /zɛd/ rather than /zi/.

> The dialect of Newfoundland varies considerably from general Canadian speech, with differences in the vowel system (e.g., merger of several vowels) and the consonant system (e.g., loss of dental fricatives). Readers should consult Wells (1982) for full details.

Caribbean English differs considerably from country to country. For example, whereas the English of Barbados is fully rhotic, the accents of Trinidad, the Bahamas, and the islands of the Leeward and Windward group are nonrhotic. Those of Jamaica and Guyana are partly rhotic. Most of Caribbean English is British-based, although American-based English is used in the US Virgin Islands. There are some general characteristics, however. First, there is the loss of the dental fricatives and their replacement by alveolar stops, although in formal styles many speakers do produce the fricatives. Second, we can consider the simplification of final clusters which occurs in those cases where an obstruent is followed by /t/ or /d/. This means that a word such as "last" will normally be pronounced as /laːs/, but a word like "lamp" has the final cluster retained. Unlike the Canadian /l/, /l/ in West Indian accents tends to be clear in all positions. Many realizational differences are found with the vowels in the different countries, but all the varieties resist the weakening of vowels in unstressed syllables common in other accents of English. Full vowels are therefore used (with the value of the vowel often predictable from the spelling), and West Indian rhythm sounds more even as a result. Stress and intonation patterns differ from country to country and generally from other forms of English as well.

> Not all the Caribbean islands have English as a first language, even if it is the official language. St. Lucia and Dominica, for example, have a French-based creole as the first language of most speakers. Conversely, many people in Surinam speak English-based creoles even though the official language is Dutch.

English in Europe

England has a large number of different regional varieties, and we can only touch on some of the major divisions here. These varieties mostly have an extra vowel compared to GA: the vowel /ɒ/, found in words such as "hot" and "cod." In terms of distributional differences, England has rhotic accents in the southwest and in a small area of the northwest near Manchester. The speech of older residents in the west and in counties bordering Wales may also be rhotic. A systemic difference is found in northern accents that lack the vowel /ʌ/, using /ʊ/ instead. A further distributional difference occurs with /æ/ and /ɑ/: northern varieties use /æ/ before fortis fricatives and nasals (e.g., in "laugh," "path," "dance"), whereas southern varieties use /ɑ/. Interestingly, midland accents share the northern loss of /ʌ/, but have the southern distribution of /æ/ and /ɑ/. In the north of England /æ/ is realized as a lower vowel than in the south (or in the United States), closer to cardinal vowel 4 [a].

> The standard accent in England is usually termed *RP*, standing for *received pronunciation.* We can interpret this term today as meaning the pronunciation received from those with no noticeable regional accent. Most Scottish and Irish speakers, however, look toward their own national standards as prestige forms of speech, rather than to RP.

Other features often noted are the loss of /h/ and the replacement of the dental fricatives by /t, d/ or /f, v/ in London English, and yod-deletion in East Anglia. This last leads to the pronunciation of "music," for example, as /ˈmuzɪk/. Both these areas make wide use of the glottal stop for noninitial /t/.

The pronunciation of English in Wales is affected by the phonology of the Welsh language, still spoken by over 20% of the population. This is perhaps most noticeable in intonation, which differs from that of RP. Although Welsh has a trilled-r, Welsh English uses the approximant-r, but is nonrhotic in postvocalic position. Welsh English /eɪ/ and /oʊ/ tend to be realized as monophthongs [e] and [o]. Northern Welsh English often uses no /z/, replacing it with /s/ (giving /ɪs/ for "is"). Welsh English is less likely than other accents of English to weaken unstressed syllables. Southern Welsh varieties have a generally palatalized voice quality (for example, /l/ is always clear), whereas northern ones have a pharyngealized quality (/l/ is always dark).

Scottish English is noted for its simplified vowel system compared to most other varieties. For example, there is no opposition between /ʊ/ and /u/ (both realized as [ʉ]), or often between /æ/ and /ɑ/ (both realized as [a]), and /eɪ/ and /oʊ/ are realized as monophthongs [e] and [o]. Scottish English is rhotic and has a trilled- or tapped-r in initial and medial position and a tapped- or approximant-r in postvocalic position. Some Scottish accents retain a palatal/velar fricative in words spelled with "gh" or "ch" (e.g., "eight" /ɛçt/, "loch" /lɔx/).

There are many distributional differences between Scottish English and other accents; e.g., "house" may be pronounced as /hus/. However, we need to note that many different accents exist in Scotland, with highland accents influenced by Scottish Gaelic (with over 70,000 speakers), and lowland accents reflecting earlier forms of English. For example, lowland accents often show very little aspiration in initial /p, t, k/, whereas highland accents show a great deal of aspiration.

Irish English (or Hiberno-English) consists of northern varieties that share many of the characteristics of lowland Scottish English, and southern varieties that do not share Scottish features (although both areas are rhotic, with approximant-r usage). Southern Irish English has a vowel system similar to that of the English of England, except that the diphthongs /aɪ/ and /ɔɪ/ merge into an intermediate form for many speakers. One of the most noticeable features is the realization of /θ, ð/ as dental plosives [t̪, d̪]. Further, intervocalically following a stressed syllable, noninitial /t/ is realized as an alveolar slit fricative (a retracted [θ̠]), and this is one of the most salient features of southern Irish English. Finally, we can note that both Scottish and Irish English tend to preserve the distinction between /w/ and /hw/ in pairs of words such as "witch" and "which."

> The first official language of the Republic of Ireland is Irish (a Celtic language), but this is only spoken as a first language by a relatively small number of people. The officially recognized areas of first language Irish are in the west of the country, and the accents of English used there reflect the influence of Irish.

Southern Hemisphere English

The forms of English spoken in South Africa, Australia, and New Zealand share some interesting characteristics, although of course they also have many individual features. South African English, for example, has a monophthong /a/ in place of the diphthong /aɪ/; Australian English is well known for its realizations of /aʊ/ and /oʊ/ ([æo] and [ʌʉ]); and New Zealand is characterized through the retention of the /w/ ~ /hw/ distinction (at least among older speakers).

> South Africa has 11 official languages, and many English speakers have another language as their mother tongue. These speakers therefore may show interference from their first language in their use of English. Apart from English, the following languages are recognized: Afrikaans, Ndebele, Northern Sotho, Sotho, Swati, Tsonga, Tswana, Venda, Xhosa, and Zulu.

Among the aspects shared by the three regions is a general raising of the front vowels. The result is that /æ/ sounds like GA /ɛ/, and /ɛ/ sounds like GA /ɪ/. In South Africa /ɪ/ in some contexts is realized as similar to /ʌ/, whereas in New Zealand it is moved to an [ɨ] or [ə] position. A second feature common to these varieties is the use of a high rising nuclear tone (often following a high head) in statements. Thus, a statement such as "I live in Melbourne" may have the intonation pattern "I ˈlive in Meľbourne" (see chap. 17 for the use of the diacritics), which can sound like a question rather than a statement to American and British listeners. High rising statement forms do, however, appear to be spreading in other English accents, as well.

REGIONAL DIFFERENCES IN AMERICAN ENGLISH

There are several different ways we can divide a map of the United States to show regional variation. The number and placement of such divisions depends on how detailed we wish to be in our analysis, of course. Even if we restrict ourselves to major divisions only, we have to remember that some varieties derive from the social or ethnic background of the speaker, rather than the geographical region. In this section we will look at two regions only, the northeast and the south (as these are the two areas most divergent from GA), but will also discuss aspects of African American English (AAE).

The Northeast

The area under consideration here is the eastern part of New England, centered on Boston. The vowel system of this accent shows systemic, distributional, and realizational differences from that of GA. First, many speakers of this variety have an additional centralized rounded vowel (/ɵ/) that contrasts with /oʊ/ in various words (there is no set patterns to which words have this vowel). For example, "rode" ~ "road" (/ɹoʊd/ ~ /ɹɵd/); and other words having /ɵ/ include "home," "smoke," "yolk," "toad," "folks," and "bone." Some speakers also have a distinction between /ɒ/ and /ɔ/, for example in "cot" versus "caught" (/kɒt/ ~ /kɔt/).

The major distributional differences include the use of a long /ɑ/ in words such as "path," "ask," and "dance"; the use of front /æ/ (with or without a pronounced /ɹ/) rather than /ɛ/ before <r> in words such as "bear" and "parents"; and the use of /ɪ/ rather than schwa in the final syllables of words such as "hunted," "waited," and "horses." We can also note a tendency to use /ʊ/ rather than /u/ in words such as "broom," "room," and "roof," and the preference for /ʌɹ/ rather than /ɝ/ in words such as "hurry." Speakers in this area also usually prefer the /ɔ/ phoneme rather than /ɑ/ in words such as "law," "call," and "caught."

The realization of many of the vowels differs from GA, also. Although /eɪ/ is usually diphthongal, /oʊ/ is more often not (so [o]); long /ɑ/ is normally very front ([a]); /ɔ/ is usually low ([ɒ]) unless a phonemic contrast exists between /ɒ/ and /ɔ/; and in some areas older speakers have a raised first element to the diphthongs /aɪ/ and /aʊ/ ([ɐɪ], [ɐʊ]).

The major difference with the consonants is the variable use of postvocalic-r. This area (and New York and New Jersey) was once nonrhotic, and many speakers still do not use a postvocalic-r. However, younger speakers have adopted the rhotic norm of GA, so this feature is no longer as strong as it was. Nonrhotic speakers have a range of centering diphthongs in contexts where GA would have a vowel plus /ɹ/. For example, "ear," "care," "door," and "poor" may be /iə/, /kæə/, /doə/, and /pʊə/. Nonrhotic speakers usually adopt r-liaison (see chap. 17) in connected speech. Many northeastern speakers also retain /j/ after /t, d, n/ and before /u/, which has been lost in GA. Thus "tune," "due," and "news," are /tjun/, /dju/, /njuz/, as in Canadian English, and as also found in most areas of Britain, Ireland, and the Southern Hemisphere dialects.

> Several northern cities (such as Detroit, Chicago, Cleveland) exhibit the "northern cities vowel shift." This shift results in /ɔ/ being realized close to [ɑ]; /ɑ/ close to [æ]; /æ/ to [eɪ]; /ɪ/ to [ɛ]; /ɛ/ to [æ] and to [ʌ]; with /ʌ/ to [ɔ].

The South

There is much regional variation in the pronunciation of English in the South, and here we include only those characteristics that are fairly widespread. The vowel system does not differ from GA in the number of phonemes (except in nonrhotic varieties described below), but there are considerable realizational, distributional, and selectional differences. Perhaps some of the most salient realizational differences include the monophthongization of /aɪ/ to [a] (although some speakers retain a diphthong before voiceless consonants), but the diphthongization of /æ/ to [æɪ], especially before /g, f, θ, s, ʃ, v, n/, as in "bath," "man," "bag," and so forth. The diphthong /ɔɪ/ also reduces (to /ɔ/) for some speakers in certain contexts. Other important patterns are the fully diphthongal nature of /eɪ/ and /oʊ/; the use of /ɔ/ rather than /ɑ/ in words such as "law," "bought," although the realization of this vowel may also be diphthongal ([ɔʊ]); conversely the use of /ɑ/ rather than /ɔ/ before /ɹ/, and the fact that lax vowels are not noticeably shorter than the tense ones.

Some interesting distributional patterns emerge from the study of the lax vowels. For example, before velars and /ʃ, ʒ/, /ɪ/ is replaced by /i/, and /ɛ/ is replaced by /eɪ/ (e.g., "dish" /diʃ/, "thing" /θiŋ/). Before nasals /ɛ/ is realized as /i/, so there may be no difference between the words "pen" and "pin." Further, before /l/, /i/ is lowered to /ɪ/, so "really" is /ˈɹɪli/. The lax vowels display several interesting realizational features. *Umlaut* refers to the effect a following vowel may have on a lax vowel. For example, /ɑ/ in "horrid" is advanced due to the /ɪ/ in the second syllable, whereas in "cellar" the /ə/ in the second syllable causes the /ɛ/ in the first to be centralized. Another pattern is *shading*, the effect of a following consonant on a preceding /ɪ/. For example, labial consonants cause a preceding /ɪ/ to centralize; others may also have this effect apart from following velars. Finally, we can note *breaking*, the addition of a schwa or /ɪ/ offglide to lax vowels. This is especially common before labial consonants in monosyllables, so "lip" with shading and breaking may be realized as [lɨəp].

Both tense /u/ and lax /ʊ/ tend to be centralized, and the latter may have little rounding, whereas the former may be somewhat diphthongal. The central vowel /ʌ/ is often pronounced as a mid central vowel, causing a virtual collapse of the distinction between /ʌ/ and /ə/. Vowels in weak syllables such as plurals and past tenses are normally /ɪ/ rather than /ə/, so "waited" is /ˈweɪtɪd/ and "horses" is /ˈhɔɹsɪz/. This can also be extended to what would be final schwa in GA, so forms such as "Texas" /ˈtɛksɪs/ and "sofa" /ˈsoʊfɪ/ can occur.

Specific patterns associated with smaller areas within the South exhibit sometimes quite different patterns. For example, in southwest Louisiana, there is a noted tendency to realize <ar> spellings as /ɔɹ/, so "park" and "pork" are homophones.

With the consonants the major issue is whether southern accents are rhotic or not. The situation is very variable both geographically and socially, and the most it is safe to state is that some southern speech is nonrhotic, at least in some contexts. For example, speakers may differentially drop /ɹ/ postvocalically in word-medial position, as compared to word-finally. There is a tendency to retain /ɝ/, even when /ɚ/ is realized as nonrhotic schwa. Finally, we can also note that intervocalic-r (as in "Carolina") may be dropped by some speakers. In nonrhotic speech, the centering diphthongs described in the previous section will be used, although r-liaison is reported less often.

Other consonantal features include the retention of /j/ after alveolars before /u/; the use of /n/ rather than /ŋ/ in "-ing" verb endings; the vocalization of dark-l or the use of a velar lateral [ʟ]; localized replacement of dental fricatives by labiodental ones; and cluster reduction of final /st, ld, nd/ clusters. Intervocalic-l is almost always clear, and vowels before dark-l often exhibit breaking. This can result in a word such as "feel" being realized as [fɪl] (lowering before /l/), whereas "fill" is realized as [fɨəl] (shading and breaking).

Finally, we can note that stress assignment in southern accents may differ from that in GA. For example, "insurance" and "reward" usually take first syllable stress.

African American English (AAE)

The patterns of vowel usage in AAE show some similarity with those in the southern forms just discussed: for example, the "pen" ~ "pin" merger, reduction of /aɪ/ and /ɔɪ/ diphthongs, and the use of centering diphthongs (because AAE is nonrhotic). Some of these centering diphthongs also show mergers, so "poor" and "door" both have /oə/ or even /oʊ/, and "fear" and "fair" both have /eə/.

AAE is nonrhotic, and the loss of /ɹ/ may not be restricted to postvocalic position; /ɹ/ may be omitted in words such as "throw," "Paris," and "secretary." As in the South, dark-l may be vocalized, realized as a velar lateral, or simply omitted. The dental fricatives are usually realized as labiodentals, but initial /ð/ is more usually /d/, and initial /θ/ is often retained.

Many of the features of AAE that are most salient are connected with syllable structure. The canonical syllable shape in natural language is CV, so any move toward that shape in English will require the simplification of clusters and the loss of final consonants. Cluster reduction in

AAE mostly affects final clusters (apart from the loss of /ɹ/ in initial clusters just noted). Final cluster reduction operates in clusters where both consonants share the same voicing, so "list," "find," "called," will be /lɪs/, /fan/, /kɔ/, this last with postvocalic-l deletion. Plurals of nouns with a deleted final consonant often do not replace that consonant: "lists" /ˈlɪsɪz/.

Apart from cluster reduction, final nasals may be deleted, with the preceding vowel being nasalized instead ("tin" /tĩ/); final alveolar stops may be deleted ("cat" /kæ/); final lenis stops may be devoiced ("hid" /hɪt/); and final stops may be replaced by glottal stops ("hid" /hɪʔ/). As in many other varieties of English, verbs ending "-ing" normally have an alveolar rather than a velar nasal at the end. We can also note a tendency to use a voiced stop rather than a voiced fricative in forms such as "isn't," "wasn't," and "even" (/ˈɪdn̩t/, /ˈwʌdn̩t/, /ˈibm̩/). Metathesis occurs with certain lexical items (a feature shared with southern varieties), the best known being "ask" /æks/.

The rhythm of AAE weakens unstressed syllables immediately before stressed ones to such an extent that syllable deletion may occur. So "about," "because," and "around" may be /baʊt/, /kʌz/, /ɹaʊn/.

Rather than view AAE as divergent from English, many researchers today prefer to characterize it as fitting to the canonical syllable structure of natural language and some make reference to the structure of West African precursor languages. Therefore, rather than using "cluster reduction" and "consonant deletion" we can think of these patterns in terms of adherence to natural syllable shape.

Although we have described AAE as if it were one homogenous variety, there is of course much internal variation, and as with other varieties of English, some speakers may use some features, but not others, depending on speech style and context.

SPANISH-INFLUENCED ENGLISH

Spanish-influenced English may be spoken by people whose first language is Spanish, or by those from the Hispanic community who speak no or little Spanish. For this reason we deal with this variety in a section separate both from varieties of English and from second language phonological features. Many of the phonological characteristics of Spanish-influenced English derive from the sound patterns of Latin American Spanish, and we can consider these in terms of the consonant system, the vowel system, and the suprasegmental system.

Spanish is the language with the greatest number of speakers in the United States after English. Recent census figures show that there are 37.4 million Hispanic people, who make up 13% of the population—although the term *Hispanic* does not imply that they speak Spanish. The Hispanic population is especially numerous in California and Texas. Two-thirds of Hispanic people come from Mexico, about 14% from other parts of Central and South America, approximately 9% from Puerto Rico, 4% from Cuba, and the remainder from elsewhere or of Spanish descent within the United States. (Statistics from U.S. Census, 2002.)

The Spanish consonant system differs from the English in lacking the velar nasal (though it has a palatal nasal), the postalveolar fricative position, and phonemic status for voiced fricatives. Spanish has a voiceless postalveolar affricate, but not a voiced one. Although European Spanish does have a voiceless dental fricative, American Spanish normally does not. Spanish has a voiceless velar fricative, unlike English. These systemic differences are complicated by a range of realizational differences. For example, Spanish has both a trilled- and a tapped-r, but not an approximant-r as in English. Furthermore, noninitial /b, d, g/ are realized as [β, ð, ɣ], and /s/ before voiced consonants is [z]. In many Latin American countries (e.g., Cuba), final /s/ is realized as [h]. We can also note that /p, t, k/ are never aspirated, and so differ in this respect from English.

Spanish-influenced English, therefore, may show some or all of the following characteristics. Fortis plosives will be unaspirated, whereas word-initial lenis plosives will be fully voiced. Word-medial and -final lenis plosives may well be weakened to the fricatives shown above. English /f/ and /s/ will be unaffected, but target /ʃ/ may be realized as the affricate /tʃ/, target /θ/ as /t/, and English /h/ may be omitted or realized as the velar fricative [x]. The voiced fricatives of English are often realized as voiced stops in word-initial position. Elsewhere, although target /ð/ may be correctly realized, target /v/ may be pronounced as [β], and /z/ as [s].

Spanish lacks a velar nasal phoneme, though [ŋ] can occur as an allophone of /n/ before velar sounds. Word-finally nasals do not contrast, and /n/ only is found (although in some dialects there is free variation between the nasals word-finally, but no contrast). These patterns may spill over into Spanish-influenced English. American Spanish has /j/ derived from European /j/ and /ʎ/. This latter is particularly prone in South America to be strengthened to [dʒ], and this realization may also be used for English /j/. Finally, as noted earlier, English /ɹ/ may be realized as a trill or tap.

Consonant clusters are restricted in Spanish, and Spanish-influenced English usually reflects this. /s/-initial clusters are usually broken up by the addition of a vowel before the /s/, so that "star" (/stɑɹ/) may be realized as [ɛstar]. Final clusters in English are nearly all problematic, and consonant deletion is often employed to simplify them, giving [las] for "lasts" and [xol] for "hold."

The Spanish vowel system is much simpler than that of English, with a five-vowel pattern /i, e, a, o, u/. Although in closed syllables slightly laxer variants of these vowels are used, Spanish speakers do not contrast tense and lax vowels and, when speaking English, are likely to merge the English tense–lax distinction, producing vowels that are nearer tense than lax. This affects the English vowel distinctions /i/~/ɪ/, /eɪ/~/ɛ/, /ɑ/~/æ/, /ou/~/ɔ/, and /u/~/ʊ/ in particular. Further, because Spanish has only one low vowel, the entire series /ɛ/~/æ/~/ʌ/~/ɑ/ is likely to be confused. Spanish also lacks any central vowels and speakers tend to give full values (as reflected by the spelling) to vowels we normally pronounce as schwa. Rhotic vowels will be pronounced as [er] (or whatever vowel is shown in the spelling) with a trilled- or tapped-r.

Spanish is a syllable-timed language (see chap. 9) and thus lacks the heavy stress and weak unstressed distinction of English. This means the tendency to reduce unstressed syllables to weak vowels is not found in Spanish and, coupled with the lack of central vowels, means that even unstressed syllables get full vowel status. Spanish stress placement is fairly regular (normally on the penultimate syllable), so there is a tendency to use this pattern in English as well.

PHONOLOGICAL PROBLEMS OF LEARNERS OF ENGLISH

In this section we will give very brief notes on some of the common pronunciation problems speakers of a variety of languages face when learning English. This is not a substitute, however, for a thorough investigation of a specific language, and speech pathologists should undertake this if working with clients with a first language other than English.

Arabic

Arabic lacks the sounds /p/ and /v/, and learners of English may substitute /b/ for /p/, and /f/ for /v/. However, Arabic does have a voicing contrast between other plosives and fricatives, and thus learners of English do not find it very difficult to acquire /p/, and especially /v/. The dental fricatives /θ, ð/ are found in Iraqi and neighboring dialects of Arabic, but are missing from most others. However, they do occur in classical Arabic, so most Arabic learners of English will have been exposed to these sounds and may be able to attempt them. Some speakers will substitute /s, z/ or /t, d/ for the dental fricatives, nonetheless. Arabic has no affricates, but does have the component parts of the /tʃ, dʒ/ affricates of English, and so speakers are normally able to pronounce them with relative ease. Arabic /r/ is a trill, which tends to be used for English /ɹ/. Consonant clusters in Arabic are restricted to final position and to two consonants only. Clusters in English, therefore, may be simplified by the use of epenthetic vowels (e.g., [laˈriniks] for /ˈlæɹɪŋks /).

The Arabic vowel system lacks the tense–lax distinction used in English, so all lax vowels may be realized as their tense counterparts. Also, Arabic has a single low vowel—/a/—and English /æ/, /ɑ/, and /ʌ/ may all be pronounced as [a]. Finally, we can note that word stress distinctions in Arabic do not result in the reduction of unstressed vowels (e.g., to schwa) that is common in English. Therefore, Arabic speakers may give full value to vowels we normally reduce.

> Arabic, and many of the other languages dealt with in this section, uses a different writing system than English. It is worth remembering, therefore, that bilingual clients may be literate only in their first language, and may not be comfortable using the Roman alphabet. Different writing systems are also used in Chinese, Japanese, Korean, and the languages of India, among those included in this section.

Chinese

Chinese consists of a large number of widely differing dialects (which many consider separate languages) with differing phonologies. We will concentrate here on Putonghua (also termed Mandarin), the national language based on northern norms, and Cantonese, a southern variety spoken in Canton in southern China and in Hong Kong.

Syllable structure in Chinese dialects is much simpler than that of English. There are no clusters, and most syllables are open (i.e., have no final consonant). In Putonghua only /n/ and /ŋ/ can end a nonopen syllable, whereas in Cantonese the possible final consonants are /m, n, ŋ, p, t, k/. The final /p, t, k/ in Cantonese are, however, always unreleased and shorter than their English equivalents. Cantonese speakers will also tend to use final unreleased /p, t, k/ for English final /b, d, g/. Chinese has a variety of fricatives and affricates, but these are all voiceless, so the fortis–lenis distinction in English fricatives and affricates may not be realized, and the pronunciation of postalveolar fricatives in English may be retroflex. Also, /θ/ may be realized as [t], [f], or [s], and /ð/ may be pronounced as [d] or [z].

Cantonese speakers may have free variation between [l] and [n] in their language, and this may spread over into their English usage as well. Confusion between /ɹ/ and /w/ or /l/ is common in Chinese-influenced English, as is that between /w/ and /v/. We mentioned earlier that no clusters are found in Chinese, so simplifications and vowel insertion are common in the English of Chinese speakers. Further, all words in Chinese consist of single syllables only, so pronouncing polysyllabic words in English (especially linking the syllables together smoothly) can be a difficulty.

The vowel system of Chinese does not distinguish between tense and lax vowels, so English lax vowels may be pronounced as their tense counterparts. Further, target English /ə/ may be pronounced as a back vowel by Putonghua speakers ([ɯ]). Because of the use of tone in Chinese (see chap. 9) and the restriction on word length, English rhythm and intonation may be especially difficult for first-language Chinese speakers.

> Remember that bilingual clients may have varying degrees of proficiency in their languages. It is important to obtain a linguistic background analysis to see how much English is spoken in the home (if any), and with children, how proficient the caregivers are in English, and what the client's dominant language is.

French

The difficulties noted in this section will be common to French speakers, whether from Europe, Canada, Louisiana, or elsewhere. The French consonant system lacks the dental fricatives, and European French speakers tend to use /s, z/ for these, whereas North American French speakers prefer /t, d/ as substitutions. French also lacks the affricates, and some speakers may use /ʃ, ʒ/ for target /tʃ, dʒ/, although, as both parts of each affricate are sounds of French, other speakers may have no difficulties with them. French plosives differ from their English counterparts in that the fortis set (/p, t, k/) are always unaspirated, and the lenis set (/b, d, g/) are always fully voiced. If /p, t, k/ are pronounced without aspiration they may sound more /b, d, g/ like to English listeners. We can also note that /t, d, n/ in French are dental, rather than alveolar, although if the English equivalents are realized as dental this will not sound greatly different from the target norm. English /ɹ/ may be realized as uvular [ʁ] or [ʀ] by standard French speakers; those from other dialects may use the alveolar trill [r]. We can also note that French lacks /h/, and orthographic <h> is not pronounced. This usually results in the omission of /h/ in English also. In French, an orthographic vowel plus single <n> is realized as a nasalized vowel without the pronunciation of the nasal stop. This practice may also be extended to the English of first-language French speakers.

The French vowel system does not distinguish between tense and lax vowels, and so tense vowels may be used for their lax counterparts. There is an especial difficulty in distinguishing between English /ɛ/, /æ/, /ʌ/, and /ɑ/. French stress operates differently than in English, and there is no vowel reduction in unstressed syllables. French intonation patterns also differ from those of English, and these suprasegmental factors may be more obvious than the segmental ones described earlier.

Hindi and Related Languages

The languages of north India and of Pakistan, Sri Lanka, and Bangladesh are all related, and much of what is included here applies to speakers of Hindi, Urdu, Panjabi, Bengali, Sinhalese, and Gujerati among others. The comments on retroflex consonants also apply to southern Indian languages such as Tamil, Telugu, Malayalam, and Kannada. Speakers of these languages tend to use their own retroflex consonants in place of English alveolar /t, d, n/. Although these languages do have nonretroflex stops, these are dental, and it seems that English alveolar stops are perceived as closer to the retroflex stops than to the dental ones. This use of retroflex consonants is very characteristic of Indian English, and the retroflex resonance is very pervasive and can cause intelligibility problems.

English aspirated /p, t, k/ may be unaspirated in Indian English. This is despite the fact that Indian languages do have aspirated stops. English aspiration is, however, much weaker than in Indian languages, so these speakers see their unaspirated stops as closest to the English target. In Indian English, labiodental approximant [ʋ] may be used for English target /v/, and [ʋ] may be used for /w/ as well. Further, the dental fricatives are not found in north Indian languages, and [t̪] and [d̪] are the usual substitutes in Indian-influenced English. Some initial and final clusters present problems and vowel epenthesis in initial position and cluster reduction in final position are common strategies.

Vowel problems are not as extensive as in some of the languages we examine in this section. Nevertheless, difficulties in distinguishing /ɛ/ and /æ/ are common, as are difficulties with the difference between /i/ and /ɛ/. Stress placement in Indian English may differ from American norms, and the use of different intonation patterns may make some Indian English speakers sound abrupt when they intend to sound polite.

> Clients with an Indian language background may very well be multilingual, speaking two or more languages of India as well as English. It is important to know whether English is the first, second, or third (or more) language of clients from India, Pakistan, Bangladesh, or Sri Lanka.

Japanese

Japanese has a very limited syllable structure: there are no clusters, and most syllables are open. Further, there is a small vowel inventory (just five vowels). All these features provide much potential for interference in Japanese speakers' second language English.

Japanese lacks /f, v/, although [v] may occur as an allophone of Japanese /b/ in intervocalic position. Japanese speakers of English, therefore, may use [b] for English /v/ and [p] for English /f/. Likewise, there are no postalveolar fricatives in Japanese, though similar (alveolopalatal) fricatives are allophones of Japanese /s, z/ before high front vowels. This results in English /ʃ, ʒ/ being pronounced as [s, z] in most contexts, but English /s, z/ sounding similar to English /ʃ, ʒ/ before /i/. Japanese has a single liquid phoneme, with variants ranging from a postalveolar lateral, through a postalveolar flap, an affricate, to an approximant-r similar to English. This results in an inability to distinguish English /l/ and /ɹ/, although the attempt may sound somewhat r-like or l-like depending on the word involved. Word-initial glides (/w-/ and /j-/) are often omitted in Japanese English.

Consonant clusters are usually broken up by the insertion of an epenthetic vowel. Moreover, as Japanese only allows a single final nasal consonant, most consonant-final words are altered through the addition of a final vowel. As with other languages we have looked at, Japanese does not have a tense–lax vowel distinction, and Japanese speakers of English have particular problems with the four low vowels. Japanese uses stress and pitch in different ways from English; there will therefore be considerable interference in prosodic aspects of Japanese English.

Korean

Korean has only two fricative phonemes (/s, z/), (with /s/ representing a voiceless fortis, aspirated fricative, and with /z/ representing a voiceless lenis, but less grooved fricative than /s/). This results in Korean speakers of English having problems with most English fricatives (including /z/). Bilabial plosives are usually substituted for /f, v/, and an affricate ([ts, dz]) for English /z/. The use of Korean [s^h] for English /s/ will result in a noticeably non-native realization. Further, [ʃ] is an allophone of Korean /s/, and Korean speakers of English may use [ʃ] for English /s/ before high front vowels. The dental fricatives are normally realized as alveolar stops: aspirated for /θ/ and unaspirated for /ð/.

Korean has plosive phonemes at the bilabial, alveolar, and velar places (as in English). However, whereas in English we have just two phonemes at each place, Korean has three: unaspirated slight voicing, heavily aspirated voiceless, and unaspirated voiceless, possibly ejective. However, these distinctions are usually neutralized in word-final position, when most plosives are simply unreleased. Korean speakers of English may not consistently produce acceptable degrees of voice or aspiration in English plosives—especially in medial and final positions.

Koreans have a single liquid phoneme, and in their English will tend to use [l] for both initial /l/ and /ɹ/ in English, although in medial position a flap-like variant may be used for both. Consonant clusters are usually broken up with epenthetic vowels both initially and finally.

Standard Korean contrasts long and short vowels, so in Korean-influenced English the lax vowels may be pronounced as shorter equivalents to the tense ones. Many varieties of Korean, however, seem to be moving toward a tense–lax distinction in their vowel system, so this may be less noticeable with younger speakers. Stress and intonation problems occur, because both Korean rhythm and intonation differ considerably from those of English.

Portuguese

Although there are differences between European Portuguese and Brazilian Portuguese, the following points hold for both varieties unless otherwise noted. Portuguese does not have phonemic affricates, so problems arise with English /tʃ, dʒ/. In European Portuguese, [ʃ] and [ʒ] are usually used for the affricates. Brazilian Portuguese has affricate allophones of /t/ and /d/ before high front vowels, but the speakers may still not be able to use the affricates in other positions, or to use [t] and [d] before the high front vowels of English. The dental fricatives of English are normally realized as /t̪/ and /d̪/. Final target /s/ in English may be realized as [ʃ], leading to confusion with final target /ʃ/. Dark-l is often pronounced as [w], but this reflects a similar change in many varieties of English. Portuguese speakers of English often delete or shorten final consonants, and may change final vowel plus nasal into a nasalized vowel alone. Some initial and final clusters may also present difficulties, with vowel insertion undertaken to split up the cluster.

Portuguese does not have the tense–lax vowel distinction, and lax vowels tend to be pronounced as their tense counterparts. There is particular difficulty with distinguishing the four low vowels of English. Portuguese word stress is regular, and therefore inaccurate stress placement may characterize Portuguese-influenced English. Further, Portuguese does not exhibit the vowel reduction found in English unstressed syllables, and so full values of vowels may be employed.

> With some clients whose English is minimal you may have to work with translators. However, this requires great care, and readers are encouraged to consult the recent book by Isaac (2002) on this topic.

Vietnamese

As in Chinese, most Vietnamese words consist of a single syllable, and clusters are not permitted. However, they do have a large vowel system and therefore experience fewer difficulties with English vowels (although the tense–lax distinction does still pose some problems). Vietnamese does not distinguish voiced from voiceless stops word-finally, allowing voiceless ones only in that position; in addition, the word-final voiceless stops are short and unreleased. Vietnamese speakers of English, therefore, have difficulty making native-like plosives of either voicing type word-finally. Further, /p/ is not found word-initially, and may be realized as [b] or [f].

Vietnamese has some fricatives (/f, v, s, z/), but these do not occur word-finally, and may be omitted in that position in Vietnamese English. Vietnamese, however, does have an affricate similar to English /tʃ/, and so Vietnamese speakers of English are often able to acquire the English affricates and postalveolar fricatives relatively easily. The English dental fricatives present problems, however, and may be replaced by plosives. Consonant clusters also are problematic, with cluster reduction through deletion a common strategy.

Vietnamese is a tone language, and the use of the English intonation system often presents problems. Also, the putting together of polysyllabic words can be difficult and affect the overall rhythm of Vietnamese-influenced English.

> If you work with many clients from a particular language background, learning the language concerned will be very useful. This will be particularly welcomed by parents of children you work with, if they themselves have limited competence of English.

BACKGROUND READING

For varieties of English around the world we strongly recommend Wells' (1982) three-volume survey of accents of English. For more detail on United States dialects readers can consult Wolfram and Schilling-Estes (1998). Southern English is described in Nagle and Sanders (2003); African American English is dealt with in detail in Green (2002). For Spanish-influenced English, specifically linked to issues in communication disorders, Centeno, Obler, and Anderson (forthcoming) is a good source. Avery and Ehrlich (1992) provides information on potential pronunciation problems in English for speakers of a wide range of languages (more than we were able to cover here). Readers may also wish to consult IPA (1999) for descriptions of the phonologies of many languages around the world.

EXERCISES

Transcription

(Answers to the transcription exercises are given at the end of the book.)

1. Which national varieties of English outside the United States might be the source of the following pronunciations?
   (a) night [nɪçt]
   (b) snow [snʌʉ]
   (c) house [hʌʊs]
   (d) chill [tʃʌl]
   (e) threat [t̪ɹɛθ̠]
   (f) better [ˈbɛʔə]
2. Which regional varieties of English inside the United States might be the source of the following pronunciations?
   (a) bone [bɵn]
   (b) sill [sɨəl]
   (c) when [wɛ̃]
   (d) sky [ska]
   (e) oil [ɔʟ]
   (f) bet [bɛ]

Review Questions

1. What are systemic, realizational, and distributional differences between accents or languages?

2. What is "Canadian raising"?
3. Which British accents are rhotic?
4. What features are shared by Southern Hemisphere English?
5. What are "breaking," "shading," and "umlaut" in southern accents?
6. What is the "northern cities vowel shift"?
7. What characteristics of African American English are linked to an optimal syllable shape?
8. List any three features of Spanish-influenced English.

Study Topics and Experiments

1. Research and make a list of all the countries you can find that have English as one of their official languages.
2. Research the phonetics and phonology of any language other than English, or the languages described in this chapter. Draw up a list of as many systemic, structural, and realization differences as you can find between that language and your variety of English.

CD

The CD has examples of a set passage (the Rainbow Passage) being read in a variety of English accents. We have not provided exercises for this chapter on the CD, but you should listen carefully to each accent, and compare the features you hear to the description in the text.

III

Disordered Speech

19

Phonological and Phonetic Disorders

INTRODUCTION

This book is intended for students who will go on to become speech-language pathologists. Therefore, although we need to provide a good basis in general phonetics and the phonetics of English, we also need to consider phonetic and phonological aspects of speech disorders. In this chapter we look first at some difficulties involved with the application of the division into phonetics and phonology to disordered speech data. Then we consider the differences between broad and narrow transcription of clinical speech samples, and we conclude with a brief overview of some typical disorder types.

THE TERMS *PHONETICS* AND *PHONOLOGY* IN THE DESCRIPTION OF DISORDERED SPEECH

The application of the binary phonetics/phonology division to disordered speech is problematic. One problem revolves around the need to discriminate between phonemic and subphonemic (i.e., allophonic) errors on the one hand, but also around whether the realization of the target sound is within or outside the target phonology (defined broadly to mean both the phonemic units and their allophonic realizations). This implies that a two-way distinction is insufficient: We need to note both whether contrastivity is lost, and whether the speaker goes beyond the target phonology or not. We suggest that two levels of decision-making are needed here: The first decision needed is whether the speaker for any particular error is using a sound from within or outside the target system; the second is whether the realization results in a loss of contrastivity or not.

For example, if the target contrast /s/–/ʃ/ is realized as [s]–[s], then we see that the speaker has stayed within the target system, but has lost contrastivity; if the same contrast is realized as [s]–[s̠] (postalveolar grooved fricative used before /ɹ/ in some varieties of English), we again see that the speaker has stayed within the target system, but this time contrastivity has been retained (even though the phonetic difference is slight). On the other hand, if target /s/–/ʃ/ is realized as [ç]–[ç], then the speaker has gone outside the target system and lost contrastivity, but if the realization is [s]–[ç], then there is use of a sound outside the target system but contrastivity is retained.

We clearly need a four-way terminology to show these distinctions, and we suggest the following, with further examples:

1. Internal allophonic: target /t/ realized as dental in all positions [t̪];
2. Internal phonemic: target /t/ realized as [d];
3. External phonetic: target /z/ realized as [ɮ];
4. External phonological: target /v/ and /ð/ realized as [β].

Also, we need to discriminate between the source of the error and the effect of the error whenever possible. In other words, we need to decide whether what we are labeling is the effect the error has on the listener in terms of loss or otherwise of contrastivity, or the site of origin of the error in terms of the components of speech organization and speech production. Of course, making this distinction is not always easy. It is relatively straightforward to provide a description of the effect speech errors have on the listener; after all, this is what most impressionistic transcription of speech does. However, an impressionistic transcription will not always disambiguate between differing articulatory gestures that result in identical or very similar percepts. Nevertheless, the great advances that we have seen in instrumental speech assessment mean that it is increasingly possible to couple impressionistic transcription with instrumental analysis that potentially can throw light on any differences between source and effect. We can illustrate the source–effect difference with some examples.

In the first example we analyze a child producing the phonological process called *velar fronting*, and transcribe target /k/ as [t], /g/ as [d], and /ŋ/ as [n]. We assume that this is a phonological disorder, because the substitutions result in a threefold loss of contrast between alveolars and velars, and occur regularly. However, electropalatography (EPG; see Hardcastle and Gibbon, 1997) shows that this is not the case. It turns out that the speaker has different tongue palate contact patterns for target alveolars and target velars, and so clearly has not merged these two target sounds. However, the release stage of the target velars result in their *sounding like* alveolars because the contact at the back of the tongue is released slightly before that at the alveolar region. Therefore, the source is a problem with coordinating articulatory gestures; the effect on the listener is a loss of phonological contrasts.

In our second example, we can imagine a child who presents with the classic characteristics of cleft palate speech: hypernasality, inability to produce plosives or fricatives, heavy use of glottal stops, and so on. The tendency would be to classify the errors as mainly phonetic, deriving from the child's physical impairments, and to assume that the target phonological system is intact.

However, then we learn that the child's cleft was repaired some time ago. The errors that we hear are "learned behavior"; that is, phonetic characteristics that were an automatic result of the cleft palate became phonologized, and are now the normal way of speaking for this client.

These two cases show that what appears to be a phonological problem to the perceiver may be a motor (phonetic) problem for the producer, and what may appear to the perceiver to be phonetic disturbances may in fact be phonological behavior for the producer.

We need a two-way terminology to show this distinction, and we suggest the following:

1. Source phonetic, effect phonological, e.g., "velar fronting";
2. Source phonological, effect phonetic, e.g., repaired cleft palate speech.

Therefore, when labeling particular speech errors in your clients, you need to be aware of the full range of phonetic and phonological criteria and to be careful about assuming that what we perceive coincides directly with what the speaker was trying to produce.

BROAD AND NARROW TRANSCRIPTION

Approaches to the task of phonetic transcription reflect different approaches to describing speech in general. Phoneticians are interested in the speech production and reception mechanisms and the acoustic signal of speech and describe these features as accurately as possible without regard to the role the sounds, themselves, play in language. Linguists—or more precisely phonologists—are, however, concerned mainly in the patterns of sound within language rather than the minutiae of the sounds themselves. This results in two different transcription traditions: that which tries to capture as much phonetic detail as possible, and that which only wishes to identify linguistically functional units. As noted in chapter 11, these two approaches have been called "phonetic" and "phonemic/phonological," and "narrow" and "broad."

However, these two pairs of labels are not totally interchangeable and are not always used in a precise way. The distinction between "phonetic" and "phonemic" should be clear: a phonetic transcription in this sense attempts to capture enough detail to mark the distinctive allophones of the phonemes of a language (therefore perhaps the term "allophonic" is better here, so we can keep "phonetic" as a general umbrella term for any kind of transcription), with "phonemic" providing only one symbol per phoneme, ignoring allophonic variation. Clearly, a phonemic transcription can only be read accurately by someone who is already acquainted with the phonology of the language and, as such, is not suitable for the purpose of illustrating a language's pronunciation to those who have no prior knowledge of the language.

"Narrow" and "broad" transcriptions as terms are, however, not necessarily tied to the notions of allophone and phoneme. They imply simply a difference between a detailed and a simple transcription. Although an allophonic transcription will tend to be detailed (and therefore "narrow"), the degree of detail will depend on whether only main allophones or all perceptible differences are being recorded. Likewise, although a phonemic transcription is bound to be broad, we may also get fairly simple transcriptions that contain some allophonic (and so not strictly "phonemic") information.

> The difference between these two terms is relevant to the use of phonetic transcription of disordered speech in the clinic. Clearly, a patient presenting with disordered speech will be demonstrating some degree of disruption (whether mild or severe) of the phonological patterns of their target accent. Because the phonology is disrupted, one cannot use a phonemic transcription, which assumes a normal phonology. We must, therefore, adopt an approach that does not record phonemic units, but attempts to describe phonetic features.

We turn, therefore, to the simple distinction in terms of amount of detail: "broad" versus "narrow." As with many clinical procedures confronting the speech-language pathologist, there is a tension here between speed and depth. It is naturally less time-consuming to undertake a transcription that involves marking the least amount of detail possible; however, the price paid for this is lack of depth in the analysis. If such lack of depth still allowed adequate classification of errors, this would not be a problem and broad transcriptions would be perfectly acceptable; however, as we will show below, lack of detail may well result in misleading analyses.

There is, however, a further consideration. Although narrow transcriptions may result in better analyses of disordered speech, the more detail that is required of a transcriber, the greater the room for transcription error and uncertainty.

We now look at some examples of clinical transcription in which the difference between broad and narrow approaches can be vital in arriving at a correct analysis (and, therefore, treatment) of the disordered phonology of the patient.

The following sample is given first in broad transcription; as all these transcriptions are non-phonemic (for reasons previously noted), square brackets are used throughout and we note which are broad and which narrow (although this is to some extent obvious from the amount of detail included).

Sample 1. Age 7;3. Broad transcription.

shop	[ʃɑp]	shoe	[ʃu]
see	[ʃi]	seat	[ʃit]
ship	[ʃɪp]	wash	[wɑʃ]
sip	[ʃɪp]	yes	[jɛʃ]
rush	[ɹʌʃ]	kiss	[kɪʃ]
cushion	[ˈkʊʃən]	messy	[ˈmɛʃi]

This sample appears to be a clear example of the loss of phonological contrast between two target phonemes of English: /s/ and /ʃ/, with [ʃ] being used for both in all places of word structure. Indeed, the minimal pair "sip" and "ship" are in the sample and appear to show a homonymic clash in this speaker's speech. However, this is a broad transcription, in which the transcriber has restricted the symbol set to those normally encountered in the transcription of adult target English phonology. In examining a narrower transcription of the same data, in which other IPA symbols are utilized, a different picture emerges:

Sample 1. Age 7;3. Narrow transcription.

shop	[ʃɑp]	shoe	[ʃu]
see	[çi]	seat	[çit]
ship	[ʃɪp]	wash	[wɑʃ]
sip	[çɪp]	yes	[jɛç]
rush	[ɹʌʃ]	kiss	[kɪç]
cushion	[ˈkʊʃən]	messy	[ˈmɛçi]

On examination of this transcription, it is seen that actually this speaker has *not* lost the contrast between target /s/ and /ʃ/. It is true that they are not realized in the standard way, but although [ç] is not a phoneme of English and will sound extremely odd being used for /s/, homonymic clashes do not result from this pronunciation and so the contrast between words will not be lost.

> The treatment approach for a patient lacking a phonological contrast will naturally differ from that needed for a patient whose phonology is intact but whose phonetic realization of some phonemes is disordered. The clinician working from the broad transcription may schedule needless time attempting to establish contrasts through minimal pair practice, when what is actually required is work on the realization of /s/ alone.

The first example involves a major simplification of the transcription process in the broad version, in that the difference between a postalveolar and a palatal fricative should be quite noticeable and is lost in the transcription simply because the transcriber chose only the English consonant set. We can demonstrate other examples in which the phonetic difference is not so great, but the importance of narrow transcription is equally clear.

Sample 2. Age 6;9. Broad transcription.

pin [pin] ten [tɛn]
bin [pin] den [tɛn]
cot [kɑt] pea [pi]
got [kɑt] bee [pi]

This data set also suggests that there is a collapse of phonological contrast: specifically the contrast between voiced and voiceless plosives in word-initial position. This clearly leads to homonymic clashes between, for example, "pin" and "bin" and "cot" and "got," respectively. Because word-initial plosives have a high functional load in English, such a loss of the voicing contrast in this context clearly requires treatment. It would appear from these data that an initial stage of treatment would concentrate on the establishment of the notion of contrast with these sounds, before going on to practice the phonetic realization of this contrast.

However, if we look at a narrow transcription of the same data, the picture alters.

Sample 2. Age 6;9. Narrow transcription.

pin [p^{h}in] ten [t^{h}ɛn]
bin [pin] den [tɛn]
cot [k^{h}ɑt] pea [p^{h}i]
got [kɑt] bee [pi]

Again it is clear from this transcription that there is not actually a loss of contrast between initial voiced and voiceless plosives. Target voiceless plosives are realized without vocal fold vibration (voice), but with aspiration on release (as are the adult target forms). The target voiced plosives are realized without aspiration (as with the adult forms), but also without any vocal fold vibration. It is this last difference that distinguishes them from the target form. For although target English "voiced" plosives are often devoiced for some of their duration in initial position, totally voiceless examples are rare. Of course, speech-language pathologists have to train themselves to hear these differences, and mustn't listen in terms of the English target system.

> The narrow transcription shows, therefore, that the difference between the speaker's pronunciation of these sounds and the target is minimal. The notion of contrast does not need to be established, and, because aspiration is the main acoustic cue used by adults to perceive the difference between these groups of plosives, the child's speech may well sound only slightly atypical for these particular sounds.

We examine one more example in which the choice of transcription suggests a more limited phonology than is the case. Here the focus is on structural rather than systemic aspects of the speaker's phonology.

Sample 3. Age 6;10. Broad transcription.

snow [hnoʊ] smile [hmaɪl]
snake [hneɪk] smoke [hmoʊk]
slow [ɬoʊ] swim [hwɪm]
slide [ɬaɪd] sweet [hwit]

This transcription presents a confusing picture of the target /s/+ sonorant clusters. It appears that in all but /sl−/ clusters, the cluster is retained with a change of target /s/ to [h] (a change incidentally quite common in historical phonology). In /sl−/ clusters there appears to be a replacement of both the /s/ and the /l/ by [ɬ]. This last might be thought of as an example of cluster reduction, although it is unclear if there is deletion of /s/ and substitution of /l/, or deletion of /l/ and substitution of /s/. This problem is clarified on examination of a narrow transcription of the same sample:

Sample 3. Age 6;10. Narrow transcription.

snow	[n̥oʊ]	smile	[m̥aɪl]
snake	[n̥eɪk]	smoke	[m̥oʊk]
slow	[ɬoʊ]	swim	[ʍɪm]
slide	[ɬaɪd]	sweet	[ʍit]

This transcription illustrates that the use of [h] in the broad transcription was an attempt to capture the voiceless nature of the sonorants. The added friction with the realization of /sl−/ clusters prompted the use of the symbol for the voiceless lateral fricative, but in the other instances, the audible voiceless breath flow was interpreted as an added /h/. This transcription also shows that the speaker was not in fact using two different strategies with these clusters and there was no /s/ → [h] change involved. In all instances, there is reduction of a two-member cluster to a single sound. This sound, however, is not one of the two target sounds, but contains features from both target sounds. This process is often called *feature synthesis*, and it can be seen that what is retained in this sample is the place and manner of the second segment (e.g., alveolar and nasal, alveolar and lateral) with the voicelessness and friction of the first segment. This results in all the subject's initial segments in this sample being voiceless and to a lesser or greater degree fricative (e.g., with considerable friction in [ɬ] and [ʍ], and audible breath with the nasals). This child, then, has actually not mastered consonant clusters (at least with these target cluster types), but has clearly attempted to produce features associated with both sounds in the target cluster.

> In normal phonological development, feature synthesis is often found just prior to the acquisition of clusters, so this would suggest an intervention strategy related to the expansion of these initial sounds into full clusters. Working from the broad transcription, however, a change from [h] to /s/ is indicated, with the /sl-/ clusters as a separate problem: In other words, the generalization that unites these pronunciations into a single phonological process is lost.

SOME TYPICAL PHONETIC-LEVEL DISORDERS

In this section we have space to look at only a few phonetic-level problems that are regularly encountered in the speech clinic. Some of the texts listed in the background reading section of this chapter will guide you further in this area. In this section we are concerned with disorders that have a phonetic source, although the effect may on occasions be phonological.

Children's Misarticulations

Common misarticulations in English child speech disorders include lisps, problems with other fricatives (especially dental fricatives), problems with the rhotic productions, and difficulties in making velar consonants.

Lisps usually affect the production of target /s/ and /z/, although the postalveolars /ʃ/ and /ʒ/ may also prove difficult and are sometimes also included under this heading. Lisps are usually divided into several main types: lateral lisps, addental lisps, dental lisps, and palatal lisps. Lateral lisps occur when target alveolar fricatives are realized as lateral fricatives (i.e., /s/ ~ /z/ → [ɬ] ~ [ɮ]); addental lisps result in dental grooved fricatives (i.e., /s/~ /z/ → [s̪] ~ [z̪]); dental lisps, on the other hand, see the use of dental slit fricatives instead of target alveolars (i.e., /s/ ~ /z/ → [θ] ~ [ð]); finally, palatal lisps result in palatalized or postalveolar realizations of the targets (i.e., /s/ ~ /z/ → [sʲ] ~[zʲ], or /s/ ~ /z/ → [ʃ] ~ [ʒ]). Lisps are relatively common, and come about because of the requirement for fine motor control over the articulators to produce both the correct tongue placement and the narrow groove needed for the airflow. The postalveolar fricatives may demonstrate addental, lateral, or palatal (i.e., /ʃ/ ~ /ʒ/ → [ç] ~ [ʝ]) realizations.

These examples show lateral lisps (including the postalveolar fricatives and affricates), and dental lisps respectively.

shops	[ɬɑpɬ]	sausages	[ˈɬɑɬɪdɮɪɮ]	chess	[tɬɛɬ]
zoos	[ɮuɮ]	station	[ˈɬteɪɬən]	splashes	[ˈɬplæɬɪɮ]
soup	[θup]	sister	[ˈθɪθtɚ]	zoos	[ðuð]
season	[ˈθiðən]	sneezes	[ˈθniðɪð]	possesses	[pɑˈðɛθɪð]

The dental fricatives /θ/ and /ð/ also require fine motor control, this time to produce a tongue placement at or between the teeth and a flattened slit fricative air channel. These sounds, too, are subject to misarticulation and the most common realizations are labiodental fricatives (i.e., /θ/ ~ /ð/ → [f]~ [v]), or alveolar plosives (i.e., /θ/ ~ /ð/ → [t] ~ [d]), or for some speakers a combination of the two. It should be recalled, that in chapter 18 we noted that such realizations are acceptable in certain regional varieties of English.

The English /ɹ/, whether the target is retroflexed or bunched, is another consonant requiring precise execution. As there is no contact between the articulators and the roof of the mouth, the production of this sound does not provide the feedback available from, for example, a stop consonant. These difficulties may result in the child using an alternative approximant consonant that has acoustic characteristics similar to those of /ɹ/. This may be the labiovelar approximant [w] (with the result that, at first sight, this may appear to be a phonological substitution), or the labiodental approximant [ʋ], or even a bilabial approximant [β̞].

Finally, we can consider problems with the velar place of articulation, briefly referred to earlier in the chapter. This has been considered a phonological disorder (that is, the loss of contrast between velars and alveolars, as target velars appear to be realized as alveolars). Recent experimental work suggests, however, that here, too, we have a problem deriving from motor control, this time of the tongue body. This work suggests that target velars are actually articulated differently from target alveolars by children who exhibit this problem, even though the resultant consonants sound the same. The target velars are articulated with the entire tongue body pressed against the roof of the mouth (they appear to be alveolars because the tongue tip is the last part of the tongue removed from the roof of the mouth following the articulation), whereas target alveolars are articulated normally with just the tongue tip and blade in use.

Adult Phonetic Problems

A wide range of phonetic problems may be manifested in disorders such as cleft palate, disfluency, and acquired neurogenic conditions (such as dysarthria). These disorders may result in speech sounds that are *atypical* (that is to say, not found in natural language; see chap. 20 for more details). For example, speakers with cleft palate may produce not only nasalized speech sounds, but sounds with audible nasal air escape (termed *nareal fricatives*), as well as nonatypical but non-English sounds such as pharyngeal fricatives and glottal stops. People with stuttering often use very strong articulations following a *block* (that is, a total stoppage of speech before a sound that is problematic for the speaker), and may use other atypical sounds during struggle behaviors. Dysarthric speakers of certain types may use very weak articulations of target sounds. All these atypical characteristics are returned to in more detail in chapter 20, where the recommended transcriptions for atypical speech are described.

SOME TYPICAL PHONOLOGICAL-LEVEL DISORDERS

In this section we will look at patterns of disordered speech that seem to derive from a disturbance in phonology rather than in articulation. These disturbances may be in the abstract level of phonology that deals with units such as syllables, or in the more applied part of phonology that deals with implementing speech patterns. We restrict ourselves here to discussion of child speech data, although some phonological level disorders can also be found, for example, in the speech of clients with various types of aphasia.

Evidence of a simplification of the phonological make-up of words can be seen in *weak syllable deletion*. This is a commonly occurring process in the speech of young children, where unstressed syllables (especially those before a stressed syllable) are omitted. If this is retained, however, it is evidence of a phonological disorder (often called a phonological delay in cases such as this, because the process is retained beyond the age it is expected to operate). Evidence of simplification of the phonological make-up of syllables can be seen in *final consonant deletion*. In phonological acquisition, syllable-initial consonants generally occur before syllable-final ones, and this reflects a universal tendency for syllable onsets to be more common than syllable codas. The deletion of final consonants, therefore, is not directly linked to the motoric difficulty of the consonant itself (because these consonants usually are realized in initial position), but to the lack of development at the syllable level of the phonology from a basic CV syllable shape to a CVC one.

These examples show context-sensitive voicing.

tag	[dæk]	thin	[ðɪn]
shows	[ʒoʊs]	choose	[dʒus]
pays	[beɪs]	flag	[vlæk]
cave	[geɪf]	sneeze	[znis]

Also connected to word shape is the process often called *context-sensitive voicing*. Here, there is a tendency to produce only voiced obstruents word-initially, and only voiceless ones word-finally (though in some cases, just the initial or just the final change is found). This again reflects universal preferences with obstruents, and also cannot be directly linked to motor problems. This is because the speakers can usually produce both voiced and voiceless obstruents—just not at the same place in word structure; and even though final obstruents may be restricted to the voiceless ones, final voiced sonorants are generally not a problem.

Finally, we can consider the simplification of consonant clusters, or *cluster reduction*. This can occur both syllable-initially and syllable-finally (although most research has centered on word-initial clusters). It is often the case that the speaker can produce the individual consonants that make up the cluster, but not the cluster itself. So, once more, it is not the motor difficulty of the individual sounds that underlies this problem, but the phonological planning of the combination of the sounds. Interestingly, when clusters are simplified in normal or delayed phonological development, the speakers usually retain the sound that is articulatorily strongest (with plosives stronger than fricatives, and fricatives stronger than approximants) and earlier in terms of normal acquisition.

Cluster reduction is also said to reflect *sonority theory.* Briefly, this theory states that the ideal syllable shape in natural language has the most sonorous (i.e., perceptually clear) sounds at the nucleus of the syllable (e.g., vowels), with the syllable onset having the least sonorous sounds (e.g., voiceless plosives) to ensure a clear difference to the listener between the onset and the nucleus of the syllable. In most cases of cluster reduction, the strongest sound in articulatory terms (that is to say, the sound usually retained) is also the lowest in sonority.

Many of the phonetic and phonological level changes we've looked at have been classed as *natural phonological processes* (see chap. 10). A full list of these processes is found in appendix 2, but remember that some of these are likely to have a phonetic level origin and some a phonological level one.

DISTURBANCES TO PROSODY

We noted in chapter 9 that prosody consisted of various aspects, such as stress, length, pitch, tempo, loudness, and voice quality. Speech-language pathologists may encounter disturbances to any of these systems in a wide range of clients including those with acquired neurogenic disorders, hearing impairment, disfluency, and voice disorders. We have the space only to look at one typical problem: intonation of the hearing-impaired. Among the findings from research on the intonation of those who have lost their hearing after acquiring English are the following features. Their intonation shows an excessive number of short intonation groups (see chap. 17); a tendency to keep nuclei at the end of the intonation group irrespective of the requirements of style or of syntax; an excessive use of level nuclei rather than rising or falling; and a paucity of the normal nuclear tone at the end of utterances (this normal end tone may be falling or rising, dependent on the variety of English concerned). Other characteristics include a general use of pitch settings that are too low (or sometimes too high) compared with the norm; excessive use of stress; speech that is too loud or too soft; and occasionally problems with voice quality and tempo.

> An example of excessive stress in a child with developmental speech disorder is given in Wells (1994). Apart from segmental problems (as seen in the transcription), the child stressed almost every syllable, though it did use an extra strong stress ([ˈˈ]) on occasion. We mark the stress on both the orthography and the phonetic transcription here.
>
> ˈme ˈmum ˈand ˈmy ˈbroˌther ˈis ˈˈdad
>
> [ˈmi ˈməm ˈʔant ˈmaĩ ˈbʊˌfə ˈʔɪs ˈˈtɛ·ʔ·hth]

The following extract shows the intonation of a 54-year-old woman from Belfast (Northern Ireland) who had lost her hearing at the age of 12. She demonstrates most of the features we noted above. It should be noted that in this variety of English final rises are expected in statements, but this speaker tends to use final level nuclei. The extract is shown using musical stave notation.

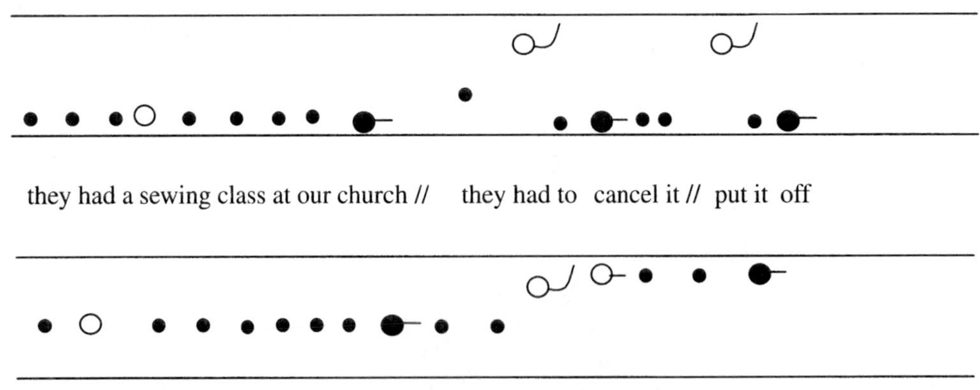

they had a sewing class at our church // they had to cancel it // put it off

//because they all wanted to see Dallas // I says // is your heads cut?

BACKGROUND READING

For a more detailed account of the use of the terms *phonetics* and *phonology* in the description of disordered speech see Ball and Müller (2002). The discussion here on broad and narrow transcriptions follows closely the contribution on this topic of the first author of this text to Ball et al. (1996). For more detail on different disorders see Bauman-Waengler (2004), or Bernthal and Bankson (2004). The examples come from Ball (1993), Ball et al. (1996), and Wells (1994) and from our files.

EXERCISES

Transcription

(Answers to the transcription exercises are given at the end of the book.)

1. What transcriptions (using either GA or RP norms) would you expect of the following target items if you were told the speaker exhibits velar fronting and a lateral lisp for alveolar fricatives?

king	sewing	zoo
game	socks	gem
vision	cogs	sagging
reason	guess	sink

2. What transcriptions (using either GA or RP norms) would you expect of the following target items if you were told the speaker exhibited cluster reduction and final consonant deletion?

strike	splash	scream
blush	prove	green
smooth	slide	snow
stop	skin	spun

Review Questions

1. How should the terms *phonetic* and *phonological* be applied to the analysis of disordered speech?

2. What is the difference between broad and narrow transcription? Why is broad transcription often insufficient in the clinic?
3. What are typical phonetic-level disorders of speech?
4. What are typical phonological-level disorders of speech?
5. What are typical prosodic disorders of speech?

Study Topics and Experiments

1. Do library research on the topic of typical phonological processes encountered in normal phonological development and in delayed phonology. Compare and contrast the process names and process groupings of at least three different authors. Which classification seems to you the best justified?
2. Make a recording (after first getting permission from the caregivers) of a young child between the ages of 2;6 and 4;0 interacting with family and/or friends. Try to get at least 10 minutes on video or good quality audio tape. Then go through the recording and note as many examples as you can of simplified pronunciations. Using the list of processes you chose in study topic 1, check how many of these occur in your data. Were there any realizations that did not fit into the list of processes? If so, list them.

CD

Listen to the examples of disordered speech and try to transcribe the test items into phonetic symbols. Answers are given at the end of the book.

20

Transcribing Atypical and Disordered Speech

ASPECTS OF ATYPICAL AND DISORDERED SPEECH

In the previous chapter we discussed the range of patterns of phonological and phonetic speech disorders that occur commonly in the clinic. We noted that many of them involved systemic simplifications, distributional restrictions, and realizational differences from the target sounds. However, in the examples we examined, the sounds used instead of the targets were always sounds of natural language, that is, sounds that have been recorded as occurring in languages, even if not in the target language itself.

However, clients in the speech clinic sometimes use sounds that have not been recorded in natural language (or extremely rarely so). These sounds constitute a group we call *atypical speech*, and in this chapter we will look at the most commonly occurring of these, and at how we might symbolize them. Because these sounds are not found in the languages of the world, there are no IPA symbols for them (because the IPA is only concerned with symbolizing the sounds of natural language). In the past, speech-language pathologists had to invent ad hoc symbols of their own to deal with atypical sounds when they occurred. Naturally, ad hoc symbols are only useful for the transcriber who invents them; anyone else reading the transcript (such as another clinician) may well not know what the symbols are supposed to represent. This is why, in the late 1980s, a group of speech-language pathologists and phoneticians drew up a set of extensions to the IPA for the transcription of atypical speech (known as the extIPA symbols). These symbols are not intended to cover every type of possible atypical sound (or even all the types ever reported by clinicians) but, rather, to provide a way of transcribing those atypical sounds that seem to occur most often.

> In this book we distinguish between *disordered speech*, which is any kind of disruption to the target speech, and *atypical speech*, which applies only to those sounds that are not found in natural language. Therefore, disordered speech may cover disruptions at the phonological or phonetic level, and if the latter, may include atypical speech as well as sounds from outside the target system but which are found in other languages.

In this chapter we will look at the extIPA symbol system in some detail, starting with the atypical places and manners of articulation that are covered. We will also look at the problem of showing how confident transcribers are with their choice of symbols, an aspect of transcription that is particularly relevant in the clinical context. Other aspects of the extIPA chart and the VoQS chart (see appendix 1) will also be covered. It should be borne in mind that, whereas consonants may be produced using a variety of atypical places and manners of articulation, atypical vowels cannot be found. This is because, by their very definition, vowels have to be made within the vowel area described in chapter 5. Because languages around the world have made use of vowels in virtually all parts of this area, any vowel encountered in the clinic (however altered from the target value) will always be a possible vowel of natural language.

Two exceptions may be argued for. First, it is possible to produce a range of vowel sounds while keeping the teeth clenched (see atypical dental places of articulation, below). The vowel sounds will be somewhat distorted, and this mode of production would appear to be atypical because it has not been reported in natural language. Second, certain vowel-like sounds can be produced even when the tongue tip and even the body are protruded from the mouth (the highest point of the tongue arch being still within the vowel area, however). In both these cases, the diacritics assigned to consonants of these types can be applied to vowel symbols.

ATYPICAL PLACES OF ARTICULATION

The extIPA chart has the following places of articulation: bilabial, labiodental, dentolabial, labioalveolar, linguolabial, interdental, bidental, alveolar, velar, and velopharyngeal. Some of these are familiar to us from the normal IPA chart and are included here because they are found with some atypical manners of articulation. We will look, then, only at some of these places in this section. Rather than devise brand-new symbols for atypical sounds, the extIPA chart mostly provides sets of diacritics to add to IPA symbols.

Atypical Labial Places of Articulation

The three places of articulation *dentolabial*, *labioalveolar*, and *linguolabial* have been encountered in atypical clinical speech. Recalling the term *labiodental* (lower lip to upper teeth), dentolabial refers to upper lip articulating against the upper edge of the lower front teeth (indeed, we may also find the label *reverse labiodental* for this place of articulation). This type of articulation can be made with a variety of consonant types: plosives, nasals, and fricatives. These sounds are transcribed through the addition of a diacritic to symbols for labial consonants, and to emphasize the dental nature of these sounds the IPA dental diacritic is adopted. However, whereas for dental articulations this diacritic is placed beneath the consonant symbol (e.g., [t̪] is a dental plosive), for dentolabial articulations the diacritic is placed above the relevant symbol: [p͆, b͆, m͆, f͆, v͆]. Figure 20.1 illustrates this place of articulation.

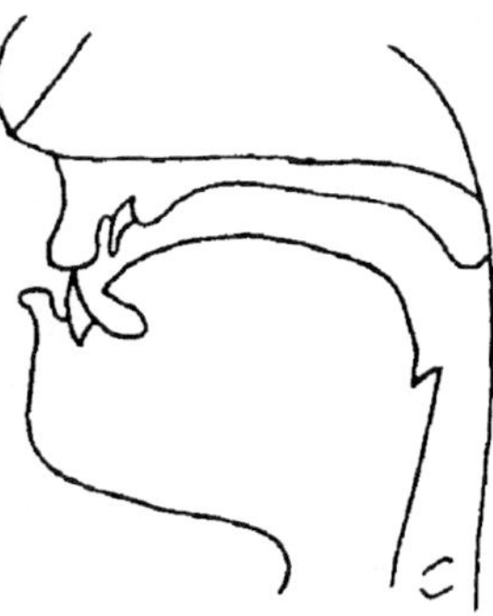

FIG 20.1. Dentolabial place of articulation.

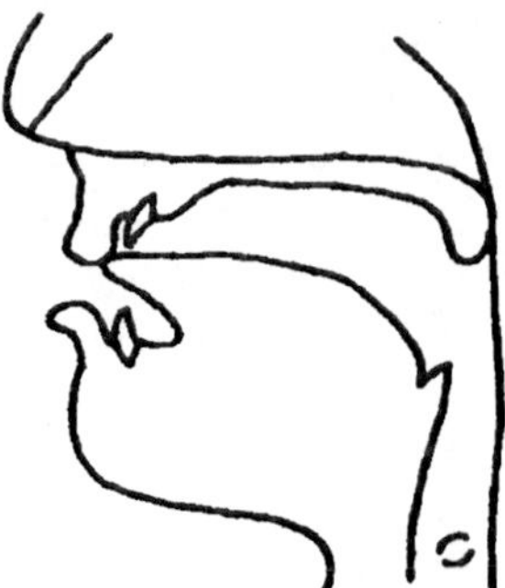

FIG 20.2. Linguolabial place of articulation.

Labioalveolar articulations can only be made easily if the speaker has an underbite. In such cases, an attempt to make a bilabial or a labiodental contact may result in the lower lip moving inside the upper lip and upper dentition and making contact with the alveolar ridge. In transcription, we assume that the target articulations in these cases are bilabial and labiodental, and so we use the symbols for these sounds to which we add the alveolar diacritic. The IPA has no diacritic for alveolar, and to fill this gap the extIPA symbols provide a subscript equals sign to represent this place of articulation. Labioalveolars can be made as plosives, nasals, and fricatives, and are transcribed as [p͇, b͇, m͇, f͇, v͇].

The linguolabial place of articulation has, in fact, been found in a few languages, but is extremely rare. Nevertheless, it is also reported reasonably often in disordered speech, so we feel it appropriate to include it here. Further, it seems that the kind of linguolabial articulations found in the clinic may involve a greater amount of tongue tip protrusion than is found in natural language (see also interdental below). As the name suggests, this place of articulation has contact between the tongue tip and the center of the upper lip, and is found with plosives, nasals, trills, fricatives, and the lateral approximant. These sounds are transcribed through the use of a diacritic designed to resemble the shape of the upper lip (though its nickname is *seagull*), which is added to alveolar symbols: [t̼, d̼, n̼, r̼, θ̼, ð̼, l̼]. Figure 20.2 shows a linguolabial articulation.

The extIPA chart also shows labiodental plosives. These sounds are rarely encountered as phonemes in the world's languages; however, they are encountered as allophones of bilabial plosives in English (and other languages), as we described in chapter 13. They are not, then, atypical sounds. Nevertheless, the extIPA chart includes them for two reasons. First, there are no IPA symbols for labiodental plosives, so there is no recognized way of symbolizing them. Second, labiodental plosives are encountered in disordered speech as misarticulations of target bilabial plosives or labiodental fricatives. They are symbolized through the addition of the dental diacritic to the bilabial plosive symbols: [p̪, b̪].

Atypical Dental Places of Articulation

Interdental, as used on the extIPA chart, is to be distinguished from dental, as found, for example, with the fricatives [θ, ð]. Although it is true that these two fricatives are often pronounced in English with a small amount of tongue-tip protrusion between the upper and lower teeth, interdental as used here refers to an excessive and visible amount of tongue protrusion involving the tip and often the blade (and sometimes even the front of the tongue body). This tongue protrusion can be found with a wide range of sounds, and we transcribe these by adding the dental diacritic both above and below the relevant symbol. This can be seen in the following

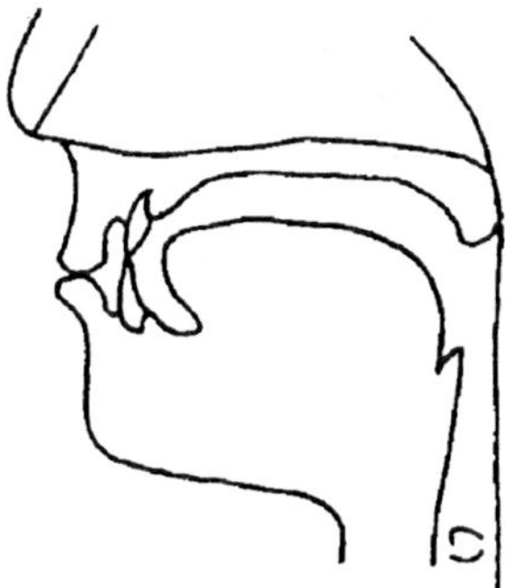

FIG 20.3. Bidental place of articulation.

examples: [t̪͆, n̪͆, θ̪͆, ð̪͆, l̪͆]. If tongue protrusion is employed as a persistent feature throughout a client's speech and irrespective of the target sound, then we can mark this over an entire stretch of speech; we show how this is done later in this chapter.

Bidental articulations involve the upper and lower teeth, and can be found with percussives (see later) or fricatives. Bidental fricatives are produced by forcing turbulent air through the slight gap between the upper and lower teeth when they are clenched together, and these fricatives are transcribed by using the symbols for the voiceless and voiced glottal fricatives with the addition of the upper and lower dental diacritics: [h̪͆, ɦ̪͆]. The choice of the glottal fricative symbols ensures that these sounds are not confused with tongue protrusion sounds, because the glottal fricatives lack any tongue involvement. As with the previous place, clinical data may show speakers using a teeth-clenched mode of articulation for all or most of their sounds on occasion; we will see below how we can mark whole stretches of speech for this feature. Figure 20.3 shows a bidental articulation.

The following client displayed both linguolabial and interdental articulations, though phonemic contrasts were actually maintained:

thin	[θ̪͆ɪn̼]	so	[s̼oʊ]
cat	[tæt̼]	foot	[ɸʊt̼]
shop	[sɑp]	dog	[d̼ɑd]
both	[boʊθ̪͆]	tease	[t̼iz̼]
that	[ð̪͆æt̼]	goose	[dus̼]

Velopharyngeal Place of Articulation

This atypical place of articulation is the velopharyngeal port (or opening) itself. As we have seen in chapter 6, the velum is lowered to allow air to flow through the nasal cavity (to produce nasal stops, nasalized vowels, and so forth). If the velum is only lowered very slightly, and air is forced through this narrow gap into the nasal cavity, then velopharyngeal friction occurs. The resultant sound (sometimes termed a *velopharyngeal snort*) is symbolized by [ʩ]. However, just as nasalization can accompany a range of other sounds, so velopharyngeal friction can be added to other vowels and consonants. To show this, we use a diacritic on the symbol of the basic sound, this diacritic being a double nasalization mark: [s͋, o͋].

> The following transcription is of an adult male speaker with disfluency. The target sentence is "the top nations of the world." He uses the velopharyngeal fricative as well as some features described in the following sections of this chapter:
>
> [ðə tˢ'\tʴ (.) {$_p$ t'\t'$_p$}ʩ\{$_f$ʩ\ʩ$_f$}\ˈt̤ɒp˺ ˈneʃənz əv ðə ˈwɝld]

ATYPICAL MANNERS OF ARTICULATION

The extIPA chart contains only three atypical manners of articulation (the other manners listed on the chart are there to illustrate the atypical places of articulation we have just described). Both diacritics and new symbols were devised for these manners.

Fricatives

In our survey of fricatives in chapter 6, we noted that central (or median) fricatives were those where the air flowed centrally along the surface of the tongue, whereas lateral fricatives were those where the air flowed sideways over the left or right side rim of the tongue. In some mis-articulations encountered in the clinic we find the use of a narrow central groove for airflow coupled with a lateral gap further around the edge of the tongue. There are, thus, two separate openings, allowing two separate airflows (both turbulent). Only alveolar lateral-median fricatives have been regularly noted, and the double articulation characteristics of these sounds is shown in transcription by using symbols that are a combination of [l] and [s] or [z] (for voiceless and voiced, respectively): [ʪ, ʫ].

The other atypical kind of fricative is the *nareal fricative*. We looked at voiced and voiceless nasal stops in chapter 6 and noted that these sounds have nonturbulent airflow (so they are classed as sonorants). It is possible, however, to produce nasal stops with turbulent airflow at the nares (the nostrils), and this is what happens with these atypical sounds. Nareal fricatives may be produced by speakers with a cleft palate in an attempt to make normal fricatives. We transcribe these sounds by adding a nareal fricative diacritic to a nasal stop symbol. As nareal friction (also called *nasal escape*) can also be made to accompany other types of sounds, this diacritic may be added to other symbols as well: [n͋, v͋].

> Nareal friction is used by this speaker with cleft palate. Notice also the widespread use of glottal stops (a common feature of cleft palate speech) and the unusual occurrence of a bilabial click:

baby	[b͋eɪbi]	toy	[ʔɔɪ]
cat	[ʔæʔʰ]	tap	[ʔæʔʘ]
bucket	[b͋ʊʔɪʔʰ]	Sue	[ç͋u]
sugar	[ç͋ɬʊʔə]	shoe	[ç͋ʷu]

Percussives

Percussives are articulations where two rigid or semirigid articulators are struck against each other to produce a short, sharp sound. Percussives are most often noted as occuring when the upper and lower teeth are brought sharply together (a bidental percussive), although the flapping together of the upper and lower lip can also produce percussive articulation (bilabial percussive). To symbolize these two percussives, the extIPA system makes use of the dental and bilabial diacritics, doubling them to represent the two sets of teeth and the two lips: [ʬ, ʭ].

Percussives are strange sounds in that it is not altogether clear whether one needs a pulmonic egressive airstream to produce them. The actual movement together of the articulators seems to produce enough airflow to allow the resultant striking together to be made audible. Percussives, therefore, may be found within a run of ordinary consonants and vowels (as substitutions for a particular sound or class of sounds), or may be used extralinguistically by a client in much the same way that speakers use clicks in English to express annoyance or encouragement.

Diacritics for Other Atypical Manners of Articulation

The extIPA chart has a boxed section beneath the main chart containing a range of diacritics. Many of these have already been described in the sections on place and manner above. There are a few diacritics—mainly connected with how articulations are carried out—that we will survey here.

Whereas the IPA provides a diacritic to show labialization, they do not have one to denote the opposite: lip-spreading. This double-headed arrow is placed beneath a symbol to show it was articulated with a spread-lip mouth shape: [s͍]. This may be useful in noting when lip-spreading was used unexpectedly by a speaker.

Strong and weak articulation diacritics are to be used when the transcriber notes a force of articulation clearly stronger or weaker than the norm for the sound in question. Strong articulations may be encountered, for example, in disfluent speech when the speaker emerges from a block (i.e., a silent period during which the speaker is struggling to produce a sound). On the other hand, weak articulations are characteristic of speakers with certain types of dysarthria where the muscles used in speech production are unable to hold an articulation as firmly as required. The strength of articulation diacritics are placed beneath the relevant symbol: [f͈, v͉].

Apart from using blocks, speakers with disfluency may also produce rapid reiterations of segments or combinations of segments. There have been numerous suggestions of how to transcribe these, from periods to hyphens. The extIPA system prefers the use of the back-slash, so a reiterated consonant would be shown as [p\p\p], while a reiterated syllable would be [pɛ\pɛ\pɛ].

> The speaker with disfluency we looked at earlier also shows examples of strong articulation and reiteration. In this example, the target utterance is "held at fourteen." The strong articulation follows a double-length pause (these are described in more detail below in the connected speech section):
>
> [(..) ˈh͈ɛld ə\ ʔat ˈf\fɔɹtin]
>
> An example of weak articulation is found in the following example from an adult male with spastic dysarthria. The target utterance is "close the window":
>
> [hloʊh ə wɪnd͉oʊ]

The diacritic for *whistled* articulation is used when a speaker creates a groove (usually for target /s/ and /z/) that is too narrow, and the resultant airflow creates a whistling sound. The diacritic (an arrow head) is placed beneath the symbol: [s͎].

The sliding articulation diacritic is for those cases where a speaker moves rapidly from one place of articulation to another, within the time slot for a single segment. This can be encountered when a client is acquiring a new place of articulation (perhaps through therapy), but still slips back into the old, substituted, place. This diacritic can only be used when the places are neighbors, and this sliding articulation should not be confused with clusters or with affricates: [θ͢s].

The remaining diacritics in this part of the chart have already been dealt with, either in this or in previous chapters.

VOICING

It may occur that we need to provide a more detailed account of vocal fold activity in a transcription than is covered by the IPA symbols and diacritics. This is especially the case when we are transcribing speech that has been analyzed through spectrographic investigation, and where we can see when the voicing starts and ends in relation to other articulatory events. The IPA provides the subscript v to mark voice, and the subscript circle to mark voicelessness, and the extIPA section on voicing expands usage patterns for these two diacritics. So, if we wish to mark that voicing started earlier than expected or lasted longer than expected we can use the subscript-v offset to the left or right of the relevant symbol: [ˬz], [zˬ]. In the same way, if we want to mark preaspiration (where aspiration commences before rather than after the release of a plosive), we can simply move the aspiration diacritic to the left of the plosive: [ʰp]. It can be noted that preaspiration is normal in some languages, but not in most varieties of English. This section of the extIPA chart also shows the unaspirated diacritic. Although lack of aspiration is often a perfectly normal feature (e.g., after /s/ in English), the IPA does not officially recognize the diacritic. As clinical phoneticians may need it to mark unexpected lack of aspiration, it is included on the extIPA chart.

Partial devoicing of target voiced sounds and partial voicing of target voiceless sounds can be shown by putting the voice and voiceless diacritics into parentheses: [z₍̥₎], [s₍̬₎]. We can even show whether the partial voicing or devoicing was at the beginning or end of the sound in question by using a single left or right bracket. This amount of detail may be difficult to discern from listening to speech but, as we noted earlier, it can be seen in acoustic analysis, which in turn may need to be included in a transcription.

RESOLVING UNCERTAINTY IN TRANSCRIPTION

We do not always have access to instrumental analyses to help us determine what the articulations are in a difficult passage of speech. This means that we cannot always be certain that the transcriptions we chose in such circumstances best represent what the speaker was doing. There may be many reasons for such uncertainty. The quality of the recording may not be good; there may be a lot of background noise, or several speakers may be speaking at once; there may be distortions to the individual sound segments due to the use of an unusual voice quality; or the individual sounds themselves may be so atypical that the transcriber is simply unsure what they are.

However, we don't want to leave blanks in a transcription if at all possible, and it may well be the case that, although we are unsure of the exact sound being used, we might be able to recognize aspects of it. For example, we may be able to tell that the sound in question is a consonant rather than a vowel; that it is a plosive rather than a fricative; that it is voiced rather than voiceless; that it is bilabial rather than velar; that it could very well be the sound [z]. The extIPA system allows us to mark these varying degrees of certainty through the use of the circle. The information one is reasonably confident about is put into the relevant place in the transcription, and then circled to show the overall uncertainty. So ◯ represents an indeterminate sound segment, and (C̲̄) an indeterminate consonant. (V̲̄) denotes an indeterminate vowel, and a (P̲̅l̲̅.v̲̅l̲̅s̲̅) voiceless plosive of indeterminate place of articulation. Finally, (z̲̅) shows the way of transcribing a sound that you think is probably [z], but about which you are not absolutely sure.

This "uncertainty" section of the chart also contains a few other symbols. A *silent articulation* or *mouthing* occurs when a speaker makes visible movements of the articulators appropriate for a particular target sound, but then omits the sound and produces the following sound in the word in question. Naturally, we can only see these silent articulations in bilabial and labiodental consonants, and perhaps dental fricatives, together with the lip rounding found with certain vowels and consonants such as English /ʃ/ and /ɹ/ (e.g., [(ʃ)]). Nevertheless, it is important to distinguish these mouthings from simple omissions of a sound: The silent articulation shows that the speaker has the sound slotted into the correct place in the syllable structure of the word, and has even got the correct articulatory configuration. The problem, therefore, lies with the instantiation of the sound. An omission implies that the sound is missing from the make-up of the target word altogether. Different therapeutic strategies will be needed to deal with these alternatives.

Finally, we can note the use of the asterisk to mark a sound that has no symbol in either the IPA or extIPA systems. The asterisk would be repeated after the transcription together with a description of the nature of the sound in question. As we noted earlier, the extIPA symbols were not designed to cover every possible atypical sound that may occur in the clinic, but only the most commonly reported. The asterisk, therefore, can fill the gap for the less common atypical sounds.

CONNECTED SPEECH

Connected speech phenomena that may need to be recorded when transcribing disordered speech include voice quality, tempo, loudness, and pausing. Some aspects of voice quality (both laryngeal and supralaryngeal) were described in chapter 4, and we take the opportunity here to revise these and add others. All the symbols needed for voice quality transcription are shown in the VoQS chart (voice quality symbols), included in appendix 1. We return below to how prosodic features can be added to a transcription.

For tempo and loudness we adopt the same terminology as used in music. On musical scores there are notations that show when a fast or slow tempo should be used, or when the musicians should play softly or loudly. These terms are taken from Italian, and include *allegro* and *lento* for fast and slow; and *piano (p)* and *forte (f)* for soft and loud, with *pp* and *ff* the abbreviations for very soft and very loud. Further terms, such as *crescendo* (getting louder) and *ralentando* (slowing down), can be used if necessary.

Pausing is often ignored in phonetic transcription. It may be assumed to be of no importance. However, in the investigation of disordered speech, the position and duration of pauses may be important in a range of disorders (such as stuttering and adult acquired disorders). There have been numerous suggestions as to how best to transcribe pauses; the extIPA system recommends periods with parentheses (to distinguish the periods from any similar diacritical marks). One, two, or three periods represent one, two, or three beats of the speaker's normal rhythm. Any pauses longer than that should be shown by placing the time elapsed within the parentheses instead of periods, e.g., (2 s).

Finally, we can consider how this connected speech information can be integrated with a segmental transcription. Any voice quality, tempo, or loudness symbols that need to be employed are linked to a pair of braces (i.e., brackets of this kind: {}). The left-hand brace shows where the feature or features commence, and the right-hand one is placed where the feature or features end. These braces are then situated within the linear transcription at the appropriate locations. For example, if during a stretch of speech, a speaker switches from normal loudness to a very soft voice, and the switches to a slightly soft voice and then back to normal loudness, this would be shown like this:

> [ðə ˈɹeɪnboʊ ɪz ə dɪˈvɪʒn̩ əv{$_{pp}$ˈwaɪt ˈlaɪt ɪntu ˈmɛni ˈbjutɪfʊl ˈkʌlɚz ðiz ˈteɪk ðə ˈʃeɪp əv ə ˈlɑŋ ˈɹaʊnd ˈɑɹtʃ$_{pp}$}{$_{p}$ wɪð ɪts ˈpæθ ˈhaɪ əˈbʌv $_{p}$} ɪts ˈtu ˈɛndz əˈpæɹəntli bəˈjɑnd ðə həˈɹaɪzn̩]

If we need to show a particular voice quality, we can adopt the same formalism. In this example, the speaker is using harsh voice quality throughout. Numerals (from 1 to 3) can be used with the voice quality symbol to show the degree of the particular voice quality; here the change in degree is signalled by the numeral alone.

> [{1V! ju ˈwɪʃt tu ˈnoʊ ˈɔl əˈbaʊt maɪ ˈgɹændfɑðɚ {2 ˈwɛl hi ɪz ˈnɪɹli ˈnaɪnti ˈθɹi 2} ˈjɝz ˈoʊld 1V!}]

It is, of course, perfectly possible to have information on voice quality, tempo, and loudness all marked in a similar way through the use of labeled braces. However, if we have too much prosodic information added to a linear transcription, it may become unreadable. In such cases, we may wish to use multilayered transcriptions, where information on segmental and suprasegmental aspects of speech (and also on gaze, gesture, and aspects of the conversation) is entered onto separate tiers.

EXAMPLE

The following example combines many of the segmental and prosodic transcription conventions discussed in this chapter. The speaker is a disfluent adult male whose target accent is Northern Irish English. See if you can identify all of the symbols for atypical speech in the sample. The speaker was recorded reading the following passage:

> The World Cup Finals of nineteen eighty-two are held in Spain this year. They will involve the top nations of the world in a tournament lasting over four weeks held at fourteen different centers in Spain. All of the first round games will be in the provincial towns, with the semifinals and final held in Barcelona and Madrid.

The transcription is as follows:

> [ð\ð:ə̤ {V̰ ə\ə\ə V̰}ˈhw̥ɝld ˈkʌp f \ˈfaɪnəlz əv ˈnaɪntin eəti {↓$_{p}$ˈtʉ $_{p}$↓} ˌɑɹ h\ˈhɛld ɪn s:p\ˈs:p\ʰe ᵊn ˈðɪs ˌjɝ (3s) ð̤:e wɪl inv\ˈv̤:ɔlv ðə tˢ\tʲ (.) {$_{p}$ t'\t'$_{p}$}fŋ\ {$_{f}$fŋ\fŋ$_{f}$} \ˈt̤ŏp̚ ˈneʃənz əv ðə ˈwɝld ɪnˑə {$_{pp}$tʰˑəʃ t ʰə\tə\ʃ$_{p}$}\ˈt̤ʉɹnəmənt ˈlastɪn ˌoʊvɚ ˈfɔɹ ˈwiks (..) ˈh̤ɛld ə\ʔat f\ˈfɔɹtin (...) {$_{pp}$ V̰ d\d\d V̰$_{pp}$}\ˈdɪfɹənt ˈsɛn{↓tɚz↓} ɪn ˈspeᵊn (3s) ə̰ (.) ˈɔl əv ðə fˑ\f ˈɔl əv ðə ˈf̤ɝst ˈɹaʉnd ˈgeᵊmz wɪl bi (.) ɪn ðə (.) w̰̆ə̰: p\pɹəv\ˈvɪnʃəl {$_{p}$ t'\t'$_{p}$} {$_{pp}$ t'\t'$_{pp}$} (.) t'\t'{$_{pp}$ t'\t'$_{pp}$} \fŋ\fŋ {↓ˈtãʉ̃nz ↓} wɪð ðə s'\s'\ˈs{↓ɛmi ˈfaɪnəlz ↓} and f\ˈfaɪnəl ˈhɛld ɪn (.) ˌbɑɹsə{$_{p}$ ˈloʊnə ənd ˈmədɹɪd $_{p}$}]

Note: Predictable vowel length is not marked; predictable consonant qualities (e.g., aspiration) are not marked on fluent items.

BACKGROUND READING

Ball et al. (1996) is a good source for material on clinical transcription; while Ball et al. (1999) describes the VoQS symbols in some detail. The examples given in this chapter are from Ball, Code, Rahilly, and Hazlitt (1994) and Ball et al. (1996) and from our own files.

EXERCISES

Transcription

(Answers to the transcription exercises are given at the end of the book.)

1. What transcriptions (using either GA or RP norms) would you expect to produce of the following target items if you were told the speaker exhibited dentolabial articulations for all target labiodental and bilabial consonants and linguolabial articulations for all target alveolars and dentals?
   thumb ten fun
   date van then
   that five teeth
   laugh thought late

2. What transcriptions (using either GA or RP norms) would you expect to produce of the following target items if you were told the speaker exhibited velopharyngeal fricatives for all target fricatives (except word-finally); velopharyngeal friction accompanying all nasal and oral stops (except word-finally); nasalization on vowels; and glottal stops for all word final consonants?
   thumb ten fun
   date van then
   that five teeth
   laugh thought late

3. What do you think the target words were for the following transcribed items? The speaker exhibits a set of problems in articulating anterior lingual fricatives. Vowels are GA norms.
   [çuʫ] [ʫil] [ˈʪæçɪʫ]
   [ʪplæç] [ʪmuð̪͆] [ʫið̪͆]
   [θ̪͆ɪmbl] [ʪaŋʫ] [hiʪ]
   [ˈçɑpɪŋ] [ð̪͆ɪʪ] [hiʫ]

Review Questions

1. What is the difference between "disordered speech" and "atypical speech"?
2. What are the main atypical places and manners of articulation?
3. How can we show in a transcription of disordered speech how certain (or uncertain) we are of the appropriateness of our choice of symbols?
4. How can the transcription of prosodic information be integrated with segmental transcription? Illustrate your answer.

Study Topics and Experiments

1. Record a natural conversation of about 6 minutes between some of your friends, and transcribe the middle 4 minutes of speech using normal orthography. Then add to the

transcription details on pausing, loudness, tempo, and voice quality using the symbols described in this chapter. Comment on the ease (or otherwise) of the task, and the amount of prosodic information you have marked. How did you deal with overlapping speech between two conversants?

2. Using the samples on the CD compare the acoustic characteristics of linguolabial fricatives with dental fricatives, and dentolabial with labiodental fricatives. Produce broad band spectrograms of the sounds, and look in detail at the noise spectra.

CD

In this section we give examples of disordered speech that contain some of the atypical sounds described in the chapter. Because many of these atypical sounds require visual as well as auditory input for adequate transcription, we have not included any exercises on the CD.

Appendix 1

THE INTERNATIONAL PHONETIC ALPHABET (revised to 1993, updated 1996)

CONSONANTS (PULMONIC)

	Bilabial	Labiodental	Dental	Alveolar	Postalveolar	Retroflex	Palatal	Velar	Uvular	Pharyngeal	Glottal
Plosive	p b			t d		ʈ ɖ	c ɟ	k ɡ	q ɢ		ʔ
Nasal	m	ɱ		n		ɳ	ɲ	ŋ	ɴ		
Trill	ʙ			r					ʀ		
Tap or Flap				ɾ		ɽ					
Fricative	ɸ β	f v	θ ð	s z	ʃ ʒ	ʂ ʐ	ç ʝ	x ɣ	χ ʁ	ħ ʕ	h ɦ
Lateral fricative				ɬ ɮ							
Approximant		ʋ		ɹ		ɻ	j	ɰ			
Lateral approximant				l		ɭ	ʎ	ʟ			

Where symbols appear in pairs, the one to the right represents a voiced consonant. Shaded areas denote articulations judged impossible.

CONSONANTS (NON-PULMONIC)

Clicks	Voiced implosives	Ejectives
ʘ Bilabial	ɓ Bilabial	ʼ Examples:
ǀ Dental	ɗ Dental/alveolar	pʼ Bilabial
ǃ (Post)alveolar	ʄ Palatal	tʼ Dental/alveolar
ǂ Palatoalveolar	ɠ Velar	kʼ Velar
ǁ Alveolar lateral	ʛ Uvular	sʼ Alveolar fricative

VOWELS

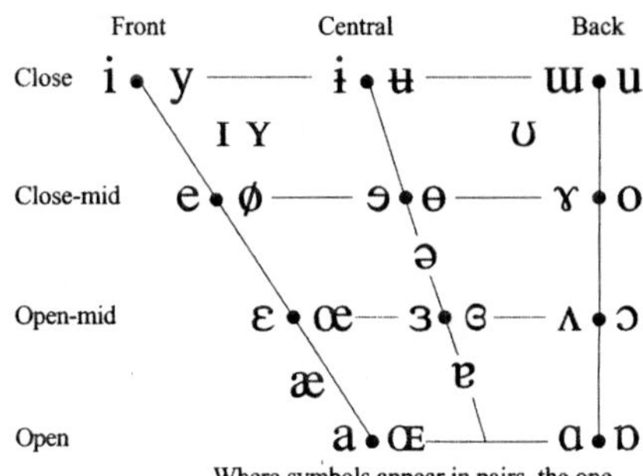

Where symbols appear in pairs, the one to the right represents a rounded vowel.

OTHER SYMBOLS

ʍ Voiceless labial-velar fricative

w Voiced labial-velar approximant

ɥ Voiced labial-palatal approximant

ʜ Voiceless epiglottal fricative

ʢ Voiced epiglottal fricative

ʡ Epiglottal plosive

ɕ ʑ Alveolo-palatal fricatives

ɺ Alveolar lateral flap

ɧ Simultaneous ʃ and x

Affricates and double articulations can be represented by two symbols joined by a tie bar if necessary. k͡p t͜s

SUPRASEGMENTALS

ˈ Primary stress

ˌ Secondary stress ˌfoʊnəˈtɪʃən

ː Long eː

ˑ Half-long eˑ

˘ Extra-short ĕ

| Minor (foot) group

‖ Major (intonation) group

. Syllable break ɹi.ækt

‿ Linking (absence of a break)

DIACRITICS Diacritics may be placed above a symbol with a descender, e.g. ŋ̊

Voiceless	n̥ d̥	Breathy voiced	b̤ a̤	Dental	t̪ d̪
Voiced	s̬ t̬	Creaky voiced	b̰ a̰	Apical	t̺ d̺
Aspirated	tʰ dʰ	Linguolabial	t̼ d̼	Laminal	t̻ d̻
More rounded	ɔ̹	Labialized	tʷ dʷ	Nasalized	ẽ
Less rounded	ɔ̜	Palatalized	tʲ dʲ	Nasal release	dⁿ
Advanced	u̟	Velarized	tˠ dˠ	Lateral release	dˡ
Retracted	e̠	Pharyngealized	tˤ dˤ	No audible release	d̚
Centralized	ë	Velarized or pharyngealized	ɫ		
Mid-centralized	e̽	Raised	e̝ (ɹ̝ = voiced alveolar fricative)		
Syllabic	n̩	Lowered	e̞ (β̞ = voiced bilabial approximant)		
Non-syllabic	e̯	Advanced Tongue Root	e̘		
Rhoticity	ɚ a˞	Retracted Tongue Root	e̙		

TONES AND WORD ACCENTS

LEVEL		CONTOUR	
e̋ or ˥	Extra high	ě or ˩˥	Rising
é ˦	High	ê ˥˩	Falling
ē ˧	Mid	e᷄ ˦˥	High rising
è ˨	Low	e᷅ ˩˨	Low rising
ȅ ˩	Extra low	e᷈ ˧˦˧	Rising-falling
↓	Downstep	↗	Global rise
↑	Upstep	↘	Global fall

extIPA SYMBOLS FOR DISORDERED SPEECH

(Revised to 2002)

CONSONANTS (other than on the IPA Chart)

	bilabial	labiodental	dentolabial	labioalv.	linguolabial	interdental	bidental	alveolar	velar	velophar.
Plosive		p̪ b̪	p͆ b͆	p̪͇ b̪͇	t̼ d̼	t̪͆ d̪͆				
Nasal			m͆	m̪͇	n̼	n̪͆				
Trill					r̼	r̪͆g				
Fricative median			f͆ v͆	f̪͇ v̪͇	θ̼ ð̼	θ̪͆ ð̪͆	h̪͆ ɦ̪͆			fŋ
Fricative lateral+median								ʪ ʫ		
Fricative nareal	m͋							n͋	ŋ͋	
Percussive	ʬ						ʭ			
Approximant lateral					l̼	l̪͆				

Where symbols appear in pairs, the one to the right represents a voiced consonant. Shaded areas denote articulations judged impossible.

DIACRITICS

͍	labial spreading	s͍	͈	strong articulation	f͈	͊	denasal	m͊
͆	dentolabial	v͆	͉	weak articulation	v͉	͌	nasal escape	v͋
̪͆	interdental/bidental	n̪͆	\	reiterated articulation	p\p\p	≈	velopharyngeal friction	s͌
͇	alveolar	t͇	↑	whistled articulation	s͎	↓	ingressive airflow	p↓
̼	linguolabial	d̼	→	sliding articulation	θ͢s	↑	egressive airflow	!↑

CONNECTED SPEECH

(.)	short pause
(..)	medium pause
(...)	long pause
f	loud speech [{$_f$ laud $_f$}]
ff	louder speech [{$_{ff}$ laudə˞ $_{ff}$}]
p	quiet speech [{$_p$ kwaɪət $_p$}]
pp	quieter speech [{$_{pp}$ kwaɪətə˞ $_{pp}$}]
allegro	fast speech [{$_{allegro}$ fast $_{allegro}$}]
lento	slow speech [{$_{lento}$ slou $_{lento}$}]
crescendo, ralentando, etc. may also be used	

VOICING

̬	pre-voicing	̬z
̬	post-voicing	z̬
₍̥₎	partial devoicing	₍z̥₎
₍̥	initial partial devoicing	₍z̥
̥₎	final partial devoicing	z̥₎
₍̬₎	partial voicing	₍s̬₎
₍̬	initial partial voicing	₍s̬
̬₎	final partial voicing	s̬₎
⁼	unaspirated	p⁼
ʰ	pre-aspiration	ʰp

OTHERS

◯, (C̲)	indeterminate sound, consonant	(( ))	extraneous noise	((2 sylls))
(V̲), (P̲l̲.̲ v̲l̲s̲)	indeterminate vowel, voiceless plosive, etc.	°	sublaminal lower alveolar percussive click	
(N̲), (v̲)	indeterminate nasal, probably [v], etc.	!¡	alveolar and sublaminal clicks (cluck-click)	
( )	silent articulation (ʃ), (m)	*	sound with no available symbol	

VoQS: Voice Quality Symbols

Airstream Types

Œ	œsophageal speech	И	electrolarynx speech
Ю	tracheo-œsophageal speech	↓	pulmonic ingressive speech

Phonation types

V	modal voice	F	falsetto
W	whisper	C	creak
V̤	whispery voice (murmur)	V̰	creaky voice
Vʰ	breathy voice	C̣	whispery creak
V!	harsh voice	V!!	ventricular phonation
V̬!!	diplophonia	V̤!!	whispery ventricular phonation
V̟	anterior or pressed phonation	W̠	posterior whisper

Supralaryngeal Settings

L̝	raised larynx	L̞	lowered larynx
Vᶱ	labialized voice (open round)	Vʷ	labialized voice (close round)
V͍	spread-lip voice	Vᶹ	labio-dentalized voice
V̺	linguo-apicalized voice	V̻	linguo-laminalized voice
V˞	retroflex voice	V̪	dentalized voice
V͇	alveolarized voice	V͇ʲ	palatoalveolarized voice
Vʲ	palatalized voice	Vˠ	velarized voice
Vʶ	uvularized voice	Vˤ	pharyngealized voice
V̝ˤ	laryngo-pharyngealized voice	Vᴴ	faucalized voice
Ṽ	nasalized voice	V͊	denasalized voice
J̞	open jaw voice	J̝	close jaw voice
J͔/J͕	right/left offset jaw voice	J̟	protruded jaw voice
◌̪͆	clenched teeth voice	Θ	protruded tongue voice

USE OF LABELED BRACES & NUMERALS TO MARK STRETCHES OF SPEECH AND DEGREES AND COMBINATIONS OF VOICE QUALITY:

[ˈðɪs ɪz ˈnɔɹməl ˈvɔɪs {3V! ˈðɪs ɪz ˈveɹi ˈhɑɹʃ ˈvɔɪs 3V} ˈðɪs ɪz ˈnɔɹməl ˈvɔɪs wʌns ˈmɔɹ {L̞ 1V! ˈðɪs ɪz ˈlɛs ˈhɑɹʃ ˈvɔɪs wɪð ˈloʊɚd ˈlæɹɪŋks 1V!L̞}]

Appendix 2

DISTINCTIVE FEATURES

The following are commonly used binary features, derived from the work of Chomsky and Halle (1968). These are the features needed for English; several other features are used for nonpulmonic sounds, for example.

Major Class Features

[± sonorant]: presence versus absence of open vocal tract. [+ sonorant] are vowels, glides, liquids, and nasals.

[± consonantal]: presence versus absence of high degree of oral obstruction. [+ consonantal] are plosives, affricates, fricatives, and nasals.

[± syllabic]: presence versus absence of ability to site the nucleus of a syllable. [+ syllabic] are vowels, syllabic liquids, and syllabic nasals. (An older label [± vocalic] with a similar definition may also be encountered.)

Place of Articulation Features

[± coronal]: use versus nonuse of the tip/blade of the tongue. [+ coronal] are dental, alveolar, and postalveolar sounds.

[± anterior]: use versus nonuse of the front of the oral cavity. [+ anterior] are bilabial, labiodental, dental, and alveolar sounds.

[± high]: use of high versus nonhigh tongue position. [+ high] are high vowels and postalveolar, palatal, and velar consonants.

[± low]: use of low versus nonlow tongue position. [+ low] are low vowels and pharyngeal and glottal consonants. Note: mid vowels are [− high, − low].

[± back]: use of back versus nonback tongue position. [+ back] are back vowels and velar, uvular, and pharyngeal consonants.

[± round]: use of rounded versus nonrounded lip shape. [+ round] are round vowels and [w].

Manner of Articulation Features

[± nasal]: use of open or closed nasal tract. [+ nasal] are the nasal stops and nasalized vowels.

[± lateral]: use or otherwise of lateral airflow. [+ lateral] are /l/ and any other lateral approximants.

[± continuant]: use or nonuse of continuing airflow through the oral cavity. [+ continuant] are vowels, glides, liquids, and fricatives. Nasals, plosives, and affricates are [− continuant].

[± delayed release] (or [± del rel]): use or otherwise of slow release of obstruction. [+ del rel] are affricates.

[± tense]: use or otherwise of muscular tension. Fortis consonants and tense vowels are [+ tense]; lenis consonants and lax vowels are [− tense].

Source Features

[± voice]: use or otherwise of vibrating vocal folds. All vowels and voiced consonants are [+ voice]; voiceless consonants are [− voice].

[± strident]: presence versus absence of noisy friction. [+ strident] are the labiodental, alveolar, and postalveolar fricatives and the postalveolar affricates.

Feature Matrices

The following feature matrices show feature values for some vowels and consonants of English.

TABLE 1
Monophthongal Vowels of English

	i	ɪ	ɛ	æ	ɑ	ɔ	ʊ	u	ʌ
son	+	+	+	+	+	+	+	+	+
cons	−	−	−	−	−	−	−	−	−
syll	+	+	+	+	+	+	+	+	+
cor	−	−	−	−	−	−	−	−	−
ant	−	−	−	−	−	−	−	−	−
high	+	+	−	−	−	−	+	+	−
low	−	−	−	+	+	+	−	−	−
back	−	−	−	−	+	+	+	+	+
round	−	−	−	−	−	+	+	+	−
tense	+	−	−	−	+	−	−	+	−

Note: Chomsky and Halle treated diphthongs as sequences of vowel + glide. Therefore, /eɪ/ would be treated as /ej/, /oʊ/ as /ow/, etc.

TABLE 2
Selected Obstruents of English

	p	b	t	g	θ	v	s	z	ʒ	tʃ	dʒ
son	−	−	−	−	−	−	−	−	−	−	−
cons	+	+	+	+	+	+	+	+	+	+	+
syll	−	−	−	−	−	−	−	−	−	−	−
cor	−	−	+	−	+	−	+	+	+	+	+
ant	+	+	+	−	+	+	+	+	−	−	−
high	−	−	−	+	−	−	−	−	+	+	+
low	−	−	−	−	−	−	−	−	−	−	−
back	−	−	−	+	−	−	−	−	−	−	−
round	−	−	−	−	−	−	−	−	−	−	−
nas	−	−	−	−	−	−	−	−	−	−	−
lat	−	−	−	−	−	−	−	−	−	−	−
cont	−	−	−	−	+	+	+	+	+	−	−
delrel	−	−	−	−	−	−	−	−	−	+	+
voice	−	+	−	+	−	+	−	+	+	−	+
strid	−	−	−	−	−	+	+	+	+	+	+

TABLE 3
Sonorants of English

	m	n	ŋ	n̩	ɹ	ɹ̩	l	l̩	w	j	h
son	+	+	+	+	+	+	+	+	+	+	+
cons	+	+	+	+	+	+	+	+	−	−	−
syll	−	−	−	+	−	+	−	+	−	−	−
cor	−	+	−	+	+	+	+	+	−	−	−
ant	+	+	−	+	−	−	+	+	−	−	−
high	−	−	+	−	−	−	−	−	+	+	−
low	−	−	−	−	−	−	−	−	−	−	+
back	−	−	+	−	−	−	−	−	+	−	−
round	−	−	−	−	−	+	−	−	+	−	−
nas	+	+	+	+	−	−	−	−	−	−	−
lat	−	−	−	−	−	−	+	+	−	−	−
cont	−	−	−	−	+	+	+	+	+	+	+
delrel	−	−	−	−	−	−	−	−	−	−	−
voice	+	+	+	+	+	+	+	+	+	+	−
strid	−	−	−	−	−	−	−	−	−	−	−

PHONOLOGICAL PRIMES FOR ENGLISH
(Adapted from Harris, 1994)

Unlike distinctive features, phonological primes (or *elements*) are pronounceable. They do not have + and − values, but are either present or absent. Where a sound has two or more primes, one may "govern" the other (as a head element), or they may be equal partners. Diphthongs and affricates are considered to be double sounds and shown in tree diagrams below; in these diagrams the "N" at the head refers to the vowel nucleus, and the "O" to the consonant onset.

Elements for Vowels

Element	Phonetic realization
[A]	[ɑ]
[I]	[i]
[U]	[u]
[@]	[ə]

Combinations for the Vowels of English
(Head Elements are Underlined)

/i/ **[I]**
/ɑ **[A]**
/ɔ/ **[A, $\underline{\text{U}}$]**
/u/ **[U]**

/ɪ/ **[I, $\underline{\text{@}}$]**
/ɛ/ **[A, I, $\underline{\text{@}}$]**
/æ/ **[I, A]**
/ʌ/ **[$\underline{\text{@}}$]**
/ə/ **[@, $\underline{\text{@}}$]**
/ɒ/ **[U, A]**
/ʊ/ **[U, $\underline{\text{@}}$]**

/eɪ/

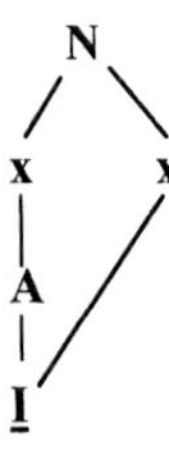

/aɪ/

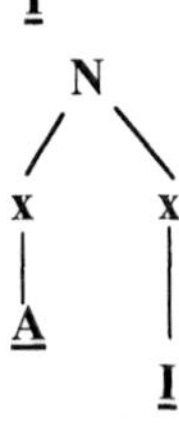

/oʊ/

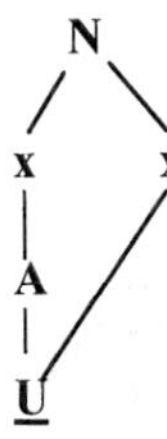

/aʊ/

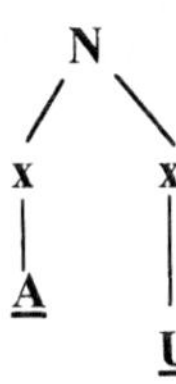

/ɔɪ/

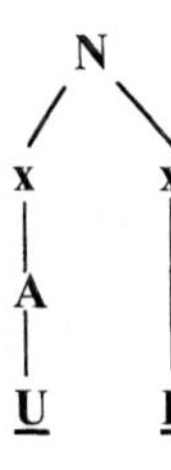

/ɚ/

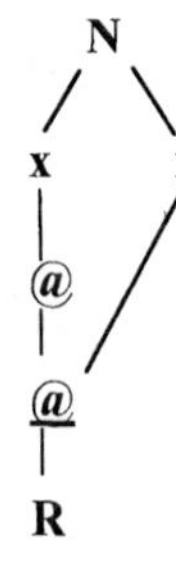

/ɝ/

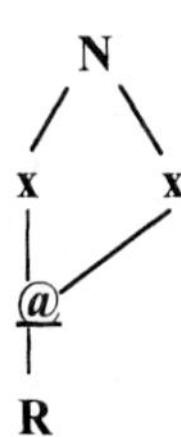

Elements for Consonants

Element	Phonetic realization
[?]	[ʔ]
[h]	[h]
[R]	[ɾ]
[I]	[j]
[U]	[w]
[@]	[ɣ]
[N]	[n]

The elements corresponding to the voiceless–voiced distinction are [**H**] and [**L**] respectively. [**H**] also implies aspiration in plosives. Because English "voiced" obstruents are rarely fully voiced, the [**L**] element is not attached to them. Because English sonorants are voiced by default, there is no need to add [**L**] to these either.

Combinations for the Consonants of English

(Head Elements are Underlined)

/p/ **[h, U, ?, H]**
/b/ **[h, U, ?]**
/t/ **[h, R, ?, H]**
/d/ **[h, R, ?]**
/k/ **[h, @, ?, H]**
/g/ **[h, @, ?]**

/f/ **[<u>h</u>, U, H]**
/v/ **[<u>h</u>, U]**
/θ/ **[h, <u>R</u>, H]**
/ð/ **[h, <u>R</u>]**
/s/ **[<u>h</u>, R, H]**
/z/ **[<u>h</u>, R]**
/ʃ/ **[<u>h</u>, R, I, H]**
/ʒ/ **[<u>h</u>, R, I]**
/h/ **[h]**

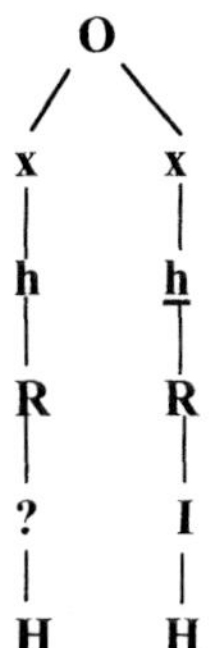

/dʒ/

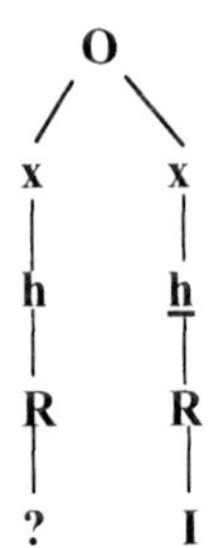

/m/ **[h, U, N, @]**
/n/ **[h, R, N, @]**
/ŋ/ **[h, @, N, @]**

/ɹ/ **[R, @]**
/l/ **[R, ?]**

/w/ **[U]**
/j/ **[I]**

NATURAL PHONOLOGICAL PROCESSES

The following are the commonly described processes adapted from the list provided by Grunwell (1987). The processes are divided into those that simplify the target phonological system, and those that simplify the target phonological structure.

We can also note the definition of a phonological process provided by Stampe (1979, p. 1): "A phonological process is a mental operation that applies in speech to substitute for a class of sounds or sound sequences presenting a common difficulty to the speech capacity of the individual, an alternative class identical but lacking the difficult property."

Processes Simplifying Structure

Weak syllable deletion; e.g., "umbrella" → [ˈbwɛlə]
Final consonant deletion; e.g., "cat" → [kæ]
Vocalization; e.g., "hill" → [hɪʊ]
Reduplication; e.g., "bottle" → [ˈbɑbɑ]
Consonant harmony; e.g., "doggy" → [ˈgɑgi] ~ [ˈdɑdi]
Cluster reduction; e.g., "scheme, cream, scream" → [kim]
Context-sensitive voicing; e.g., "cat" → [gæt]; "dog" → [dɑk]

Processes Simplifying System

Velar fronting; e.g., "gawking" → [ˈdɔtɪn]
Fricative stopping; e.g., "fish" → [pɪt]; "this" → [dɪt]
Fricative simplification; e.g., "fish" → [fɪs]; "this" → [vɪs]
Glottal replacement; e.g., "begin" → [ˈʔəʔɪʔ]

Answers to Transcription Exercises

Examples from other languages in the transcription exercises both in the book and on the CD are taken from Maddieson (1984), Laver (1994), Ladefoged and Maddieson (1996), the *Handbook of the IPA* (1999), Ball and Rahilly (1999) and the authors' own files. English examples are from the authors' own knowledge and with help from Cruttenden (2001) and Wells (1982, 2000). Examples from disordered speech are generally derived from the authors' own experience, but for ethical reasons are not identical to original sources except where cited in publications.

CHAPTER 11

1. GA

(a) need /nid/ (b) writ /ɹɪt/
(c) door /dɔɹ/ (d) cool /kul/
(e) foot /fʊt/ (f) kept /kɛpt/
(g) bat /bæt/ (h) stop /stɑp/
(i) tune /tun/ (j) meat /mit/
(k) head /hɛd/ (l) paw /pɑ/~/pɔ/
(m) lamb /læm/ (n) build /bɪld/
(o) put /pʊt/ (p) hot /hɑt/

RP

(a) need /nid/ (b) writ /ɹɪt/
(c) door /dɔ/ (d) cool /kul/
(e) foot /fʊt/ (f) kept /kɛpt/
(g) bat /bæt/ (h) stop /stɒp/
(i) tune /tjun/ (j) meat /mit/
(k) head /hɛd/ (l) paw /pɔ/
(m) lamb /læm/ (n) build /bɪld/
(o) put /pʊt/ (p) hot /hɒt/

2. GA

(a) feed [fiːd] (b) feat [fiˑt]
(c) queen [kwĩːn] (d) boot [buˑt]
(e) fool [fuᵊl] (f) bell [bɛᵊl]
(g) bat [bæ̆t] (h) bad [bæd]
(i) booed [buːd] (j) tin [tɪ̃n]
(k) spoon [spũːn] (l) awl [ɑᵊl]~[ɔᵊl]
(m) send [sɛ̃nd] (n) build [bɪᵊld]
(o) feel [fiᵊl] (p) hill [hɪᵊl]

RP

(a)	feed	[fɪːd]	(b)	feat	[fɪˑt]
(c)	queen	[kwɪ̃ːn]	(d)	boot	[buˑt]
(e)	fool	[fuᵊl]	(f)	bell	[bɛᵊl]
(g)	bat	[bæ̆t]	(h)	bad	[bæd]
(i)	booed	[buːd]	(j)	tin	[tɪ̃n]
(k)	spoon	[spũːn]	(l)	awl	[ɔᵊl]
(m)	send	[sɛ̃nd]	(n)	build	[bɪᵊld]
(o)	feel	[fɪᵊl]	(p)	hill	[hɪᵊl]

3.

(a)	/nɑt/	not, knot	(b)	/sin/	seen, scene
(c)	/lɛd/	led, lead	(d)	/flu/	flue, flu, flew
(e)	/ænt/	ant, aunt	(f)	/wʊd/	wood, would
(g)	/nɪt/	nit, knit	(h)	/sɔɹ/	soar, sore

CHAPTER 12

1. GA

(a)	purred	/pɝd/	(b)	cut	/kʌt/
(c)	why	/waɪ/	(d)	join	/dʒɔɪn/
(e)	loud	/laʊd/	(f)	stay	/steɪ/
(g)	slow	/sloʊ/	(h)	player	/pleɪɚ/
(i)	attend	/ətɛnd/	(j)	curse	/kɝs/
(k)	mower	/moʊɚ/	(l)	tailor	/teɪlɚ/
(m)	mother	/mʌðɚ/	(n)	kite	/kaɪt/
(o)	louse	/laʊs/	(p)	annoy	/ənɔɪ/

RP

(a)	purred	/pɜd/	(b)	cut	/kʌt/
(c)	why	/waɪ/	(d)	join	/dʒɔɪn/
(e)	loud	/laʊd/	(f)	stay	/steɪ/
(g)	slow	/sləʊ/	(h)	player	/pleɪə/
(i)	attend	/ətɛnd/	(j)	curse	/kɜs/
(k)	mower	/məʊə/	(l)	tailor	/teɪlə/
(m)	mother	/mʌðə/	(n)	kite	/kaɪt/
(o)	louse	/laʊs/	(p)	annoy	/ənɔɪ/

2. GA

(a)	bide	[baːɪd]	(b)	spurt	[spɝˑt]
(c)	turn	[tɝ̃ːn]	(d)	foal	[foᶷəl]
(e)	owl	[aᶷəl]	(f)	town	[tãʊ̃ːn]
(g)	bite	[baˑɪt]	(h)	loud	[laːʊd]
(i)	state	[steˑɪt]	(j)	isle	[aᶦəl]
(k)	lout	[laˑʊt]	(l)	stun	[stʌ̃n]
(m)	spurred	[spɝːd]	(n)	staid	[steːɪd]
(o)	spoil	[spɔᶦəl]	(p)	pail	[peᶦəl]

RP

(a)	bide	[baːɪd]	(b)	spurt	[spɜˑt]
(c)	turn	[tɜ̃ːn]	(d)	foal	[fəᶷəl]
(e)	owl	[aᶷəl]	(f)	town	[tãʊ̃ːn]
(g)	bite	[baˑɪt]	(h)	loud	[laːʊd]
(i)	state	[steˑɪt]	(j)	isle	[aᶦəl]
(k)	lout	[laˑʊt]	(l)	stun	[stʌ̃n]
(m)	spurred	[spɜːd]	(n)	staid	[steːɪd]
(o)	spoil	[spɔᶦəl]	(p)	pail	[peᶦəl]

3.

(a)	/ɹaɪt/	right, write	(b)	/baʊ/	bough, bow
(c)	/hɝd/	herd, heard	(d)	/steɪd/	staid, stayed
(e)	/moʊn/	mown, moan	(f)	/əsɜnt/	assent, ascent
(g)	/mænɚ/	manner, manor	(h)	/kɔɪ/	coy, koi
			(i)	/ɹʌf/	rough, ruff

CHAPTER 13

1. GA

(a)	bead	/bid/	(b)	get	/gɛt/
(c)	took	/tʊk/	(d)	pipe	/paɪp/
(e)	chew	/tʃu/	(f)	deep	/dip/
(g)	cog	/kɑg/	(h)	jaw	/dʒɑ/~/dʒɔ/
(i)	tube	/tub/	(j)	peat	/pit/
(k)	dead	/dɛd/	(l)	kit	/kɪt/
(m)	gap	/gæp/	(n)	boot	/but/
(o)	jab	/dʒæb/	(p)	chop	/tʃɑp/

RP

(a)	bead	/bid/	(b)	get	/gɛt/
(c)	took	/tʊk/	(d)	pipe	/paɪp/
(e)	chew	/tʃu/	(f)	deep	/dip/
(g)	cog	/kɒg/	(h)	jaw	/dʒɔ/
(i)	tube	/tjub/	(j)	peat	/pit/
(k)	dead	/dɛd/	(l)	kit	/kɪt/
(m)	gap	/gæp/	(n)	boot	/but/
(o)	jab	/dʒæb/	(p)	chop	/tʃɒp/

2. GA

(a)	type	[tʰaɪp*ʰ*]	(b)	spike	[sp⁼aɪk*ʰ*]
(c)	church	[tʃ*ʷ*ɝtʃ*ʷ*]	(d)	Bobby	[b̥ɑbi]
(e)	pike	[pʰaɪk*ʰ*]	(f)	goat	[g̊ʷoʊt*ʰ*]
(g)	madder	[mædɚ]	(h)	cope	[kʰʷoʊp*ʰ*]
(i)	stew	[st⁼ʷu]	(j)	judge	[d̥ʒʌdʒ̊]
(k)	cat	[kʰæt*ʰ*]	(l)	two	[tʰʷu]
(m)	mugger	[mʌgɚ]	(n)	scoot	[sk⁼ʷut*ʰ*]
(o)	deed	[d̥id̥]	(p)	bike	[b̥aɪk*ʰ*]

RP

(a) type	[tʰaɪp*ʰ*]	(b) spike	[sp⁼aɪk*ʰ*]
(c) church	[tʃ*ʷ*ɜtʃ*ʷ*]	(d) Bobby	[b̥ɒbi]
(e) pike	[pʰaɪk*ʰ*]	(f) goat	[g̊əʊt*ʰ*]
(g) madder	[mædə]	(h) cope	[kʰəʊp*ʰ*]
(i) stew	[st⁼ju]	(j) judge	[d̥ʒʌdʒ̊]
(k) cat	[kʰæt*ʰ*]	(l) two	[tʰʷu]
(m) mugger	[mʌgə]	(n) scoot	[sk⁼ʷut*ʰ*]
(o) deed	[d̥id̥]	(p) bike	[b̥aɪk*ʰ*]

Note: Symbols in italics are optional variants; final fortis stops could be marked as unreleased (e.g., [p̚]) rather than aspirated.

3.

(a) /taɪd/	tide, tied	(b) /dʒæm/	jam, jamb
(c) /bit/	beat, beet	(d) /ki/	key, quay
(e) /gɹeɪz/	graze, grays	(f) /deɪz/	days, daze
(g) /tʃuz/	choose, chews	(h) /pliz/	pleas, please

4.

(a) matter	flap	(b) retake	plosive
(c) pretend	plosive	(d) pretty	flap
(e) citizen	flap	(f) detach	plosive

CHAPTER 14

1. GA

(a) fees	/fiz/	(b) show	/ʃoʊ/
(c) zoos	/zuz/	(d) heave	/hiv/
(e) these	/ðiz/	(f) vase	/veɪs/~/veɪz/~/vɑz/
(g) heath	/hiθ/	(h) thief	/θif/
(i) seizure	/siʒɚ/	(j) hush	/hʌʃ/
(k) shove	/ʃʌv/	(l) fuss	/fʌs/
(m) father	/fɑðɚ/	(n) ether	/iθɚ/
(o) seas	/siz/	(p) Asia	/eɪʃə/~/eɪʒə/

RP

(a) fees	/fiz/	(b) show	/ʃəʊ/
(c) zoos	/zuz/	(d) heave	/hiv/
(e) these	/ðiz/	(f) vase	/vɑz/~/veɪz/
(g) heath	/hiθ/	(h) thief	/θif/
(i) seizure	/siʒə/	(j) hush	/hʌʃ/
(k) shove	/ʃʌv/	(l) fuss	/fʌs/
(m) father	/fɑðə/	(n) ether	/iθə/
(o) seas	/siz/	(p) Asia	/eɪʃə/~/eɪʒə/

2. GA

(a)	those	[ð̥ʷoʊz̥]	(b)	seat	[sit]
(c)	foot	[fʷʊt]	(d)	that	[ð̥æt]
(e)	whose	[hʷuz̥]	(f)	veal	[v̥il]
(g)	dove	[d̥ʌv̥]	(h)	sore	[sʷɔɹ]
(i)	zeal	[z̥il]	(j)	beige	[b̥eɪʒ̊]
(k)	zoos	[z̥ʷuz̥]	(l)	feet	[fit]
(m)	shoes	[ʃʷuz̥]	(n)	soothe	[sʷuð̥]
(o)	voice	[v̥ʷɔɪs]	(p)	thorn	[θʷɔɹn]

RP

(a)	those	[ð̥əʊz̥]	(b)	seat	[sit]
(c)	foot	[fʷʊt]	(d)	that	[ð̥æt]
(e)	whose	[hʷuz̥]	(f)	veal	[v̥il]
(g)	dove	[d̥ʌv̥]	(h)	sore	[sʷɔ]
(i)	zeal	[z̥il]	(j)	beige	[b̥eɪʒ̊]
(k)	zoos	[z̥ʷuz̥]	(l)	feet	[fit]
(m)	shoes	[ʃʷuz̥]	(n)	soothe	[sʷuð̥]
(o)	voice	[v̥ʷɔɪs]	(p)	thorn	[θʷɔn]

3.

(a)	/faɪl/	file, phial	(b)	/veɪn/	vain, vein
(c)	/ʃu/	shoe, shoo	(d)	/fɹiz/	freeze, frieze
(e)	/θɹu/	through, threw	(f)	/wɛðɚ/	weather, whether, wether
(g)	/si/	see, sea	(h)	/hiɹ/	here, hear

CHAPTER 15

1. GA

(a)	among	/əmʌŋ/	(b)	wall	/wɑl/~/wɔl/
(c)	kneel	/nil/	(d)	wing	/wɪŋ/
(e)	year	/jɝ/	(f)	wrung	/ɹʌŋ/
(g)	numb	/nʌm/	(h)	leer	/lɪɹ/
(i)	young	/jʌŋ/	(j)	real	/ɹil/
(k)	maul	/mɑl/~/mɔl/	(l)	yellow	/jɛloʊ/
(m)	runner	/ɹʌnɚ/	(n)	lung	/lʌŋ/
(o)	limb	/lɪm/	(p)	near	/nɪɹ/

RP

(a)	among	/əmʌŋ/	(b)	wall	/wɔl/
(c)	kneel	/nil/	(d)	wing	/wɪŋ/
(e)	year	/jɜ/	(f)	wrung	/ɹʌŋ/
(g)	numb	/nʌm/	(h)	leer	/lɪə/
(i)	young	/jʌŋ/	(j)	real	/ɹil/
(k)	maul	/mɔl/	(l)	yellow	/jɛləʊ/
(m)	runner	/ɹʌnə/	(n)	lung	/lʌŋ/
(o)	limb	/lɪm/	(p)	near	/nɪə/

2. GA

(a)	slow	[sl̥ʷoʊ]	(b)	goal	[g̊ʷoʊɫʷ]
(c)	pool	[pʷuɫʷ]	(d)	twice	[tʷw̥aɪs]
(e)	snail	[sn̥eɪɫ]	(f)	riddle	[ɹɪdɫ̩]
(g)	clay	[kl̥eɪ]	(h)	loom	[lʷum]
(i)	smile	[sm̥aɪɫ]	(j)	fuel	[fjʷuɫʷ]
(k)	noodle	[nʷudɫ̩]	(l)	lean	[lʲin]
(m)	pure	[pj̊ʊɹ]	(n)	news	[njʷuz̥]~[nʷuz̥]
(o)	rude	[ɹʷud̥]	(p)	crane	[kɹ̥eɪn]

RP

(a)	slow	[sl̥əʊ]	(b)	goal	[g̊əʊɫʷ]
(c)	pool	[pʷuɫʷ]	(d)	twice	[tʷw̥aɪs]
(e)	snail	[sn̥eɪɫ]	(f)	riddle	[ɹɪdɫ̩]
(g)	clay	[kl̥eɪ]	(h)	loom	[lʷum]
(i)	smile	[sm̥aɪɫ]	(j)	fuel	[fjʷuɫʷ]
(k)	noodle	[nʷudɫ̩]	(l)	lean	[lʲin]
(m)	pure	[pj̊ʊə]	(n)	news	[njʷuz̥]
(o)	rude	[ɹʷud̥]	(p)	crane	[kɹ̥eɪn]

3.

(a)	/læm/	lamb, lam	(b)	/naɪt/	night, knight
(c)	/mid/	mead, Mede	(d)	/ɹɛtʃ/	retch, wretch
(e)	/bɪld/	build, billed	(f)	/wʌn/	won, one
(g)	/plʌm/	plum, plumb	(h)	/hju/	hue, hew, Hugh

CHAPTER 16

1.

(a)	ˈgrassˌhopper	(b)	ˈbachelor
(c)	perˌsonifiˈcation	(d)	ˌindiˈstinguishable
(e)	ˌinterˌnationaliˈzation	(f)	reˈlation
(g)	phoˈtography	(h)	ˈproˌgram
(i)	ˌincaˈpaciˌtate	(j)	ˈborderˌline
(k)	ˌobjecˈtivity	(l)	ˌdiploˈmatic

2. GA

		Verb	Noun/adj
(a)	abstract	/ˌæbˈstɹækt /	/ˈæbˌstɹækt /
(b)	digest	/ˌdaɪˈdʒɛst /	/ˈdaɪˌdʒɛst /
(c)	torment	/ˌtɔɹˈmɛnt /	/ˈtɔɹˌmɛnt /
(d)	require	n/a	
(e)	transfer	/tɹənsˈfɝ /	/ˈtɹænsˌfɝ /
(f)	absent	/ˌæbˈsɛnt /	/ˈæbsənt /
(g)	defend	n/a	
(h)	segment	/ˌsɛgˈmɛnt /	/ˈsɛgmənt /
(i)	subject	/səbˈdʒɛkt /	/ˈsʌbˌdʒɛkt /
(j)	produce	/pɹəˈdus /	/ˈpɹɑˌdus /~/ˈpɹoʊˌdus /

RP

	Verb	Noun/adj
(a) abstract	/ˌæbˈstɹækt/	/ˈæbˌstɹækt/
(b) digest	/ˌdaɪˈdʒɛst/	/ˈdaɪˌdʒɛst/
(c) torment	/ˌtɔˈmɛnt/	/ˈtɔˌmɛnt/
(d) require	n/a	
(e) transfer	/tɹənsˈfɜ/	/ˈtɹænsˌfɜ/
(f) absent	/ˌæbˈsɛnt/	/ˈæbsənt/
(g) defend	n/a	
(h) segment	/ˌsɛgˈmɛnt/	/ˈsɛgmənt/
(i) subject	/səbˈdʒɛkt/	/ˈsʌbˌdʒɛkt/
(j) produce	/pɹəˈdjus/	/ˈpɹɒˌdjus/

3.

(a) would	/wʊd/	/wəd, əd, d/
(b) am	/æm/	/m, əm/
(c) have	/hæv/	/həv, əv, v/
(d) had	/hæd/	/həd, əd, d/
(e) is	/ɪz/	/z, s/
(f) must	/mʌst/	/məst, məs/
(g) to	/tu/	/tə/
(h) should	/ʃʊd/	/ʃəd/
(i) has	/hæz/	/həz, əz, z, s/
(j) some	/sʌm/	/səm/

4. GA

(a) Joan and Cathy wouldn't be walking in this weather
/ˈdʒoʊn əŋ ˈkæθi wəbm̩p bi ˈwɑkɪŋ ɪn ˈðɪs ˈwɛðɚ/

(b) She put her handbag on the brown box
/ʃi ˈpʊt ɚ ˈhæmbæg ɑn ðə ˈbɹaʊm ˈbɑks/

(c) He walked back to his car to fetch his coat
/hi ˈwɑk ˈbæk tə hɪz ˈkɑɹ tə ˈfɛtʃ ɪz ˈkoʊt/

(d) Last month Vicky had a good many customers in the store
/ˈlæs ˈmʌnʔθ ˈvɪki əd ə ˈgʊb ˈmɛni ˈkʌstəmɚz ɪn ðə ˈstɔɹ/

(e) They couldn't go any faster than they were
/ðeɪ ˈkʊgŋk ˈgoʊ ˈɛni ˈfæstɚ ðən ðeɪ ˈwɝ/

(f) Fred gulped down seven bottles of beer and a ham sandwich
/ˈfɹɛd ˈgʌlpt daʊn ˈsɛvəm ˈbɑɾl̩z əv ˈbɪɹ ənd ə ˈhæm ˈsæmwɪtʃ/

RP

(a) Joan and Cathy wouldn't be walking in this weather
/ˈdʒəʊn əŋ ˈkæθi wəbm̩p bi ˈwɔkɪŋ ɪn ˈðɪs ˈwɛðə/

(b) She put her handbag on the brown box
/ʃi ˈpʊt ə ˈhæmbæg ɒn ðə ˈbɹaʊm ˈbɒks/

(c) He walked back to his car to fetch his coat
/hi ˈwɔk ˈbæk tə hɪz ˈkɑ tə ˈfɛtʃ ɪz ˈkəʊt/

(d) Last month Vicky had a good many customers in the store
/ˈlɑs ˈmʌn*t*θ ˈvɪki əd ə ˈgʊb ˈmɛni ˈkʌstəməz ɪn ðə ˈstɔ/

(e) They couldn't go any faster than they were
/ðeɪ ˈkʊgŋk ˈgəʊ ˈɛni ˈfɑstə ðən ðeɪ ˈwɜ/

(f) Fred gulped down seven bottles of beer and a ham sandwich
/ˈfɹɛd ˈgʌlpt daʊn ˈsɛvəm ˈbɒtl̩z əv ˈbɪə ənd ə ˈhæm ˈsæmwɪdʒ/

CHAPTER 17

1.

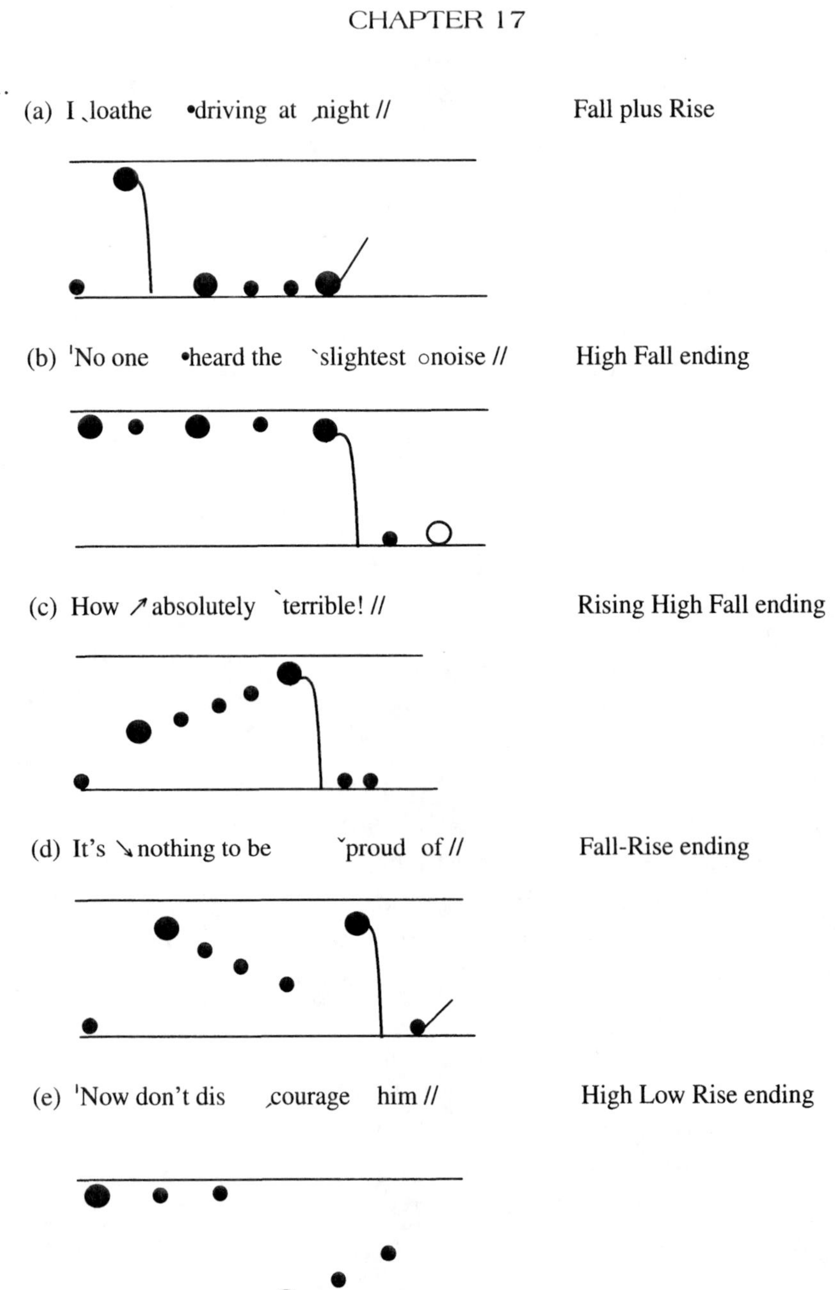

(a) I ˎloathe •driving at ˏnight //
Fall plus Rise
(b) ˈNo one •heard the ˋslightest ∘noise //
High Fall ending
(c) How ↗absolutely ˋterrible! //
Rising High Fall ending
(d) It's ↘nothing to be ˇproud of //
Fall-Rise ending
(e) ˈNow don't dis ˏcourage him //
High Low Rise ending

2.

(a) ˈWho does he need to ˏspeak to? // — High Low Rise ending
(b) I've ˈnever seen anything ˆlike them // — Rise-Fall ending
(c) I'm ˈonly too ˋhappy to do it // — High Fall ending
(d) ˈSomewhere in ˋOregon would be nice this ˏyear // — Fall plus Rise
(e) Well ˈgive him a >dollar / (and send him off to the mall) // — Mid-Level ending

CHAPTER 18

1.

(a) night [nɪçt] Scottish
(b) snow [snʌʉ] Australian
(c) house [hʌʊs] Canadian
(d) chill [tʃʌl] South African
(e) threat [t̪ɹ̝εθ̠] southern Irish/Hiberno-English
(f) better [ˈbεʔə] London England

2.

(a) bone [bɵn] Northeastern
(b) sill [sɪəl] South
(c) when [wε̃] African American English
(d) sky [ska] South
(e) oil [ɔʟ] South
(f) bet [bε] African American English

Notes: (b), (d), and (e) can also be found in AAE.

CHAPTER 19

1. GA

king	[tɪn]	sewing	[ˈɬoʊɪn]	zoo	[ɮu]
game	[deɪm]	socks	[ɬɑtɬ]	gem	[dʒεm]
vision	[ˈvɪɮən]	cogs	[tɑdɮ]	sagging	[ˈɬædɪn]
reason	[ˈɹiɮən]	guess	[dεɬ]	sink	[ɬɪnt]

RP

king	[tɪn]	sewing	[ˈɬəʊɪn]	zoo	[ɮu]
game	[deɪm]	socks	[ɬɒtɬ]	gem	[dʒεm]
vision	[ˈvɪɮən]	cogs	[tɒdɮ]	sagging	[ˈɬædɪn]
reason	[ˈɹiɮən]	guess	[dεɬ]	sink	[ɬɪnt]

2. GA

strike	[taɪ]	splash	[pæ]	scream	[ki]
blush	[bʌ]	prove	[pu]	green	[gi]
smooth	[mu]	slide	[saɪ]	snow	[noʊ]
stop	[tɑ]	skin	[kɪ]	spun	[pʌ]

RP

strike	[taɪ]	splash	[pæ]	scream	[ki]
blush	[bʌ]	prove	[pu]	green	[gi]
smooth	[mu]	slide	[saɪ]	snow	[nəʊ]
stop	[tɒ]	skin	[kɪ]	spun	[pʌ]

CHAPTER 20

1. GA

thumb	[θ̼ʌm̄]	ten	[t̼ɛn̼]	fun	[f̄ʌn̼]
date	[d̼eɪt̼]	van	[¯væn̼]	then	[ð̼ɛn̼]
that	[ð̼æt̼]	five	[f̄aɪv̄]	teeth	[t̼iθ̼]
laugh	[l̼æf̄]	thought	[θ̼ɔt̼]	late	[l̼eɪt̼]

RP

thumb	[θ̼ʌm̄]	ten	[t̼ɛn̼]	fun	[f̄ʌn̼]
date	[d̼eɪt̼]	van	[¯væn̼]	then	[ð̼ɛn̼]
that	[ð̼æt̼]	five	[f̄aɪv̄]	teeth	[t̼iθ̼]
laugh	[l̼ɑf̄]	thought	[θ̼ɔt̼]	late	[l̼eɪt̼]

2. GA

thumb	[fŋʌ̃m̃̃]	ten	[t̃ɛ̃ñ̃]	fun	[fŋʌ̃ñ̃]
date	[d̃ẽĩʔ]	van	[fŋæ̃ñ̃]	then	[fŋɛ̃ñ̃]
that	[fŋæ̃ʔ]	five	[fŋãĩʔ]	teeth	[t̃iʔ]
laugh	[læ̃ʔ]	thought	[fŋɔ̃ʔ]	late	[lẽĩʔ]

RP

thumb	[fŋʌ̃m̃̃]	ten	[t̃ɛ̃ñ̃]	fun	[fŋʌ̃ñ̃]
date	[d̃ẽĩʔ]	van	[fŋæ̃ñ̃]	then	[fŋɛ̃ñ̃]
that	[fŋæ̃ʔ]	five	[fŋãĩʔ]	teeth	[t̃iʔ]
laugh	[lɑ̃ʔ]	thought	[fŋɔ̃ʔ]	late	[lẽĩʔ]

3. GA

[çuʫ]	shoes	[ʫil]	zeal	[ˈʪæçɪʫ]	sashes
[ʪplæç]	splash	[ʪmuð̥̄]	smooth	[ʫið̥̄]	these
[ˈθ̥̄ɪmbl̩]	thimble	[ʪɑŋʫ]	songs	[hɪʪ]	hiss
[ˈçɑpɪŋ]	shopping	[ð̥̄ɪʪ]	this	[hɪʫ]	his

RP

[çuʫ]	shoes	[ʫil]	zeal	[ˈʪæçɪʫ]	sashes
[ʪplæç]	splash	[ʪmuð̥̄]	smooth	[ʫið̥̄]	these
[ˈθ̥̄ɪmbl̩]	thimble	[ʪɒŋʫ]	songs	[hɪʪ]	hiss
[ˈçɒpɪŋ]	shopping	[ð̥̄ɪʪ]	this	[hɪʫ]	his

Answers to Audio CD Transcription Exercises

CHAPTER 1

Exercise 1.1

	Number of sounds	*Number of letters*
thinking	6	8
ballet	4	6
examine	7	7
attack	4	6
sheets	4	6
dress	4	5
sneeze	4	6
whose	3	5
philosophy	8	10
brushes	6	7

CHAPTER 2

Exercise 2.1

	Number of syllables
imply	2
rehabilitate	5
helicopter	4
embargo	3
prism	2
photograph	3
walks	1
unreal	2 (3 for some speakers who add vowel before "l")
rhinoceros	4 (3 for some speakers who delete third vowel)
capitalize	4

CHAPTER 3

Exercise 3.1

[p'ɑ]	[ɑtɑ]	[f'ɑ]
[k'ɑs']	[sɑf']	[kɑt']
[ɑfɑ]	[ɑt'ɑf']	[s'ɑpɑ]

Exercise 3.2

[dɑ]	[ɑɓɑ]	[ɗɑ]
[bɑʛ]	[gɑd]	[ɓaɗ]
[ɑɗɑ]	[ɑʛɑɓ]	[dɑbɑ]

Exercise 3.3

[k'ɑb]	[s'ɑɓɑ]	[t'ɑɗ]
[fɑf']	[sɑg]	[ʛɑt']
[ɑpɑɓ]	[ɑtɑf']	[kɑp'ɑ]

Exercise 3.4

[|ɑ]	[ɑ‖ɑ]	[ʘɑ]
[!ɑ‖]	[‖ɑd]	[|ɑ!]
[ɑ|ɑ]	[ɑʘɑ‖]	[‖ɑ!ɑ]

Exercise 3.5

[|ɑ]	[t'ɑ]	[s'ɑ]
[t'ɑ|]	[tɑ|]	[|ɑs']
[s'ɑ|ɑ]	[t'ɑ|ɑs']	[|ɑsɑ]

CHAPTER 4

Exercise 4.1

(a) voiceless; voiced	(b) voiced; voiced	(c) voiceless; voiced
(d) voiceless; voiceless	(e) voiceless; voiced	(f) voiced; voiced
(g) voiced; voiceless	(h) voiced; voiced	(i) voiced; voiceless

Exercise 4.2

[ˈð	W
ɪ	W
s	Vls
ɪ	W
z	W
ˈw	W
ɪ	W
s	Vls
p	Vls
ɚ	W
d	W
f	Vls
oʊ	W
ˈn	W
eɪ	W
ʃ	Vls
n]	W

Exercise 4.3

[ˈk	Vls
ɹ	C
i	C
k	Vls
f	Vls
oʊ	C
ˈn	C
eɪ	C
ʃ	Vls
n	C
ɪ	C
z	C
ˈk	Vls
w	C
aɪ	C
t	Vls
ˈk	Vls
ɑ	C
m	C
ə	C
n]	C

Exercise 4.4

(a) Vls (b) V (c) V
(d) V (e) W (f) Vls
(g) V (h) W (i) C
(j) C (k) Vls (l) W

Exercise 4.5

(a) Hypernasal voice
(b) Ventricular voice
(c) Hypernasal ventricular voice
(d) Breathy voice
(e) Diplophonia
(f) Murmur

CHAPTER 5

Exercise 5.1

(a) [mize] (d) [sakɛ] (g) [ɑsne] (i) [iglɔ]
(b) [ɛfli] (e) [lɑfu] (h) [volɔ] (k) [dukɛ]
(c) [ponɑ] (f) [timu] (i) [femɔ] (l) [alzɑ]

Exercise 5.2

(a) [bønɤ] (d) [mytʌ] (g) [ɒgœs] (j) [mɶzɯ]
(b) [lœby] (e) [ɯvdø] (h) [kelɛ] (k) [lyze]
(c) [pøzo] (f) [ɑmnɔ] (i) [fugɯ] (l) [yvif]

Exercise 5.3

(a) [dɛgɜ]	(d) [ɨfla]	(g) [usɵn]	(j) [lɜsy]
(b) [kotʉ]	(e) [ɑvze]	(h) [ʉzlø]	(k) [nɨti]
(c) [bɒnʉ]	(f) [ɯvmɨ]	(i) [ɵdmʌ]	(l) [wɜpɔ]

Exercise 5.4

(a) [aɪ]	(d) [øʏ]	(g) [ɛɪ]
(b) [oʊ]	(e) [ɛə]	(h) [ɑʊ]
(c) [ʊə]	(f) [ɔʊ]	(i) [ɪə]

CHAPTER 6

Exercise 6.1

(a) affricate	(d) plosive	(g) plosive
(b) fricative	(e) fricative	(h) fricative
(c) fricative	(f) affricate	(i) plosive
		(j) lateral fricative

Exercise 6.2

(a) trill	(d) nasal	(g) central approximant
(b) lateral approximant	(e) tap	(h) nasal
(c) central approximant	(f) lateral approximant	(i) trill
		(j) tap

Exercise 6.3

(a) fricative	[βɑ]	(d) nasal	[ɳɑ]	(g) central approximant	[ʋɑ]
(b) trill	[ʙɑ]	(e) lateral fricative	[ɮɑ]	(h) affricate	[pɸɑ]
(c) plosive	[cɑ]	(f) lateral approximant	[lɑ]	(i) fricative	[ʒɑ]
				(j) plosive	[ʔɑ]

CHAPTER 7

Exercise 7.1

(a) retroflex	(d) labiodental	(g) bilabial
(b) labiodental	(e) alveolar	(h) postalveolar
(c) dental	(f) postalveolar	(i) retroflex
		(j) postalveolar

Exercise 7.2

(a) uvular	(d) velar	(g) palatal
(b) uvular	(e) glottal	(h) velar
(c) pharyngeal	(f) palatal	(i) velar
		(j) glottal

Exercise 7.3

(a) [ɢɑ]	(e) [xu]	(i) [ɹe]
(b) [ra]	(f) [θɑ]	(j) [ʔɛ]
(c) [ɭɔ]	(g) [çɛ]	(k) [ʃɑ]
(d) [me]	(h) [ɦi]	(l) [ħo]

CHAPTER 8

Exercise 8.1

(a) [mɛtəl]	central release
(b) [ʃɪp^{h}]	full release
(c) [ɹætl̩]	lateral release
(d) [pʌdl̩]	lateral release
(e) [næp˺]	non-release
(f) [ɹɛdn̩]	nasal release
(g) [pæt^{s}]	affricated release
(h) [sneɪk˺]	non-release
(i) [hʊk^{x}]	affricated release
(j) [kɪtən]	oral release
(k) [meɪk^{h}]	full release
(l) [ɹɪtn̩]	nasal release

Exercise 8.2

(a) [ɥe]	(e) [jeʒu]	(i) [ɣɑjɔ]
(b) [wɑ]	(f) [θɑʋi]	(j) [lywu]
(c) [ji]	(g) [ɥɛŋu]	(k) [ʀeɥa]
(d) [ʋɛ]	(h) [ɬowɛ]	(l) [ʋowo]

Exercise 8.3

(a) [ɑʃ^{ʕ}ɑ]	pharyngealization
(b) [t^{j}e]	palatalization
(c) [di]	no secondary articulation
(d) [ɛs^{w}u]	labialization
(e) [ɑni]	no secondary articulation
(f) [al^{ɣ}o]	velarization
(g) [s^{j}i]	palatalization
(h) [f^{ɣ}u]	velarization
(i) [s^{ʕ}a]	pharyngealization

CHAPTER 9

Exercise 9.1

Test item	*Stress*	*Language*	*Meaning*
(a) mynyddoedd	second	Welsh	mountains
(b) παρακαλῶ (parakalo)	last	Modern Greek	please
(c) follasach	first	Irish	clear
(d) Geschwindigkeit	second	German	speed
(e) yliopisto	first	Finnish	university
(f) Übernachtung	third	German	overnight stay
(g) hunangofiant	third	Welsh	autobiography
(h) καλημέρα (kalimera)	third	Modern Greek	good morning

Exercise 9.2

Test item	*Length*	*Language*	*Meaning*
(a) llyn	neither	Welsh	lake
(b) fatto	long C	Italian	made
(c) täällä	both	Finnish	here
(d) llun	long V	Welsh	picture
(e) otto	long C	Italian	eight
(f) kissa	long C	Finnish	cat
(g) fato	neither	Italian	fate
(h) hen	long V	Welsh	old

Exercise 9.3

(a) [dà]	high falling	大	meaning "big"
(b) [tǎ]	low dipping	塔	meaning "tower" among others
(c) [wā]	high level	蛙	meaning "frog"
(d) [pá]	high rising	爬	meaning "climb" among others
(e) [bà]	high falling	爸	meaning "father" among others
(f) [yā]	high level	鸭	meaning "duck"

(Thanks to Liang Chen for suggesting these items.)

CHAPTER 10

Exercise 10.1

(a) [!o]	(d) [kɑɓo]	(g) [da‖ɛɗa]
(b) [p'ɛ]	(e) [‖et'u]	(h) [ʛɑkegu]
(c) [ɗu]	(f) [ʃ'itʃ'o]	(i) [tʃiʘok'u]
		(j) [t'u|ɔs'o]

Exercise 10.2

(a) [qu]
(b) [ɖɑ]
(c) [k͡xi]
(d) [d͡zɛʈu]
(e) [ʔiɟa]
(f) [ɢɑgo]
(g) [dɑp͡ɸeɖɛ]
(h) [cakɛqu]
(i) [quɟɔti]
(j) [g͡ɣoʔupɔ]

Exercise 10.3

(a) [ʂu]
(b) [çy]
(c) [χɑ]
(d) [βeħa]
(e) [ɮɛɣo]
(f) [θɔʝi]
(g) [ʁuxɔʐø]
(h) [ɸiʔoðɯ]
(i) [ɬœçeʂu]
(j) [xɑχɛɦa]

Exercise 10.4

(a) [ŋɑ]
(b) [ɲe]
(c) [ɳo]
(d) [ɱœŋa]
(e) [niɴɔ]
(f) [mɯɓo]
(g) [t'yçeɳa]
(h) [quɣeɱo]
(i) [ɖɑɬɛǁø]
(j) [ɲeŋuɴɑ]

Exercise 10.5

(a) [lø]
(b) [ʋe]
(c) [ɥi]
(d) [jaʎo]
(e) [ŋɛɰa]
(f) [ɭaɹy]
(g) [ʈoʟeʋa]
(h) [jiɥɛɭɔ]
(i) [ʋewuɥɛ]
(j) [ʎijɔqɯ]

Exercise 10.6

(a) [rø]
(b) [ʙy]
(c) [ʀɑ]
(d) [quɾa]
(e) [ɟeɽo]
(f) [rɯɾɛ]
(g) [gaʙiɢu]
(h) [ʀɑceɾɔ]
(i) [rœɾuɽa]
(j) [ɖurɔoʙø]

Exercise 10.7

(a) [quʐeʎyk']
(b) [ʘɯroçeɖ]
(c) [ʔɑxɛʋir]
(d) [ɥɛcaʂɔɲ]
(e) [ɓuɣøwɑɭ]
(f) [jaɾœβɔʈ]
(g) [ɹyʝeɢɑɴ]
(h) [ɰɔχuħɑp']
(i) [ŋak͡xoʃuʁ]
(j) [ɟɛɽaɸød͡ʒ]

CHAPTER 11

Exercise 11.1

	GA	RP	RP only	
meat	/mit/	/mit/	loll	/lɒl/
smell	/smɛl/	/smɛl/	pod	/pɒd/
teen	/tin/	/tin/		
look	/lʊk/	/lʊk/		
lore	/lɔɹ/	/lɔ/		
sill	/sɪl/	/sɪl/		
loot	/lut/	/lut/		
hen	/hɛn/	/hɛn/		
fool	/ful/	/ful/		
spa	/spɑ/	/spɑ/		
teal	/til/	/til/		
worn	/wɔɹn/	/wɔn/		
mead	/mid/	/mid/		
hand	/hænd/	/hænd/		
food	/fud/	/fud/		

Exercise 11.2

	GA	RP	RP only	
meat	[miˑt]	[miˑt]	loll	[lɒᵊl]
smell	[smɛᵊl]	[smɛᵊl]	pod	[pɒd]
teen	[tĩːn]	[tĩːn]		
look	[lŭk]	[lŭk]		
lore	[lɔːɹ]	[lɔː]		
sill	[sɪᵊl]	[sɪᵊl]		
loot	[luˑt]	[luˑt]		
hen	[hɛ̃n]	[hɛ̃n]		
fool	[fuːᵊl]	[fuːᵊl]		
spa	[spɑː]	[spɑː]		
teal	[tiːᵊl]	[tiːᵊl]		
worn	[wɔ̃ːɹn]	[wɔ̃ːn]		
mead	[miːd]	[miːd]		
hand	[hæ̃nd]	[hæ̃nd]		
food	[fuːd]	[fuːd]		

CHAPTER 12

Exercise 12.1

	GA	RP	RP only	
diver	/daɪvɚ/	/daɪvə/	leers	/lɪəz/
but	/bʌt/	/bʌt/	toured	/tʊəd/
apply	/əplaɪ/	/əplaɪ/	hair	/hɛə/
earn	/ɝn/	/ɜn/		
round	/ɹaʊnd/	/ɹaʊnd/		

road	/ɹoʊd/	/ɹəʊd/
I'm	/aɪm/	/aɪm/
rain	/ɹeɪn/	/ɹeɪn/
roam	/ɹoʊm/	/ɹəʊm/
rate	/ɹeɪt/	/ɹeɪt/
height	/haɪt/	/haɪt/
nail	/neɪl/	/neɪl/
rote	/ɹoʊt/	/ɹəʊt/
toil	/tɔɪl/	/tɔɪl/
hide	/haɪd/	/haɪd/

Exercise 12.2

	GA	RP	RP only	
diver	[daːɪvɚ]	[daːɪvə]	leers	[lɪːəz]
but	[bʌ̆t]	[bʌ̆t]	toured	[tʊːəd]
apply	[ə̆plaːɪ]	[ə̆plaːɪ]	hair	[hɛːə]
earn	[ɝ̃ːn]	[ɜ̃ːn]		
round	[ɹaːʊ̃nd]	[ɹaːʊ̃nd]		
road	[ɹoːʊd]	[ɹəːʊd]		
I'm	[aːĩm]	[aːĩm]		
rain	[ɹeːĩn]	[ɹeːĩn]		
roam	[ɹoːʊ̃m]	[ɹəːʊ̃m]		
rate	[ɹeˑɪt]	[ɹeˑɪt]		
height	[haˑɪt]	[haˑɪt]		
nail	[neːˈəl]	[neːˈəl]		
rote	[ɹoˑʊt]	[ɹəˑʊt]		
toil	[tɔːˈəl]	[tɔːˈəl]		
hide	[haːɪd]	[haːɪd]		

CHAPTER 13

Exercise 13.1

	GA	RP
padded	/pædɪd/	/pædɪd/
cadge	/kædʒ/	/kædʒ/
gouging	/gaʊdʒɪŋ/	/gaʊdʒɪŋ/
scoop	/skup/	/skup/
bidden	/bɪdn̩/~/bɪdən/	/bɪdn̩/
jabbed	/dʒæbd/	/dʒæbd/
got	/gɑt/	/gɒt/
tact	/tækt/	/tækt/
ditch	/dɪtʃ/	/dɪtʃ/
speed	/spid/	/spid/
totter	/tɑɾɚ /	/tɒtə/
stoop	/stup/	/stup/
backer	/bækɚ /	/bækə/
checked	/tʃɛkt/	/tʃɛkt/
cuddle	/kʌdl̩/~/kʌdəl/	/kʌdl̩/

Exercise 13.2

	GA	RP
padded	[p^{h}ædɪd̥]	[p^{h}ædɪd̥]
cadge	[k^{h}ædʒ̊]	[k^{h}ædʒ̊]
gouging	[g̊aʊdʒɪŋ]	[g̊aʊdʒɪŋ]
scoop	[sk$^{=}$up^{h}]	[sk$^{=}$up^{h}]
bidden	[b̥ɪd^{n}n̩]~[b̥ɪɾən]	[b̥ɪd^{n}n̩]
jabbed	[dʒ̊æb̚d̥]	[dʒ̊æb̚d̥]
got	[g̊ɑt^{h}]	[g̊ɒt^{h}]
tact	[t^{h}æk̚t^{h}]	[t^{h}æk̚t^{h}]
ditch	[d̥ɪtʃ]	[d̥ɪtʃ]
speed	[sp$^{=}$id̥]	[sp$^{=}$id̥]
totter	[t^{h}ɑɾɚ]	[t^{h}ɒt^{h}ə]
stoop	[st$^{=}$up^{h}]	[st$^{=}$up^{h}]
backer	[b̥æk^{h}ɚ]	[b̥æk^{h}ə]
checked	[tʃɛk̚t^{h}]	[tʃɛk̚t^{h}]
cuddle	[k^{h}ʌd^{l}l̩]~[k^{h}ʌɾəl]	[k^{h}ʌd^{l}l̩]

CHAPTER 14

Exercise 14.1

	GA	RP
favor	/feɪvɚ/	/feɪvə/
thrive	/θɹaɪv/	/θɹaɪv/
beige	/beɪʒ/	/beɪʒ/
suffers	/sʌfɚz/	/sʌfəz/
phases	/feɪzɪz/	/feɪzɪz/
shoes	/ʃuz/	/ʃuz/
bathers	/beɪðɚz/	/beɪðəz/
heath	/hiθ/	/hiθ/
savers	/seɪvɚz/	/seɪvəz/
rehash	/ɹihæʃ/	/ɹihæʃ/
vision	/vɪʒn̩/	/vɪʒn̩/
these	/ðiz/	/ðiz/

Exercise 14.2

	GA	RP
favor	[feɪvɚ]	[feɪvə]
thrive	[θɹaɪv̥]	[θɹaɪv̥]
beige	[b̥eɪʒ̊]	[b̥eɪʒ̊]
suffers	[sʌfɚz̥]	[sʌfəz̥]
phases	[feɪzɪz̥]	[feɪzɪz̥]
shoes	[ʃuz̥]	[ʃuz̥]
bathers	[b̥eɪðɚz̥]	[b̥eɪðəz̥]
heath	[hiθ]	[hiθ]

savers	[seɪvɚz̥]	[seɪvəz̥]
rehash	[ɹiɦæʃ]	[ɹiɦæʃ]
vision	[v̥ɪʒn̩]	[v̥ɪʒn̩]
these	[ð̥iz̥]	[ð̥iz̥]

CHAPTER 15

Exercise 15.1

	GA	RP
snail	/sneɪl/	/sneɪl/
fume	/fjum/	/fjum/
ring	/ɹɪŋ/	/ɹɪŋ/
mule	/mjul/	/mjul/
drain	/dɹeɪn/	/dɹeɪn/
plea	/pli/	/pli/
queen	/kwin/	/kwin/
small	/smɑl/	/smɔl/
train	/tɹeɪn/	/tɹeɪn/
wrong	/ɹɑŋ/	/ɹɒŋ/
cram	/kɹæm/	/kɹæm/
hewn	/hjun/	/hjun/
rung	/ɹʌŋ/	/ɹʌŋ/
prune	/pɹun/	/pɹun/
cling	/klɪŋ/	/klɪŋ/

Exercise 15.2

	GA	RP
snail	[sn̥eɪɫ]	[sn̥eɪɫ]
fume	[fj̊um]	[fj̊um]
ring	[ɹɪŋ]	[ɹɪŋ]
mule	[mjuɫ]	[mjuɫ]
drain	[dɹ̝eɪn]	[dɹ̝eɪn]
plea	[pl̥i]	[pl̥i]
queen	[kw̥in]	[kw̥in]
small	[sm̥ɑɫ]	[sm̥ɔɫ]
train	[tɹ̝̊eɪn]	[tɹ̝̊eɪn]
wrong	[ɹɑŋ]	[ɹɒŋ]
cram	[kɹ̥æm]	[kɹ̥æm]
hewn	[hj̊un]~[çun]	[hj̊un]~[çun]
rung	[ɹʌŋ]	[ɹʌŋ]
prune	[pɹ̥un]	[pɹ̥un]
cling	[kl̥ɪŋ]	[kl̥ɪŋ]

CHAPTER 16 (GA)

Exercise 16.1

(a) imply [ɪmˈplaɪ]
(b) rehabilitate [ˌɹi.əˈbɪlɪˌteɪt]
(c) helicopter [ˈhɛliˌkɑptɚ]
(d) embargo [ɛmˈbɑɹˌgoʊ]
(e) chasm [ˈkæzm̩]
(f) photograph [ˈfoʊɾəˌgɹæf]
(g) walks [ˈwɑks]
(h) unreal [ˌʌnˈɹil]
(i) rhinoceros [ˌɹaɪˈnɑsəɹəs]
(j) capitalize [ˈkæpəɾəˌlaɪz]

Exercise 16.2

(a) "John was reading the book"
/ˈdʒɑn wəz ˈɹidɪŋ ðə ˈbʊk/

(b) "The girl was talking to the therapist"
/ðə ˈgɝl wəz ˈtɑkɪŋ tə ðə ˈθɛɹəpɪst/

(c) "We all want to go to the movies tonight"
/wi ˈɔl ˈwɑnt tə ˈgoʊ tə ðə ˈmuviz təˈnaɪt/

(d) "What is the name of the singer, Mark?"
/ˈwɑt ɪz ðə ˈneɪm əv ðə ˈsɪŋɚ ˈmɑɹk/

(e) "Phonetics is easy if you study hard"
/fəˈnɛɾɪks ɪz ˈizi ɪf ju ˈstʌdi ˈhɑɹd/

Exercise 16.3

(a) "Where's my best dress?"
/ˈwɛɹz maɪ ˈbɛs ˈdɹɛs/

(b) "Please put my brown case here"
/ˈpliz ˈpʊp maɪ ˈbɹaʊŋ ˈkeɪs ˈhɪɹ/

(c) "John's better off in Canada"
/ˈdʒɑnz ˈbɛɾɚ ɑf ɪŋ ˈkænədə/

(d) "He's eating a ham sandwich"
/hiz ˈiɾɪŋ ə ˈhæm ˈsæmwɪtʃ/

(e) "Next week I'm going to Spain"
/ˈnɛks ˈwik aɪm ˈgoʊɪŋ tə ˈspeɪn/

(f) "What do you think we should do this evening?"
/ˈwɑdʒə ˈθɪŋk wi ʃʊd ˈdu ðəs ˈivnɪŋ/

(g) "I wonder if we should go to the theater?"
/aɪ ˈwʌndɚ ɪf wi ʃʊg ˈgoʊ tə ðə ˈθi.əɾɚ/

(h) "John and Keith'll be over in a minute"
/ˈdʒɑn ŋ ˈkiθ l̩ bi ˈoʊvɚ ɪn ə ˈmɪnɪt/

(i) "Last night it poured from midnight to five o'clock"
/ˈlæs ˈnaɪt ɪp ˈpɔɹd fɹəm ˈmɪdnaɪt tə ˈfaɪv əˈklɑk/

(j) "Don't be so eager to go"
/ˈdoʊmp bi soʊ ˈigɚ tə ˈgoʊ/

CHAPTER 16 (RP)

Exercise 16.1

(a) imply [ɪmˈplaɪ]
(b) rehabilitate [ˌɹi.əˈbɪlɪˌteɪt]
(c) helicopter [ˈhɛliˌkɒptə]
(d) embargo [ɛmˈbɑˌgəʊ]
(e) chasm [ˈkæzm̩]
(f) photograph [ˈfəʊtəˌgɹɑf]
(g) walks [ˈwɔks]
(h) unreal [ˌʌnˈɹil]
(i) rhinoceros [ˌɹaɪˈnɒsəɹəs]
(j) capitalize [ˈkæpɪtəˌlaɪz]

Exercise 16.2

(a) "John was reading the book"
/ˈdʒɒn wəz ˈɹidɪŋ ðə ˈbʊk/

(b) "The girl was talking to the therapist"
/ðə ˈgɜl wəz ˈtɔkɪŋ tə ðə ˈθɛɹəpɪst/

(c) "We all want to go to the movies tonight"
/wi ˈɔl ˈwɒnt tə ˈgəʊ tə ðə ˈmuviz təˈnaɪt/

(d) "What is the name of the singer, Mark?"
/ˈwɒt ɪz ðə ˈneɪm əv ðə ˈsɪŋə ˈmɑk/

(e) "Phonetics is easy if you study hard"
/fəˈnɛtɪks ɪz ˈizi ɪf ju ˈstʌdi ˈhɑd/

Exercise 16.3

(a) "Where's my best dress?"
/ˈwɛəz maɪ ˈbɛs ˈdɹɛs/

(b) "Please put my brown case here"
/ˈpliz ˈpʊp maɪ ˈbɹaʊŋ ˈkeɪs ˈhɪə/

(c) "John's better off in Canada"
/ˈdʒɒnz ˈbɛtəɹ ɒf ɪŋ ˈkænədə/

(d) "He's eating a ham sandwich"
/hiz ˈitɪŋ ə ˈhæm ˈsæmwɪdʒ/

(e) "Next week I'm going to Spain"
/ˈnɛks ˈwik aɪm ˈgəʊɪŋ tə ˈspeɪn/

(f) "What do you think we should do this evening?"
/ˈwɒdʒə ˈθɪŋk wi ʃʊd ˈdu ðəs ˈivnɪŋ/

(g) "I wonder if we should go to the theater?"
/aɪ ˈwʌndəɹ ɪf wi ʃʊg ˈgəʊ tə ðə ˈθiətə/

(h) "John and Keith'll be over in a minute"
/ˈdʒɒn ŋ ˈkiθ l̩ bi ˈəʊvəɹ ɪn ə ˈmɪnɪt/

(i) "Last night it poured from midnight to five o'clock"
/ˈlɑs ˈnaɪt ɪp ˈpɔd fɹəm ˈmɪdnaɪt tə ˈfaɪv əˈklɒk/

(j) "Don't be so eager to go"
/ˈdəʊmp bi səʊ ˈigə tə ˈgəʊ/

CHAPTER 17

Exercise 17.1

(a) It's how tall? — High Rise Ending

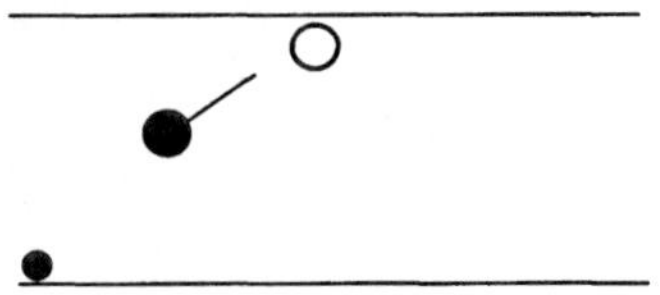

(b) But they haven't brought it! — Rise-Fall Ending

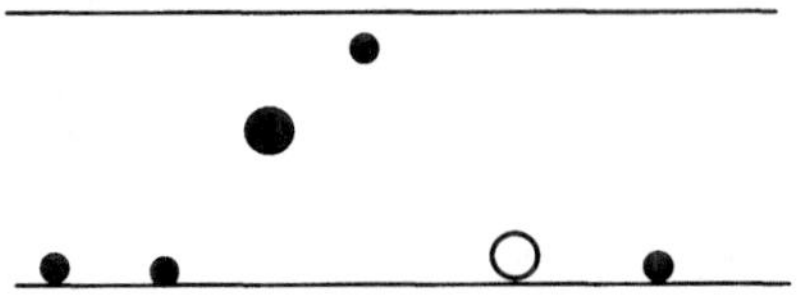

(c) She may not have meant to say it. — Fall-Rise Ending

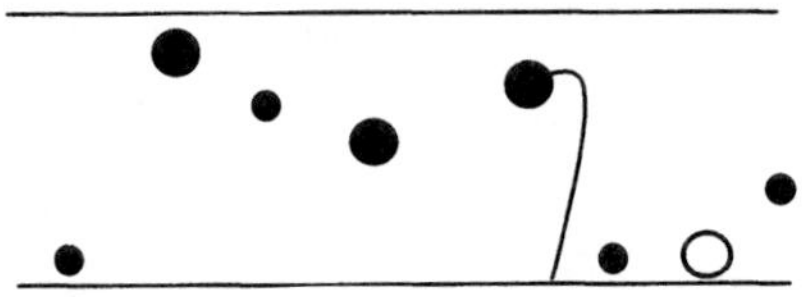

(d) Are you sure this is the right road? — Low Rise Ending

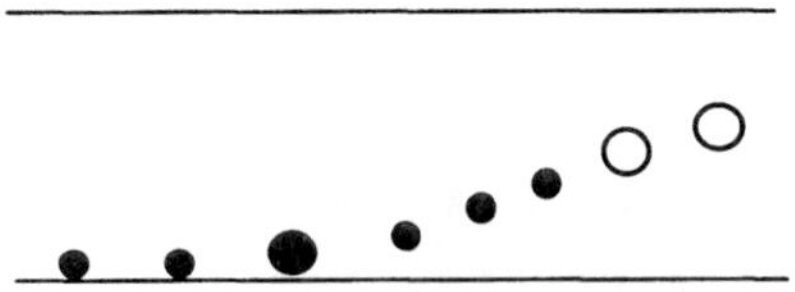

(e) I can hardly believe it. — High Fall Ending

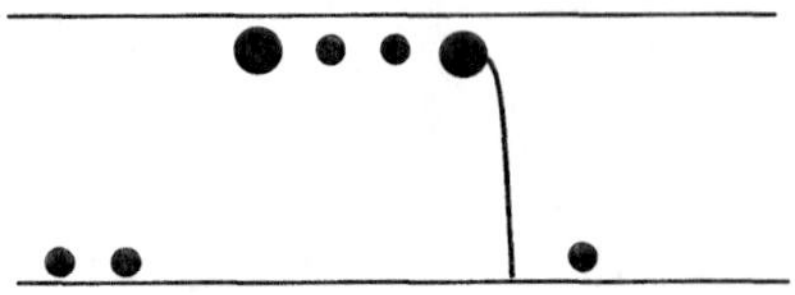

(f) We could go at five o' clock [or at six. . .] — Mid-Level Ending

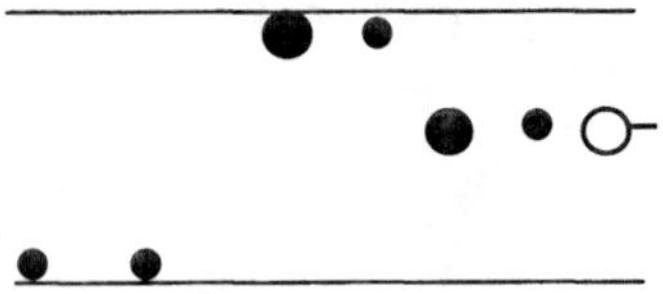

(g) We'll be far too early. — Rise-Fall Ending

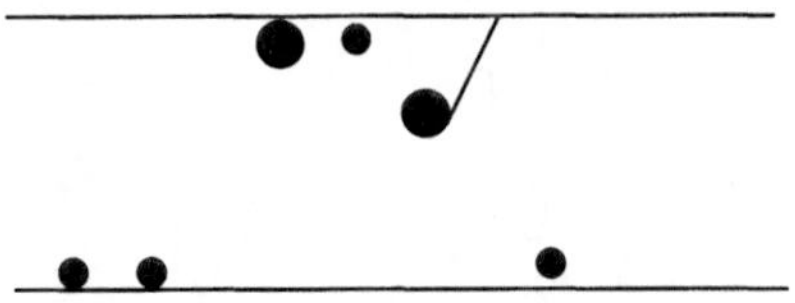

(h) Send it to Arthur. Low Fall Ending

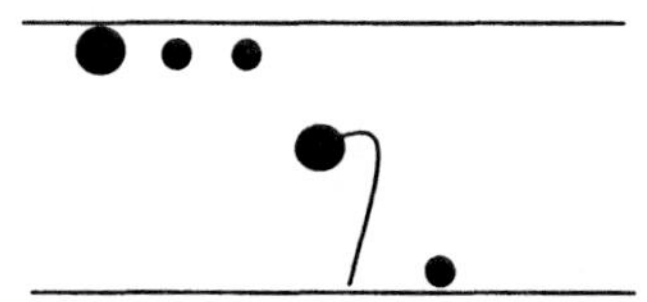

(i) It might be possible. Fall-Rise Ending

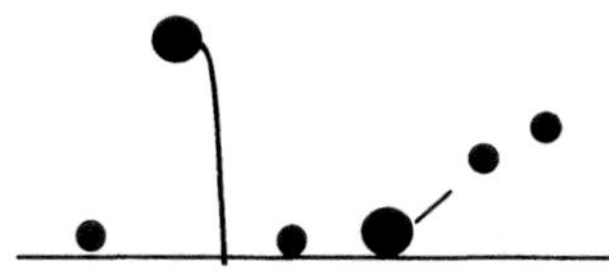

(j) Peter's going to do it. Low Fall Ending

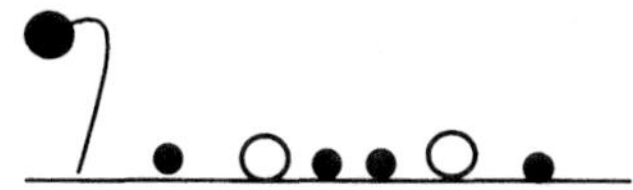

CHAPTER 19

Exercise 19.1

(a) creaking crane [ˈtwitɪn ˈtweɪn]
(b) stripey tiger [ˈdaɪpi ˈdaɪdə]
(c) five fishes [ˈpaɪb ˈpɪtɪd]
(d) roaring lion [ˈwɔwɪn ˈjaɪən]
(e) yellow lily [ˈjɛjoʊ ˈjɪji]
(f) red robin [ˈʋɛd ˈʋɑbɪn]

Exercise 19.2

(a) shoe shop [ˈçu ˈçɑp]
(b) sizzling [ˈɬɪɮɪŋ]
(c) sister [ˈθɪθtɚ]
(d) slush [ʃlʌç]
(e) Susie [ˈɬuɮi]
(f) zebras [ˈðibɹəð]

Exercise 19.3

(a) snowman [ˈn̥oʊmæ̃]
(b) elephant [ˈɛz̡əɸəmp]
(c) christmas tree [ˈcɥɪçməç ˈcɥi]
(d) dolly house [ˈd͡zɒʎi ˈʔaʊʔ]
(e) television [ˈʔɛləʋɪçə̃]
(f) strawberry jam [ˈt̪͡θɔbwi ˈd̪͡ðæm]
(g) happy snake [ˈxæʔi ˈn̥eɪʔ]
(h) magic dragon [ˈmæɟɪc ˈdɮæɟəɲ]
(i) jigsaw puzzle [ˈdɪd̪θɔ ˈpʌd̪͡ðəl]
(j) nasty noise [ˈnæ̃nĩ nɔ̃ĩʔ]

References

Abberton, E., & Fourcin, A. (1997). Electrolaryngography. In M. J. Ball & C. Code (Eds.), *Instrumental clinical phonetics* (pp. 119–148). London: Whurr.

Avery, P., & Ehrlich, S. (1992). *Teaching American English pronunciation.* Oxford: Oxford University Press.

Ball, M. J. (1993). *Phonetics for speech pathology* (2nd ed.). London: Whurr.

Ball, M. J., Code, C., Rahilly, J., & Hazlett, D. (1994). Non-segmental aspects of disordered speech: Developments in transcription. *Clinical Linguistics and Phonetics, 8*, 67–83.

Ball, M. J., Esling, J., & Dickson, C. (1999). Transcription of voice. In R. D. Kent & M. J. Ball (Eds.), *Voice quality measurement* (pp. 49–58). San Diego: Singular.

Ball, M. J., & Kent, R. D. (Eds.). (1997). *The new phonologies: Developments in clinical linguistics.* San Diego: Singular.

Ball, M. J., & Müller, N. (2002). The use of the terms phonetics and phonology in the description of disordered speech. *Advances in Speech-Language Pathology, 4*, 95–108.

Ball, M. J., & Rahilly, J. (1999). *Phonetics: The science of speech.* London: Arnold.

Ball, M. J., Rahilly, J., & Tench, P. (1996). *The phonetic transcription of disordered speech.* San Diego: Singular.

Barlow, S. (1999). *Handbook of clinical speech physiology.* San Diego: Singular.

Bauman-Waengler, J. (2004). *Articulatory and phonological impairments: A clinical focus* (2nd ed.). Boston: Allyn & Bacon.

Bedore, L., Leonard, L., & Gandour, J. (1994). The substitution of a click for sibilants: A case study. *Clinical Linguistics and Phonetics, 8*, 283–293.

Bernthal, J., & Bankson, N. (2004). *Articulation and phonological disorders* (5th ed.). Boston: Allyn & Bacon.

Bolinger, D. (1986). *Intonation and its parts: Melody in spoken English.* Stanford, CA: Stanford University Press.

Bolinger, D. (1989). *Intonation and its uses: Melody in grammar and discourse.* Stanford, CA: Stanford University Press.

Borden, G., Harris, K., & Raphael, L. (1994). *Speech science primer: Physiology, acoustics and perception of speech* (3rd ed.). Baltimore: Lippincott, Williams, & Wilkins.

Catford, J. (1977). *Fundamental problems in phonetics.* Edinburgh: Edinburgh University Press.

Centeno, J., Obler, L., & Anderson, R. (Eds.). (forthcoming). *Studying communication disorders in Spanish speakers: Theoretical, research, and clinical aspects.* Clevedon, UK: Multilingual Matters.

Chomsky, N., & Halle, M. (1968). *The sound pattern of English.* Cambridge, MA: MIT Press.

Clark, J., & Yallop, C. (1995). *An introduction to phonetics and phonology* (2nd ed.). Oxford: Blackwell.

Cruttenden, A. (1986). *Intonation.* Cambridge: Cambridge University Press.

Cruttenden, A. (2001). *Gimson's pronunciation of English* (6th ed.). London: Arnold.

Culbertson, W., & Tanner, D. (1997). *Introductory speech and hearing anatomy and physiology workbook.* Boston: Allyn & Bacon.

Delattre, P. (1965). *Comparing the phonetic features of English, German, Spanish and French.* Heidelberg: Julius Groos Verlag.

Denes, P., & Pinson, E. (1973). *The speech chain* (2nd ed.). New York: Anchor.

Deterding, D. (1997). The formants of monophthong vowels in standard southern British English pronunciation. *Journal of the International Phonetic Association, 27*, 47–55.

Edwards, H. (2003). *Applied phonetics: The sounds of American English* (3rd ed.). Clifton Park, NY: Thomson Delmar Learning.

Fry, D. (1947). The frequency of occurrence of speech sounds in southern English. *Archives Néerlandaises de Phonétique Expérimentale*, 20.

Fudge, E. (1984). *English word stress.* London: Allen & Unwin.

Green, L. (2002). *African American English: A linguistic introduction.* Cambridge: Cambridge University Press.

Grunwell, P. (1987). *Clinical phonology* (2nd ed.). Baltimore: Williams & Wilkins.

Halliday, M. A. K. (1970). *A course in spoken English: Intonation.* Oxford: Oxford University Press.

Hardcastle, W., & Gibbon, F. (1997). Electropalatography and its clinical applications. In M. J. Ball & C. Code (Eds.), *Instrumental clinical phonetics* (pp. 149–193). London: Whurr.

Harris, J. (1994). *English sound structure.* Oxford: Blackwell.

Heselwood, B. (1997). A case of nasal clicks for target sonorants: A feature geometry account. *Clinical Linguistics and Phonetics, 11*, 43–61.

Hillenbrand, J., Getty, L., Clark, M., & Wheeler, K. (1995). Acoustic characteristics of American English vowels. *Journal of the Acoustical Society of America, 97*, 3099–3111.

Hixon, T. J. (1973). Respiratory function in speech. In F. D. Minifie, T. J. Hixon, & F. Williams (Eds.), *Normal aspects of speech, hearing and language* (pp. 73–125). Englewood Cliffs, NJ: Prentice–Hall.

IPA [=International Phonetic Association] (1999). *Handbook of the International Phonetic Association.* Cambridge: Cambridge University Press.

Isaac, K. (2002). *Speech pathology in cultural and linguistic diversity.* London: Whurr.

Johnson, K. (1997). *Acoustic and auditory phonetics.* Oxford: Blackwell.

Kahane, J., & Folkins, J. (1984). *Atlas of speech and hearing anatomy.* Columbus, OH: Bell & Howell.

Kent, R. D. (1997). *The speech sciences.* San Diego: Singular.

Kent, R. D., & Ball, M. J. (Eds.). (1999). *Voice quality measurement.* San Diego: Singular.

Kent, R. D., & Read, C. (1992). *The acoustic analysis of speech.* San Diego: Singular.

Ladefoged, P. (1962). *Elements of acoustic phonetics.* Chicago: University of Chicago Press.

Ladefoged, P. (1993). *A course in phonetics* (3rd ed.). New York: Harcourt Brace.

Ladefoged, P., & Maddieson, I. (1996). *The sounds of the world's languages.* Oxford: Blackwell.

Landau, S. (2000). *Cambridge dictionary of American English.* Cambridge: Cambridge University Press.

Laver, J. (1980). *The phonetic description of voice quality.* Cambridge: Cambridge University Press.

Laver, J. (1994). *Principles of phonetics.* Cambridge: Cambridge University Press.

Maddieson, I. (1984). *Patterns of sounds.* Cambridge: Cambridge University Press.

Nagle, S., & Sanders, S. (Eds.). (2003). *English in the southern United States.* Cambridge: Cambridge University Press.

O'Connor, J., & Arnold, G. (1973). *Intonation of colloquial English* (2nd ed.). London: Longmans.

Perkins, W., & Kent, R. D. (1986). *Textbook of functional anatomy of speech, language and hearing.* London: Taylor & Francis.

Peterson, G., & Barney, H. (1952). Control methods in a study of the vowels. *Journal of the Acoustical Society of America, 24*, 175–184.

Pickett, J. M. (Ed.). (1999). *The acoustics of speech communication.* Boston: Allyn & Bacon.

Pike, K. (1945). *Intonation of American English.* Ann Arbor, MI: University of Michigan Press.

Seikel, J. A., King, D. W., & Drumright, D. G. (2000). *Anatomy and physiology for speech and language* (2nd ed.). San Diego: Singular.

Shriberg, L., & Kent, R. (2003). *Clinical phonetics* (3rd ed.). Boston: Allyn & Bacon.

Small, L. (1999). *Fundamentals of phonetics: A practical guide for students.* Boston: Allyn & Bacon.

Speaks, C. (1999). *Introduction to sound* (3rd ed.). San Diego: Singular.

Stampe, D. (1979). *A dissertation on natural phonology.* New York: Garland.

Stevens, K. (1998). *Acoustic phonetics.* Cambridge, MA: MIT Press.

Wells, J. (1982). *Accents of English* (vols. 1–3). Cambridge: Cambridge University Press.

Wells, J. (2000). *Longman pronunciation dictionary* (2nd ed.). London: Longman.

Wells, W. (1994). Junction in developmental speech disorder: A case study. *Clinical Linguistics and Phonetics, 8*, 1–25.

Wolfram, W., & Schilling-Estes, N. (1998). *American English: Dialects and variation.* Oxford: Blackwell.

Zajac, D., & Yates, C. (1997). Speech aerodynamics. In M. J. Ball and C. Code (Eds.), *Instrumental clinical phonetics* (pp. 87–118). London: Whurr.

Index